Advances in Melanoma

Guest Editor

DAVID E. FISHER, MD, PhD

T0372046

HEMATOLOGY/ONCOLOGY CLINICS OF NORTH AMERICA

www.hemonc.theclinics.com

June 2009 • Volume 23 • Number 3

SAUNDERS an imprint of ELSEVIER, Inc.

W.B. SAUNDERS COMPANY
A Division of Elsevier Inc.

1600 John F. Kennedy Blvd. • Suite 1800 • Philadelphia, PA 19103-2899

http://www.theclinics.com

HEMATOLOGY/ONCOLOGY CLINICS OF NORTH AMERICA Volume 23, Number 3
June 2009 ISSN 0889-8588, ISBN 13: 978-1-4377-0488-4, ISBN 10: 1-4377-0488-3

Editor: Kerry Holland

Hematology/Oncology Clinics (ISSN 0889-8588) is published bimonthly by Elsevier Inc., 360 Park Avenue South, New York, NY 10010-1710. Months of issue are February, April, June, August, October, and December. Business and Editorial Offices: 1600 John F. Kennedy Blvd., Suite 1800, Philadelphia, PA 19103-2899. Customer Service Office: 11830 Westline Industrial Drive, St. Louis, MO 63146. Periodicals postage paid at New York, NY and additional mailing offices. Subscription prices are $283.00 per year (domestic individuals), $439.00 per year (domestic institutions), $141.00 per year (domestic students/residents), $321.00 per year (Canadian individuals), $537.00 per year (Canadian institutions) $382.00 per year (international individuals), $537.00 per year (international institutions), and $191.00 per year (international and Canadian students/residents). International air speed delivery is included in all *Clinics* subscription prices. All prices are subject to change without notice. **POSTMASTER:** Send address changes to *Hematology/Oncology Clinics of North America*, 11830 Westline Industrial Drive, St. Louis, MO 63146. Customer Service (orders, claims, online, change of address): Elsevier Periodicals Customer Service, 11830 Westline Industrial Drive, St. Louis, MO 63146. Tel: 1-800-654-2452 (U.S. and Canada). Fax: 314-523-5170. E-mail: journalscustomerservice-usa@elsevier.com (for print support); journalsonlinesupport-usa@elsevier.com (for online support).

Reprints. For copies of 100 or more, of articles in this publication, please contact the Commercial Reprints Department, Elsevier Inc., 360 Park Avenue South, New York, New York 10010-1710; Tel.: 212-633-3813, Fax: 212-462-1935, E-mail: reprints@elsevier.com.

Hematology/Oncology Clinics of North America is covered in *MEDLINE/PubMed (Index Medicus)*, *EMBASE/Excerpta Medica*, and *BIOSIS*.

Printed and bound by CPI Group (UK) Ltd, Croydon, CR0 4YY

Transferred to Digital Print 2011

Contributors

GUEST EDITOR

DAVID E. FISHER, MD, PhD
Chief, Department of Dermatology; and Director, Cutaneous Biology Research Center; and Director, Melanoma Program in Medical Oncology; and Edward Wigglesworth Professor of Dermatology, Massachusetts General Hospital, Harvard Medical School, Boston, Massachusetts

AUTHORS

RAVI K. AMARAVADI, MD
Assistant Professor of Medicine, Department of Medicine, Division of Hematology and Oncology, Abramson Cancer Center, University of Pennsylvania, Philadelphia, Pennsylvania

MICHAEL F. BERGER, PhD
The Broad Institute of MIT and Harvard, Cambridge, Massachusetts

PAUL B. CHAPMAN, MD
Melanoma/Sarcoma Service, Department of Medicine, Memorial Sloan-Kettering Cancer Center; Professor of Medicine, Weill Medical College of Cornell University, New York, New York

NATHALIE DHOMEN, BSc, PhD
Section of Cell and Molecular Biology, Institute of Cancer Research, London, United Kingdom

LYN MCDIVITT DUNCAN, MD
Associate Professor of Pathology, Department of Pathology, Harvard Medical School; and Chief, MGH Dermatopathology Unit, Massachusetts General Hospital, Boston, Massachusetts

ALEXANDER M.M. EGGERMONT, MD, PhD
Head and Professor, Department of Surgical Oncology, Erasmus University MC–Daniel den Hoed Cancer Center, Rotterdam, The Netherlands

LESLIE A. FECHER, MD
Assistant Professor of Medicine, Department of Medicine, Division of Hematology and Oncology, Abramson Cancer Center, University of Pennsylvania, Philadelphia, Pennsylvania

DAVID E. FISHER, MD, PhD
Chief, Department of Dermatology; and Director, Cutaneous Biology Research Center; and Director, Melanoma Program in Medical Oncology; and Edward Wigglesworth Professor of Dermatology, Massachusetts General Hospital, Harvard Medical School, Boston, Massachusetts

KEITH T. FLAHERTY, MD
Assistant Professor of Medicine, Department of Medicine, Division of Hematology and Oncology, Abramson Cancer Center, University of Pennsylvania, Philadelphia, Pennsylvania

LEVI A. GARRAWAY, MD, PhD
The Broad Institute of MIT and Harvard, Cambridge; Department of Medical Oncology, Dana-Farber Cancer Institute; Center for Cancer Genome Discovery, Dana-Farber Cancer Institute, Boston, Massachusetts

ALAN C. GELLER, MPH, RN
Senior Research Scientist, Division of Public Health Practice, Harvard School of Public Health, Landmark Center, Boston, Massachusetts

ALLAN C. HALPERN, MD
Dermatology Service, Department of Medicine, Memorial Sloan-Kettering Cancer Center, New York, New York

RICHARD MARAIS, BSc, PhD
Professor of Molecular Oncology, Cancer Section of Cell and Molecular Biology, Institute of Cancer Research, London, United Kingdom

ALEXANDER G. MARNEROS, MD, PhD
Member, Cutaneous Biology Research Center, Massachusetts General Hospital, Charlestown; Department of Dermatology, Harvard Medical School, Boston, Massachusetts

MARTIN C. MIHM, Jr, MD
Professor of Pathology and Dermatology, Department of Pathology and Dermatopathology, Massachusetts General Hospital, Harvard Medical School, Boston, Massachusetts

DEVARATI MITRA
Student, Biology and Biomedical Sciences Program, Cutaneous Biology Research Center, Harvard Medical School, Charlestown, Massachusetts

ADRIANO PIRIS, MD
Instructor in Pathology, Department of Pathology, Massachusetts General Hospital, Harvard Medical School, Boston, Massachusetts

DIRK SCHADENDORF, MD, PhD
Director, Chair, and Professor, Department of Dermatology, University Hospital Essen, Essen, Germany

LYNN M. SCHUCHTER, MD
Professor of Medicine, Department of Medicine, Division of Hematology and Oncology, Abramson Cancer Center, University of Pennsylvania, Philadelphia, Pennsylvania

KENNETH TANABE, MD
Associate Professor of Surgery, Department of Surgery, Harvard Medical School; Chief of Surgical Oncology, Division of Surgical Oncology, Department of Surgery, Massachusetts General Hospital, Boston, Massachusetts

VITALY TERUSHKIN, BS
Dermatology Service, Department of Medicine, Memorial Sloan-Kettering Cancer Center, New York, New York

HENSIN TSAO, MD, PhD
Department of Dermatology, Wellman Center for Photomedicine, Harvard Medical School; The Melanoma and Pigmented Lesion Center, Massachusetts General Hospital, Boston, Massachusetts

MARGARET A. TUCKER, MD
Director, Human Genetics Program; and Chief, Genetic Epidemiology Branch, Division of Cancer Epidemiology and Genetics, National Cancer Institute, Bethesda, Maryland

DURGA UDAYAKUMAR, PhD
Department of Dermatology, Wellman Center for Photomedicine, Harvard Medical School, Massachusetts General Hospital, Boston, Massachusetts

JENNIFER A. WARGO, MD
Instructor in Surgery, Department of Surgery, Harvard Medical School; Assistant in Surgery, Division of Surgical Oncology, Department of Surgery, Massachusetts General Hospital, Boston, Massachusetts

ARVIN S. YANG, MD, PhD
Medical Oncology Fellow, Melanoma/Sarcoma Service, Department of Medicine, Memorial Sloan-Kettering Cancer Center, New York, New York

Contents

metastatic melanoma. It has become increasingly clear that a therapeutic approach that combines angiogenesis inhibitors with cytotoxic agents or other treatment modalities is more likely to result in a clinical benefit for patients rather than antiangiogenesis treatments alone. However, a targeted treatment approach with antiangiogenic agents needs to be based on an in-depth understanding of the complex mechanisms involved in melanoma tumor angiogenesis.

Transcriptional regulation in melanoma is a complex process that tends to hijack the normal melanocyte signaling pathways involved in melanocyte development, pigmentation, and survival. At the center of these often overlapping networks of transcriptional activation and repression is microphthalmia-associated transcription factor (MITF), a melanocyte lineage marker that increases pigment production and exhibits diverse effects on cell survival, proliferation, and cell cycle arrest. The particular conditions that allow MITF to produce these potentially contradictory roles have not yet been fully elucidated, but analysis of the pathways involved provides opportunities to learn about new therapeutic strategies.

This article reviews the main aspects of the histopathology of cutaneous melanoma with emphasis on recent advances in the morphological evaluation of these lesions. The limitations of morphology for the "so called" borderline lesions are briefly discussed, with a list of diagnostic criteria to help predict behavior for these challenging lesions. The prognostic factors are described with emphasis on the ones that are currently being used by the American Joint Committee on Cancer staging system. Ancillary tests, such as immunohistochemistry and molecular techniques, are also briefly touched upon as complimentary tools to help understand the biology of malignant melanoma. The conclusion is that an accurate morphological evaluation remains the most efficient approach to establish the diagnosis and predict behavior of this challenging neoplasm.

Recognizing early forms of melanoma may have significant impact on decreasing mortality from this malignancy. As a result, multiple efforts have focused on developing new and improving current early detection strategies. These include educating patients about the importance of performing skin self-examination, increasing rates of complete skin examinations by physicians in the context of routine care, initiating mass screening campaigns, creating specialized skin cancer clinics, and developing better diagnostic tools through advances in technology. In this article, the current state of these efforts is reviewed.

Forty years ago, a clinical and histological classification scheme and prognostic factors were described for cutaneous melanoma. This scheme included the subtypes superficial spreading, nodular and lentigo maligna, and prognostic factors including tumor thickness, ulceration, and mitotic activity. There have been some tweaks to the classification scheme, but these basic findings form the foundation for melanoma diagnosis and staging today. Currently, no molecular marker or target has proved reliably useful in the staging or treatment of melanoma. Measurement with a simple ruler serves as the basis for the staging of primary cutaneous melanoma, while the recognition of primary tumor mitotic activity and ulceration also remain significant factors. Recently, mutational analysis has revealed a correlation of activating mutations with the morphological descriptors from decades ago. Future classification schemes may have more power in predicting response to therapy by integrating specific genomic and intra-tumoral expression profiles with histologic findings.

Many deaths of melanoma can be prevented through identification and screening of persons at greatest risk of disease. Herein, we discuss various strategies to reduce avoidable mortality—including targeted screening of persons with changing moles and middle-aged and older men of lower socioeconomic status. We also propose the framework for a randomized screening trial for melanoma.

The RAS/RAF/MEK/ERK signaling pathway has emerged as a major player in the induction and maintenance of melanoma, particularly the protein kinase BRAF, mutated in approximately 44% of melanoma cases. The availability of new drugs affecting the components of this pathway and pathways that may cooperate with MAPK signaling, means that targeted therapies are fast becoming a real option in the clinical management of melanoma. The authors discuss what they learned from clinical trials using first- and second-generation inhibitors to this pathway.

About 20% of all primary melanomas will spread. The likelihood of metastatic behavior correlates with prognostic factors such as tumor thickness, mitotic index, presence of ulceration, lymphocyte infiltration, age, gender, and anatomic site. Immunotherapies are developed for melanoma patients in stage IV who have distant metastases and in stage II to III patients in the adjuvant micrometastatic setting, where only a fraction of patients have widespread (microscopic) disease.

Melanoma is an increasing health care problem worldwide. Up to 80,000 cases of melanoma are diagnosed per year and it is the sixth leading cause of cancer death in the United States. The lifetime risk is estimated to be 1 in 75 individuals for the development of melanoma. Surgery remains the mainstay of treatment of melanoma, and in most cases it is curative. Several important surgical issues are discussed in this review, including the extent of surgical margins, Mohs micrographic surgery for melanoma in situ, the use of sentinel lymph node biopsy, the usefulness of lymphadenectomy, isolated limb perfusion, and the role of metastasectomy.

Melanoma is considered a chemotherapy-resistant cancer, but in reality there are several chemotherapy drugs with significant single-agent activity. Response rates to combination regimens are reproducibly higher than with standard dacarbazine, but of the randomized trials comparing combination regimens with dacarbazine, none were of sufficient size to detect a realistic effect on survival. Similarly, adjuvant chemotherapy has not had a realistic test in melanoma. Response to chemotherapy is associated reproducibly with better survival rates suggesting that regimens with higher response rates are needed. Recent observations suggest that combining antiangiogenic agents with either dacarbazine or temozolomide can double response rates. These combinations are worthy of further investigation and might serve as a foundation on which to build a combination regimen that improves overall survival in metastatic melanoma patients.

Melanoma continues to be one of the most aggressive and morbid malignancies once metastatic. Overall survival for advanced unresectable melanoma has not changed over the past several decades. However, the presence of some long-term survivors of metastatic melanoma highlights the heterogeneity of this disease and the potential for improved outcomes. Current research is uncovering the molecular and genetic scaffolding of normal and aberrant cell function. The known oncogenic pathways in melanoma and the attempts to develop therapy for them are discussed. The targeting of certain cellular processes, downstream of the common genetic alterations, for which the issues of target and drug validation are somewhat distinct, are also highlighted.

THE CLINICS ARE NOW AVAILABLE ONLINE!

Access your subscription at:
www.theclinics.com

Preface

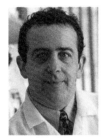

David E. Fisher, MD, PhD
Guest Editor

Melanoma incidence continues to climb at unprecedented rates. Risk factors for melanoma are thought to be largely impacted by a key environmental exposure: ultraviolet radiation. Despite this information, strategies to diminish melanoma mortality via prevention, early detection, or enhanced therapy have not yet come to light.

It is clear that the foundation of our understanding of melanoma is beginning to shift—in a good way. From better knowledge about the incidence and epidemiology of the disease, to improving technologies aimed at early detection, to enhanced histopathologic diagnostic tools, the definition of the disease and the factors that participate in its formation are being redefined in ways that are much more likely to impact patient outcomes. Oncogene discovery has not only permitted reclassification of melanoma subtypes, but also has greatly spurred the discovery and application of targeted therapies; and importantly, first glimpses of clinical success have been seen: drug-induced suppression of mutant c-KIT has produced dramatic clinical responses in patients who have metastatic melanoma harboring activating mutations within that oncogenic receptor. The importance of this finding is several-fold; it will likely enhance patient survival in this disease subset, and it provides proof-of-principal that identification of drugable oncogenic lesions can produce dramatic clinical effects, even in melanoma. Thus molecular reclassification of melanoma is extremely important, and so is perseverance with attempts to further develop clinical agents against additional oncogenic lesions in melanoma.

Immunotherapy strategies have a longer history of efficacy in subgroups of melanoma patients, and significant strides have been made in understanding mechanisms of tolerance and breaking them. How will these approaches best be applied to melanoma patients? Who benefits and who does not? How much is determined by the host and the tumor? Numerous key questions remain, but there is compelling evidence that these questions are bringing us closer and closer to major clinical impact, some of which is already evident. Even the use of cytotoxic chemotherapy—often considered ineffective, yet still very commonly employed—is worthy of thorough review for the sake of patients here and now.

Hematol Oncol Clin N Am 23 (2009) xiii–xiv
doi:10.1016/j.hoc.2009.03.014
0889-8588/09/$ – see front matter © 2009 Elsevier Inc. All rights reserved.
hemonc.theclinics.com

The convergence of so many technologies is affording us better opportunities to prevent, diagnose early, or cure melanoma. This issue of *Hematology/Oncology Clinics of North America* brings together thought leaders from many of these complementing disciplines. While significant work remains before melanoma mortality truly declines, many of the barriers to that goal are in better focus now than ever before. The success of these efforts may appear incremental, as with c-KIT, but systematic and creative building on these gains makes the eventual cure or prevention of melanoma seem ultimately inevitable.

David E. Fisher, MD, PhD
Department of Dermatology
Cutaneous Biology Research Center
Melanoma Program in Medical Oncology
Massachusetts General Hospital
Harvard Medical School
Building 149, 13th Street
Charlestown, MA 02129, USA

E-mail address:
dfisher3@partners.org (D.E. Fisher)

Melanoma Epidemiology

Margaret A. Tucker, MD[a,b,*]

KEYWORDS

- Melanoma • Risk factors • Nevi • UV • Genetics

With the rapid increases in the incidence of melanoma in the United States, Australia, and Europe during the last decades, melanoma has been considered an epidemic cancer in these areas. Many epidemiologic studies have been conducted to evaluate the etiology of melanoma. These studies have included descriptive population registry-based studies, which yield important information about trends in specific areas but usually do not have individual-level information; analytic studies, often case control, which may include not only individual exposure information but also host factors and phenotype; and family studies, which may be phenotype intensive, designed in large part to identify susceptibility genes. Most recently, with the advent of genome-wide association studies, agnostic assessment of genetic variation across the genome as risk factors for melanoma has been possible. A comprehensive review of all of these results is not feasible within the limits of this article; only recent advances based on epidemiologic studies will be included.

US POPULATION MELANOMA RATES

Melanoma incidence has continuously increased in the Surveillance, Epidemiology, and End Results (SEER) program during the last 30 years (**Table 1**)[1]. In 2005, the age-adjusted incidence was 24.6 per 100,000 for men and 15.6 per 100,000 for women. There is a well-described lag in reporting of melanomas,[2] so the estimates in **Table 1** reflect delay-adjusted incidence. In the 1970s the rate of increase was higher, but the estimated annual percent change (EAPC) is currently 2.9%/y overall in the United States. This overall rate of increase, however, disguises the extensive variability in incidence. Melanoma, similar to other adult-onset cancers, is a complex, heterogeneous cancer. Incidence rates differ between genders, ages, ethnic groups,

This work was supported by the Intramural Research Program, NCI, NIH.

[a] Human Genetics Program, Division of Cancer Epidemiology and Genetics, National Cancer Institute, 6120 Executive Boulevard, Room 7122, Bethesda, MD 20892-7236, USA

[b] Genetic Epidemiology Branch, Division of Cancer Epidemiology and Genetics, National Cancer Institute, 6120 Executive Boulevard, Room 7122, Bethesda, MD 20892-7236, USA

* Genetic Epidemiology Branch, Division of Cancer Epidemiology and Genetics, National Cancer Institute, 6120 Executive Boulevard, Room 7122, Bethesda, MD 20892-7236, USA.
E-mail address: tuckerp@mail.nih.gov

Table 1
Joinpoint analysis of surveillance, epidemiology, and end results of melanoma age-adjusted and delay-adjusted incidence trends over time

Both Sexes, All Races		Males		Females	
Trend	Period	Trend	Period	Trend	Period
6.0 (P<.05)	1975–1981	5.4 (P<.05)	1975–1985	5.4 (P<.05)	1975–1980
2.9 (P<.05)	1981–2005	3.4 (P<.05)	1985–2000	2.5 (P<.05)	1980–2005
		−0.2	2000–2003		
		7.7 (P<.05)	2003–2005		

and regions. Before age 40 years, the incidence is higher in each age category in young women; after age 40 years, the incidence increases rapidly in men, but the rate of increase slows dramatically in women.[3] This unusual incidence pattern has led to hypotheses about hormonal influences in melanoma etiology, which have been investigated in numerous studies.[4,5] More recently, using newer analytic methods, the population patterns have been explored as manifestations of the heterogeneity in melanoma.[3,6] Lachiewicz and colleagues assessed patterns of melanoma by age, gender, and anatomic site. Within anatomic site (trunk and face/ears), they also compared superficial spreading and nodular melanomas. They found different age-specific patterns consistent with divergent causal pathways.[6] Anderson and colleagues recently evaluated age of onset of melanoma by gender, histopathologic classification, and anatomic site.[3] Gender, histopathology, and anatomic site were age-specific effect modifiers for melanoma. The crossing of the incidence curves of males and females at age 40 years is consistent with bimodal age distributions. Age-period-cohort models were used to simultaneously assess age, calendar period, and cohort effects by gender. A combination of female, lower-extremity site, and superficial spreading melanoma was mostly early onset in age, but the combination of male, head and neck or upper-extremity site and lentigo maligna melanomas was mostly late-onset in age.[3] These groups are 2 that could be clearly differentiated among likely many subgroups that can be variously categorized. Another aspect of heterogeneity in melanoma is reflected in the differing histologic subtypes and anatomic distributions of melanoma across ethnicities in the United States.[1,7] Little is known about the etiology of melanoma in these groups, but among Hispanics in California, the rates appear to be increasing in all tumor thicknesses.[8]

Purdue and colleagues[9] recently evaluated the incidence and mortality patterns of melanoma in teenagers and young adults younger than 40 years of age from 1973 to 2004. The incidence rate in young men increased substantially between 1973 and 1980 (EAPC 6.6%; $P = .0010$), but it has been relatively flat since (EAPC 0.4%; $P = .35$). There is some hint that the rates may be beginning to increase again in the last few years. In young women, however, from 1973 to 1978, the increase was quite steep (EAPC 9.2%; P<.0001). From 1978 to 1987 the rate of increase was less (EAPC 2.6%; $P = .0001$). The incidence then stabilized for several years. Since 1992, the incidence has increased steadily at the earlier pace (EAPC 2.7%; P<.0001). The incidence rates rose for both thicker and thin melanomas and for both localized and regional/distant disease. These patterns are suggestive of a gender-specific change in exposure patterns.

Melanoma mortality rates have not increased as dramatically as the incidence rates.[1] The mortality rates are based on the entire US population, not just the areas covered by the SEER registries. From 1975 to 1989, the overall mortality increased (EAPC 1.6% P<.05) but has been stable since (EAPC -0.1%). For men, the mortality rates increased from 1975 to 1990 (EAPC 2.2%; *P*<.05) but flattened from 1990 to 2005 (EAPC 0.1%). The modeled age-adjusted mortality rate for men in 2005 is 3.9 per 100,000. For women, the mortality rate increased more slowly than for men from 1975 to1988 (EAPC 0.8%; *P*<.05) but then decreased from 1988 to 2005 (EAPC -0.6%; *P*<.05). The 2005 mortality rate for women is 1.7 per 100,000 and has essentially returned to the 1976 mortality rate.

The discrepancy in the rate of increase in the incidence and mortality has led to the hypothesis of "nonmetastasizing melanoma."[10] The argument is that there is over-diagnosis or misdiagnosis of early lesions that are not biologically significant, leading to an inflation of the incidence.[11,12] Against this, however, is the concurrent increase in thicker, more advanced lesions,[9] especially in those of lower socioeconomic status.[13] Another interpretation of the discrepancy between the incidence and mortality is that with greater awareness of melanoma, thinner lesions are being found earlier at a curative stage, resulting in lower mortality. This issue is likely not going to be resolved until there are better prognostic markers for excised lesions and better identification of lesions to excise.

ANALYTIC STUDIES OF MELANOMA ETIOLOGY

Most of the individual analytic studies have not been large enough to have sufficient power to evaluate subgroups of melanoma, however defined. There is also great heterogeneity in study designs, definition of risk factors, collection of data, and extent of phenotyping (eg, self-reports to physician examinations). It is therefore difficult to pool data, conduct meta-analyses, or directly compare results across studies. Meta-analyses use aggregate data; pooled analyses need to "harmonize" the individual-level data, usually not at the finest level of detail for exposures or phenotypes. Therefore, risks that are seen in these combined analyses are likely to be lower than that in the more pristine studies. Despite these difficulties, clear risk factors have evolved during the past several decades. Increased number of nevi, no matter how evaluated, is an important risk factor. Other host factors with consistently demonstrated risks include complexion, tanning ability, extent of freckling, and family history of melanoma. Most studies also find that ultraviolet exposure is the most important environmental factor related to melanoma risk.

Most of the studies assessing number of nevi combine all nevus types; some separate nevi by size; few classify and enumerate total body dysplastic nevi and common nevi. In general, studies with only combined nevus counts report odds ratios on the order of 4 to 6 for the highest count category. When only common acquired nevi are included, the risks are on the order of 2 to 4.[14] In a recent meta-analysis of 47 studies including 10,499 cases and 14,256 controls, Gandini and colleagues[15] were able to extend distribution of risks across finer categories. Among the 26 studies with whole-body counts of common nevi, the relative risks (RRs) rose from 1.47 (95% confidence intervals [CI], 1.36–1.59) for 16 to 40 nevi to 6.89 (95% CI, 4.63–10.25) for 101–120. There have also been 2 recent pooled analyses of nevi as a risk factor for melanoma.[16,17] There is major overlap of the studies in the 2 analyses (2 of 10 in Olsen's study are not included in Chang's study), but somewhat different endpoints were assessed. Olsen was testing the hypotheses that increased number of nevi would be related to melanomas arising in areas of less sun exposure and higher nevus counts such as the back and that nevi would be less strong risk factors for melanomas arising on constantly exposed skin, such as the head and neck. Analyses included women only (2406 cases and 3119 controls); the pooled dataset had been created to evaluate reproductive factors. As a surrogate for *MC1R* variation, they also analyzed the combined effect of nevus number, hair color, and freckling. The most frequent nevus variable assessed was the count of nevi on the arm(s). Only two studies had observer-counted nevi on most of the body. They found that the risk of melanoma related to the highest number of nevi was strongest for trunk (5-fold increased) melanomas and limb (legs 3-fold; arms 4-fold increased) melanomas. The association was less strong, and not statistically significant, for head and neck melanomas. These findings are consistent with their hypothesis. When freckling and red hair were combined with the nevus variable, the pooled odds ratio (pOR) rose from 4.5 (95% CI, 1.3–15.7) in the highest nevus category without freckling or red hair to 7.3 (95% CI, 2.7–19.7) with high nevus counts and freckling to 14.4 (95% CI, 2.0–102) in the small group (24 cases; 8 controls) with high nevus counts and red hair, with or without freckling. Site-specific melanoma risks could not be addressed in the analyses including the red hair variable in this large dataset.

The hypothesis of Chang and colleagues[17] was that melanoma risk associated with nevi might vary by latitude. Latitude was considered in two levels: northern region (latitude $\geq$50N) and southern region (latitude <50N). The pooled dataset included 15 case-control studies (5421 melanoma cases and 6966 controls), 5 of which had health care provider-observed total body nevus counts. Three had atypical or dysplastic nevus counts. Because of the diverse data, nevus counts were considered in four strata for arm and total body counts separately in two age groups, <50 and $\geq$50. The pORs for the highest categories ranged from 4.0 (95% CI 2.5-6.4) for arm counts in those older than age 50 to 69 years (95% CI 4.4-11.2) for whole-body counts in those younger than age 50 years. Variation in the studies using arm nevus counts was greater than that in the studies reporting total body nevus counts. The pORs across latitudes were relatively similar. In the small number of studies with atypical nevi noted, any atypical nevi conferred a 4-fold increased risk of melanoma (95% CI, 2.8–5.8).

Relatively fewer studies have reported the risks of melanoma associated with dysplastic nevi and common nevi.[18] These studies with careful phenotyping are much more expensive to conduct because of the associated costs of professional examinations. In addition, with the falling response rates in epidemiologic studies, accruing sufficient numbers of truly representative controls who are willing to dedicate the time and effort to participate has become increasingly difficult. Despite the relatively few studies, it is clear that clinically identified dysplastic nevi are important risk factors for melanoma. The usual clinical criteria include two obligate features: size greater than 5 mm in the largest diameter and a prominent flat component; and two of three additional features: irregular, asymmetric outline, indistinct borders, and variable pigmentation.[14] The histologic features include the presence of a disordered or immature growth pattern with a lymphocytic host response and random cytologic atypia in melanocytes.[19] Based on the findings from several case-control studies, these lesions are relatively common (about 10% [range, 7%–24%] of adults) in populations of northern European descent.[18] The risks conferred by dysplastic nevi are much greater than those conferred by increased number of common nevi.[14] Among studies evaluating the role of dysplastic nevi in melanoma, dysplastic nevi are reported in 34% to 56% of melanoma cases.[18] Gandini and colleagues[15] also evaluated the risks of melanoma associated with dysplastic nevi in their meta-analysis. Among 13 studies with dichotomous data, any dysplastic nevi conferred a 10-fold increased risk of melanoma (95% CI, 5.04–20.32). Among 15 studies with continuous data on number of dysplastic nevi, the risk rose from 1.6 (95% CI, 1.38–1.85) for individuals with 1 dysplastic nevus to 10-fold increased (95% CI, 5.05–21.76) with five or more dysplastic nevi. There are likely population differences in the prevalence of dysplastic nevi; again, few studies have been conducted. A joint case-control study of melanoma in which nevi were assessed in the United Kingdom and Australia found that dysplastic nevi were three times more frequent in the Australian controls (6%) than in the British controls (2%), but the prevalence of nevi on non-sun-exposed areas was the same.[20]

The etiology of nevi in general, and dysplastic nevi in particular, is not well characterized. There is evidence from twin studies of a genetic component to the etiology of nevus counts.[21–24] Candidate regions have been evaluated, but no causal or susceptibility genes have been confirmed to date.[25] There are increasing data that sun exposure is important in the pattern of development and number of nevi.[26–28] Limited data exist for dysplastic nevi. Although common acquired nevi occur predominantly in intermittently sun-exposed areas, dysplastic nevi also occur on areas with little or no sun exposure.

Virtually all studies of melanoma have demonstrated that light skin color (RR, 2.06; 95% CI, 1.68–2.52), poor tanning ability (RR, 2.09; 95% CI, 1.67–2.58), and light eye (RR, 1.47; 95% CI, 1.28–1.69) and hair (RR, 1.78; 95% CI, 1.63–1.95) color are risk factors for melanoma and are highly correlated.[29] These complexion measures confer a relatively low risk, especially when the presence and number of nevi are adjusted for.[14] Red hair usually confers a higher risk (RR, 3.64; 95% CI, 2.56–5.37),[29] which likely reflects the presence of variation in *MC1R*. Freckling, a complex phenotype that represents not only susceptibility to sun and frequent *MC1R* variation but also extent of sun exposure, is measured in many ways across studies. Despite this heterogeneity in assessment, freckling is almost always associated with risk of melanoma (RR, 2.1; 95% CI, 1.8–2.45).[29]

The major environmental risk factor for melanoma is UV radiation (UVR). Sun exposure as a risk factor for melanoma has been extensively evaluated for decades; more recently, sun-bed exposure has also been assessed. In 1992, the International Agency for Research on Cancer concluded that there was sufficient evidence in humans for the carcinogenicity of sun exposure.[30] Several questions about the relationship of UVR to melanoma risk remain. It is difficult to collect lifetime history of a universal exposure. Earlier, English and colleagues assessed the reproducibility of recall of sun exposures at different ages among adults. They found that adult exposures appeared more reproducible than childhood exposures. Total sun exposure was also more reproducible than intermittent exposures.[31] In 2009, Yu and colleagues[32] compared time-based (hours outdoors in the middle of the day) and activity-based (time outdoors according to specific activities) responses to self-administered questionnaires. They found that the responses for childhood periods were similar for either method. For adult exposure, however, the activity-based approach was more reliable than the time-based approach (intraclass correlation coefficient, 0.69 vs 0.43; P = .003). There were distinct differences in the patterns for men and women; much of the improvement in the activity-based approach was in the women respondents. The men reported more time outdoors in both childhood and adult years. Few studies of sun exposure as a risk factor for melanoma have assessed the exposure patterns of men and women separately.[33] Fears and colleagues[34] reported very different patterns of exposure between men and women; exposure patterns also varied by skin tanning ability, age, and geographic location. Even among individuals who tanned well, melanoma risk increased with increasing time outdoors.

Despite the difficulties in estimating exposure, meta-analysis of sun exposure in analytic studies has demonstrated increased risks.[33] For the purposes of this meta-analysis, "intermittent" exposure was largely recreational and elicited in most studies by asking about high-exposure activities, such as sunbathing, water sports, and sunny vacations. "Chronic" exposure was essentially occupational exposure. "Total" exposure was a combination of both chronic and intermittent. In the meta-analyses, genders were combined, and individual-level data on exposure or phenotype were not available. Childhood (age, <15 years) and adult (age, >19 years) sunburns were also separated. Overall, total sun exposure was associated with a modest risk (RR, 1.34; 95% CI, 1.02–1.77). There was heterogeneity in the studies included in this analysis, which was explained partially by year of publication. Studies published before 1990 had lower risks (RR, 0.92; 95% CI, 0.59–1.42) than those published later (RR, 1.75; 95% CI, 1.31–2.35). Intermittent sun exposure also conferred somewhat higher risk (RR, 1.61; 95% CI, 1.31–1.99), again with significant heterogeneity. This heterogeneity was attributed to variation in definitions of intermittent exposure, country of origin, and adjustment for phenotype or phototype. Chronic sun exposure, however, was not significantly associated with melanoma risk (RR, 0.95; 95% CI, 0.87–1.04), but again, there was evidence of heterogeneity. Two of the factors in the heterogeneity were controls with dermatologic conditions and latitude of the study.[33] At higher latitudes, there was a greater association between chronic exposure and melanoma (P = .031). Sunburns conferred an increased risk in almost all of the studies included (RR, 2.03; 95% CI, 1.73–2.37). For history of sunburns, latitude affected risk estimates. Above 46° (average latitude), the estimates were higher (RR, 2.54; 95% CI, 1.99–3.24) than those in lower latitudes (RR, 1.91; 95% CI, 1.58–2.31). Timing of the sunburns, childhood or adult, varied somewhat, but both appeared important and were not significantly different. In another meta-analysis of sunburns and melanoma risk, Dennis and colleagues[35] found evidence for a dose-response relationship with number of sunburns and melanoma risk across childhood, adolescence, and adulthood. Although childhood exposure is clearly important for melanoma risk, growing evidence suggests that sun exposure during all age periods affects melanoma risk.

Two recent meta-analyses have evaluated the risk of melanoma associated with sun-bed use.[36,37] There is a major overlap between the studies included in the two analyses. Not surprisingly, the findings were quite similar. Ever/never use of sunlamps/sun beds was associated with melanoma in both (RR, 1.25; 95% CI, 1.05–1.49; RR, 1.15; 95% CI, 1.00–1.31). Young age at first exposure conferred a somewhat higher risk (RR, 1.69; 95% CI, 1.32–2.18; RR, 1.75; 95% CI, 1.35–2.26). Gallagher and colleagues[36] also evaluated the longest duration or highest frequency of use and found similar risks (RR, 1.61; 95% CI, 1.21–2.12). Given the frequency of sun-bed use in adolescents,[38] and the ready availability of indoor tanning facilities in the United States,[39] the increase in melanoma noted in young women by Purdue and colleagues[9] may be a sentinel finding for a persistent future increase in young adults.

There are also biologic data and limited epidemiologic data that suggest a role of redox-active metals in melanoma risk.[40] Most of the epidemiologic data derive from exposure cohorts, such as occupational cohorts or joint-replacement cohorts. Neither group of cohorts has adequate sun exposure information to control for this major risk factor or to explore interactions with metal exposure. Despite the limitations, the role of metals in melanoma risk is intriguing and should be pursued.

Screening for melanoma remains controversial.[41] Fears and colleagues[42] developed a melanoma risk assessment tool for primary care providers to identify individuals who might benefit from screening. They first developed parsimonious RR models within a large case-control study, which yielded attributable risks of 86% for men and 89% for women. Non-Hispanic whites who had no personal history of melanoma or nonmelanoma skin cancers or family history of melanoma were included. Other ethnicities were excluded, because the numbers were too sparse. Individuals with previous skin cancer or family history of melanoma should already be in skin screening programs as part of accepted best practices. Fears and colleagues then used SEER gender-, age-, and location-specific incidence rates to estimate a 5-year absolute risk for an individual using age, gender, location, and limited phenotype markers accessible on the back (freckling, complexion, solar damage, number of nevi). These phenotypic makers are a measure of both susceptibility and exposure. The tool is available at http://www.cancer.gov/melanomarisktool/, but it needs to be validated in different groups. If validated, it could be useful as an early screening tool to decide who is at sufficient risk to warrant full skin examination.

FAMILY AND GENETIC SUSCEPTIBILITY STUDIES

Family history of melanoma confers approximately two-fold increased risk of melanoma.[29,43,44] Family history of one relative is moderately frequent in the United States; one large study found that 8% of cases had such a history.[44] Much more infrequent are families with three or more living members with melanoma; these are the families in which identification of high-risk susceptibility genes is possible. In the same study, only 0.4% of cases reported two or more relatives previously diagnosed with melanoma.

Familial melanoma is also heterogeneous. Two major susceptibility genes have been identified: CDKN2A and CDK4. CDKN2A codes for two different proteins, p16 (in the retinoblastoma pathway) and p14ARF (in the p53 apoptosis pathway). CDK4 is also in the retinoblastoma pathway. CDKN2A mutations are identified in 39% of 385 melanoma-prone families from Australia, North America, Europe, and Israel.[45] The prevalence of mutations varied by continent, with the lowest prevalence in Australia (20%); intermediate in North America (45%); and highest in Europe (57%). Goldstein and colleagues examined several features previously associated with CDKN2A mutations as predictors of mutation status across the different geographic areas. In Australia, the presence of multiple primary melanomas in two or more family members, median age of diagnosis less than or equal to age 40 years, and six or more individuals in the family with melanoma was associated with mutations in CDKN2A. In North America, families with at least one individual with multiple primary melanomas and median age at diagnosis less than or equal to 40 years were more likely to have mutations. In Europe, four or more individuals with melanoma in the family, one or more with multiple primary melanomas, age 50 years or lesser at diagnosis of melanoma, and history of pancreatic cancer in a family member predicted mutation status. These findings are consistent with the lower population rates of melanoma in Europe and higher rates of melanoma in North America and Australia. The lack of pancreatic cancer association in Australia could be due to the spectrum of mutations.[45] The penetrance of CDKN2A mutations also varies across the continents. The overall cumulative risk of melanoma by age 80 years among mutation carriers from families with CDKN2A mutations is 0.67 (95% CI, 0.31–0.96), but it ranged from 0.58 in Europe to 0.76 in the United States to 0.91 in Australia.[46] Population rates of melanoma were associated with the variation; this implies that factors important in determining melanoma in the general population are also important in high-risk families. The penetrance of melanoma by age 80 years among individuals with CDKN2A mutations unselected for family history of melanoma from Australia, the United States and Europe has been estimated to be 0.28 (95% CI, 0.18–0.40).[47] The difference in penetrance among individuals in high-risk families and those unselected for family history suggests that additional risk factors may be involved in the families with many affected individuals.

The frequency of mutations in CDK4 is much lower than the frequency of CDKN2A mutations. Among 466 families identified by GenoMEL, a consortium comprising melanoma genetics research groups from North America, Europe, Australia, and Asia, the prevalence of CDKN2A and CDK4 mutations was evaluated.[48] Mutations in *CDKN2A* that affected only p14ARF (exon 1β and large deletions), the alternative reading frame of *CDKN2A,* were considered separately from those that affect p16. Overall, 41% of families (n = 190) had mutations; 178 of these affected p16. Of the remaining 12 mutations identified, 5 (1.8%) affected *CDK4* and 7 (2.5%) affected p14ARF. Founder mutations in *CDKN2A* were the most frequent mutations in specific geographic locales (the Netherlands, Sweden, United Kingdom). The median age at diagnosis differs by mutation status within the families. In families with no mutation detected, the median age was 45 years; in those with *CDKN2A* mutations, 36 years; in those with p14ARF, 30 years; and in those with *CDK4,* 32 years. The occurrence of tumors other than melanoma in family members was compared across the families with different mutations. As previously noted,[49] there was a strong relationship between pancreatic cancer and *CDKN2A* mutations (P<.001); the risk of pancreatic cancer also varied by specific mutations.[48] In contrast, no families with p14ARF mutations or *CDK4* mutations had pancreatic cancer. Families with p14ARF mutations (exon 1β or large deletions) had a marginally significant association with neural tumors (n = 2/7; P = .05); inclusion of families with *CDKN2A* mutations that altered both p16 and p14ARF changed the association (9/99; P = .12). No families with *CDK4* mutations had neural tumors. No significant association with uveal melanomas was found in any of the mutation groups.

Variations in *MC1R* are important components of pigment diversity.[50] Multiple variants have been described, and allele frequencies differ across populations; some variants are associated with red hair (RHC) and some are not (rhc). Variants differ in their associations with melanoma and nonmelanoma skin cancer, but rhc variants as well as RHC variants confer increased risk. A recent meta-analysis of 22 studies that evaluated the association of 9 common *MC1R* variants (pV60L, pD84E, pV92M, pR142H, pR151C, pI155T, pR160W, pR163Q, and pD294H) and melanoma risk summarized the risks of melanoma for each variant.[51] Risks ranged from 1.15 (95% CI, 0.92–1.43) for pV60L to 2.45 (95% CI, 1.32–4.55) for pI155T. All but two, pV60L and pV92M, were significantly associated with melanoma risk. The five variants with significant association with red hair (pD84E, pR124H, pR151C, pR160W, and pD294H) conferred melanoma risks from 1.43 (95% CI, 1.20–1.70) to 2.40 (1.50-3.84). Two others (pV92M, pI155T) were not associated with red hair; pV92M was also not significantly associated with melanoma risk (RR, 1.22; 95% CI, 0.99–1.50). The other two variants (pV60L, pR163Q) were inversely associated with red hair; pR163Q was associated with melanoma risk (RR, 1.42 [1.09–1.85]).[51] Germline *MC1R* variation has been associated with somatic *BRAF* mutant melanomas, but not *BRAF* wild type.[52,53] These findings are consistent with the hypothesis that variants in *MC1R* affect melanoma risk by other mechanisms than just pigmentation pathways.

Within melanoma-prone families, *MC1R* variation increases the risk of melanoma in families without *CDKN2A* mutation[54] and modifies the risk of melanoma associated with *CDKN2A* mutations.[55] Most cases in the *CDKN2A* mutation-positive families had at least one *MC1R* variant. Among *CDKN2A* carriers, after adjustment for age, nevi, and pigmentation, multiple *MC1R* variants conferred a seven-fold (95% CI, 1.6–33.2) increased risk of melanoma. Individuals with multiple primary melanomas were significantly more likely to carry multiple *MC1R* variants. Age of onset was also younger for those with multiple *MC1R* variants.[55] To explore the effects of *MC1R* variants on the risk of melanoma in carriers of one *CDKN2A* founder mutation dating back approximately 97 generations, pG101W, Goldstein and colleagues[56] evaluated melanoma-prone families from France, Italy, Spain, and the United States. Overall, the risk of developing melanoma associated with multiple *MC1R* variants was very similar (RR, 7.2; 95% CI, 2.3–23.1). There was also a similar pattern of more frequent multiple *MC1R* variants in multiple primary cases, but the association was weaker when the American families (included in the previous analysis) were removed. Most of the overall effect derived from the multiplex families. Two or more *MC1R* variants were also associated with earlier age of onset in the individuals with multiple primary melanomas. The Italian families were significantly different from the other groups. There were fewer individuals with *MC1R* variants and no association between number of *MC1R* variants and melanoma risk.

As noted above, although high-risk susceptibility genes *CDKN2A* and *CDK4* have been identified, they explain less than half of familial melanoma. It is unlikely that additional high-risk susceptibility genes with a larger effect will be found, because multiple groups have been searching diligently since *CDK4* was identified in 1996.[57] To identify additional lower-risk susceptibility genes by an agnostic approach, genome-wide association studies have been conducted by several groups. In a genome-wide scan of 864 melanoma cases and 864 controls from Australia, two single nucleotide polymorphisms (SNPs) of interest were identified, rs17305657 ($P = 2.56 \times 10^{-7}$) and rs4911442 ($P = 2.39 \times 10^{-6}$).[58] These SNPs are approximately 1.5 Mb apart on chromosome 20q. Replication of 33 SNPs selected for fine mapping across a 2.78-Mb region on 20q was done in three sets of melanoma cases and controls totaling 2019 cases and 2105 controls. Two of the fine mapping SNPs (rs910873 and rs1885120) yielded a higher significance than the original SNPs ($P < 1 \times 10^{-15}$). The effects of these 2 SNPs could not be separated and were not related to 2 candidate genes of interest in the region, *E2F1* and *ASIP*. The authors also explored per allele risk according to age at onset and found some evidence of a stronger effect in patients 40 years old and younger. The Icelandic group originally conducted a genome-wide scan of pigmentation characteristics in 2986 Icelandic individuals and identified 6 areas of interest.[59] They then replicated nine SNPs in the six areas in 2718 additional Icelandic and 1214 Dutch individuals. They found a highly significant association of rs4785763 (OR, 5.6; $P = 3.2 \times 10^{-56}$) located in *MC1R* for red hair. They also identified a novel region on 6p25.3 best characterized by rs1540771 (OR, 1.4, $P = 1.9 \times 10^{-9}$) related to freckling and rs1042602 in tyrosinase also related to freckling ($P = 1.5 \times 10^{-11}$). Three SNPs in the first exons of *SLC24A4* were significantly associated with hair color and eye color ($P < 1.9 \times 10^{-8}$). SNPs in the known pigmentation gene *OCA2* were significantly associated with eye and hair color; rs1667394 showed the strongest risk (OR, 35, $P = 1.4 \times 10^{-124}$ for blue vs brown eyes). The final SNP was rs12821256 on 12q21.33, which was significantly related to blond versus brown hair ($P = 3.8 \times 10^{-30}$). The nearest gene to this SNP is *KITLG*. They then increased the sample size of the full scan to 5130 and replicated additional SNPs in 2116 Icelandic and 1214 Dutch individuals.[60] They found significant association ($P = 3.9 \times 10^{-9}$) with burning and freckling with 6 SNPs in linkage disequilibrium on 20q11.22. A 2-SNP haplotype, which they called the *ASIP* haplotype, accounts for the association and is highly significant in the combined analysis ($P < 10^{-24}$). Two coding SNPs in *TPCN2* were associated with blond versus brown hair ($P < 10^{-16}$). One SNP in a linkage disequilibrium block that includes *TYRP1* was significantly related to eye color ($P = 5.9 \times 10^{-17}$). The 11 SNPs identified in these two studies and *MC1R* variants were then tested for association with melanoma in three groups from Iceland, Sweden, and Spain.[61] A total of 1586 invasive and 407 in situ melanomas and 40,094 controls were included. In the combined melanoma cases, there was a significant association with the *ASIP* haplotype (OR, 1.45; 95% CI, 1.29–1.64; $P = 1.2 \times 10^{-9}$). The effect was stronger in the invasive than the in situ cases. There was also a significant association with the rs1126809[A] variant of *TYR* (OR, 1.21; 95% CI, 1.13–1.30; $P = 2.8 \times 10^{-7}$). Any *MC1R* variant conferred significant risk (OR, 1.24;

Table 2
Summary of risks for melanoma by identified risk factors

Risk Factor	Risk Quantification Method	Summary Estimates (Ref)
CDKN2A mutation, high-risk family	Penetrance at 80	0.67 (0.31–0.96)[46]
Europe		0.58
United States		0.76
Australia		0.91
CDKN2A mutation, unselected	Penetrance at 80	0.28 (0.18–0.40)[47]
MC1R RHC	RR	1.4–2.4[51]
rhc	RR	1.15 (NS)–2.5
Nevi (total body)		
16–40	RR	1.47 (1.36–1.59)[15]
101–120	RR	6.89 (4.63–10.25)
Dysplastic nevi (dichotomous)	RR	10 (5.0–20)[15]
1 DN	RR	1.6 (1.38–1.85)
5+DN	RR	10 (5.1–22)
Light skin color	RR	2.06 (1.68–2.52)[29]
Poor tanning ability	RR	2.09 (1.67–2.58)
Light eye color	RR	1.47 (1.28–1.69)
Light hair color	RR	1.78 (1.63–1.95)
Freckling	RR	2.1 (1.8–2.5)
Total sun exposure	RR	1.34 (1.01–1.77)[33]
Sunburns	RR	2.03 (1.73–2.37)
Sun-bed use	RR	1.25 (1.05–1.49)[36]

Abbreviation: DN, dysplastic nevi.

95% CI, 1.17–1.32; $P = 1.6 \times 10^{-11}$). The effect was higher and more significant with RHC variants. Thus, to date, most of the loci identified in genome-wide association studies seem related to pigmentation. Ongoing studies may yield additional informative loci.

With all of the epidemiologic studies in the past several decades (**Table 2**), we can now identify individuals at increased risk of melanoma and exposures related to melanoma. It is time to consider translating this knowledge to appropriate interventions to decrease melanoma risk in the susceptible subgroups.

REFERENCES

1. Ries LAG, Melbert D, Krapcho M, et al. SEER Cancer statistics review, 1975–2005. Bethesda (MD): National Cancer Institute; 2008.
2. Clegg LX, Feuer EJ, Midthune DN, et al. Impact of reporting delay and reporting error on cancer incidence rates and trends. J Natl Cancer Inst 2002;94(20):1537–45.
3. Anderson WF, Pfeiffer RM, Tucker MA, et al. Divergent cancer pathways for early-onset and late-onset cutaneous malignant melanoma. Cancer, in press.
4. Karagas MR, Zens MS, Stukel TA, et al. Pregnancy history and incidence of melanoma in women: a pooled analysis. Cancer Causes Control 2006;17(1):11–9.
5. Lea CS, Holly EA, Hartge P, et al. Reproductive risk factors for cutaneous melanoma in women: a case-control study. Am J Epidemiol 2007;165(5):505–13.

6. Lachiewicz AM, Berwick M, Wiggins CL, et al. Epidemiologic support for melanoma heterogeneity using the surveillance, epidemiology, and end results program. J Invest Dermatol 2008;128(5):1340–2.

7. Bradford PT, Goldstein AM, McMaster ML, et al. Acral lentiginous melanoma: incidence and survival patterns in the United States, 1986–2005. Arch Dermatol, in press.

8. Cockburn MG, Zadnick J, Deapen D. Developing epidemic of melanoma in the Hispanic population of California. Cancer 2006;106(5):1162–8.

9. Purdue MP, Freeman LE, Anderson WF, et al. Recent trends in incidence of cutaneous melanoma among US Caucasian young adults. J Invest Dermatol 2008; 128(12):2905–8.

10. Burton RC, Armstrong BK. Non-metastasizing melanoma? J Surg Oncol 1998; 67(2):73–6.

11. Swerlick RA, Chen S. The melanoma epidemic: more apparent than real? Mayo Clin Proc 1997;72(6):559–64.

12. Welch HG, Woloshin S, Schwartz LM. Skin biopsy rates and incidence of melanoma: population based ecological study. BMJ 2005;331(7515):481–4.

13. Linos E, Swetter SM, Cockburn MG, et al. Increasing burden of melanoma in the United States. J Invest Dermatol 2009 [epub ahead of print].

14. Tucker MA, Halpern A, Holly EA, et al. Clinically recognized dysplastic nevi. A central risk factor for cutaneous melanoma. JAMA 1997;277(18):1439–44.

15. Gandini S, Sera F, Cattaruzza MS, et al. Meta-analysis of risk factors for cutaneous melanoma: I. Common and atypical naevi. Eur J Cancer 2005;41(1):28–44.

16. Olsen CM, Zens MS, Stukel TA, et al. Nevus density and melanoma risk in women: a pooled analysis to test the divergent pathway hypothesis. Int J Cancer 2009; 124(4):937–44.

17. Chang YM, Newton-Bishop JA, Bishop DT, et al. A pooled analysis of melanocytic nevus phenotype and the risk of cutaneous melanoma at different latitudes. Int J Cancer 2009;124(2):420–8.

18. Tucker MA, Goldstein AM. Melanoma etiology: where are we? Oncogene 2003; 22(20):3042–52.

19. Elder DE, Clark WH Jr, Elenitsas R, et al. The early and intermediate precursor lesions of tumor progression in the melanocytic system: common acquired nevi and atypical (dysplastic) nevi. Semin Diagn Pathol 1993;10(1):18–35.

20. Bataille V, Grulich A, Sasieni P, et al. The association between naevi and melanoma in populations with different levels of sun exposure: a joint case-control study of melanoma in the UK and Australia. Br J Cancer 1998;77(3):505–10.

21. Falchi M, Spector TD, Perks U, et al. Genome-wide search for nevus density shows linkage to two melanoma loci on chromosome 9 and identifies a new QTL on 5q31 in an adult twin cohort. Hum Mol Genet 2006;15(20):2975–9.

22. Zhu G, Montgomery GW, James MR, et al. A genome-wide scan for naevus count: linkage to CDKN2A and to other chromosome regions. Eur J Hum Genet 2007;15(1):94–102.

23. Barrett JH, Gaut R, Wachsmuth R, et al. Linkage and association analysis of nevus density and the region containing the melanoma gene CDKN2A in UK twins. Br J Cancer 2003;88(12):1920–4.

24. Zhu G, Duffy DL, Turner DR, et al. Linkage and association analysis of radiation damage repair genes XRCC3 and XRCC5 with nevus density in adolescent twins. Twin Res 2003;6(4):315–21.

25. Celebi JT, Ward KM, Wanner M, et al. Evaluation of germline CDKN2A, ARF, CDK4, PTEN, and BRAF alterations in atypical mole syndrome. Clin Exp Dermatol 2005;30(1):68–70.

26. Gallagher RP, Rivers JK, Lee TK, et al. Broad-spectrum sunscreen use and the development of new nevi in white children: a randomized controlled trial. JAMA 2000;283(22):2955–60.
27. Oliveria SA, Satagopan JM, Geller AC, et al. Study of Nevi in Children (SONIC): baseline findings and predictors of nevus count. Am J Epidemiol 2009;169(1): 41–53.
28. Wachsmuth RC, Turner F, Barrett JH, et al. The effect of sun exposure in determining nevus density in UK adolescent twins. J Invest Dermatol 2005;124(1):56–62.
29. Gandini S, Sera F, Cattaruzza MS, et al. Meta-analysis of risk factors for cutaneous melanoma: III. Family history, actinic damage and phenotypic factors. Eur J Cancer 2005;41(14):2040–59.
30. IARCIn: IARC Monographs on the Evaluation of Carcinogenic Risks to Humans: Solar and Ultraviolet Radiation, vol. 55. Lyon (France): IARC Monographs on the Evaluation of Carcinogenic Risks to Humans; 1992.
31. English DR, Armstrong BK, Kricker A. Reproducibility of reported measurements of sun exposure in a case-control study. Cancer Epidemiol Biomarkers Prev 1998; 7(10):857–63.
32. Yu CL, Li Y, Freedman DM, et al. Assessment of lifetime cumulative sun exposure using a self-administered questionnaire: reliability of two approaches. Cancer Epidemiol Biomarkers Prev 2009;18(2):464–71.
33. Gandini S, Sera F, Cattaruzza MS, et al. Meta-analysis of risk factors for cutaneous melanoma: II. Sun exposure. Eur J Cancer 2005;41(1):45–60.
34. Fears TR, Bird CC, Guerry D, et al. Average midrange ultraviolet radiation flux and time outdoors predict melanoma risk. Cancer Res 2002;62(14):3992–6.
35. Dennis LK, Vanbeek MJ, Beane Freeman LE, et al. Sunburns and risk of cutaneous melanoma: does age matter? A comprehensive meta-analysis. Ann Epidemiol 2008;18(8):614–27.
36. Gallagher RP, Spinelli JJ, Lee TK. Tanning beds, sunlamps, and risk of cutaneous malignant melanoma. Cancer Epidemiol Biomarkers Prev 2005;14(3):562–6.
37. IARC Working Group on artificial ultraviolet (UV) light and skin cancer. The association of use of sunbeds with cutaneous malignant melanoma and other skin cancers: a systematic review. Int J Cancer 2007;120(5):1116–22.
38. Cokkinides V, Weinstock M, Lazovich D, et al. Indoor tanning use among adolescents in the US, 1998 to 2004. Cancer 2009;115(1):190–8.
39. Hoerster KD, Garrow RL, Mayer JA, et al. Density of indoor tanning facilities in 116 large U.S. cities. Am J Prev Med 2009;36(3):243–6.
40. Meyskens FL Jr, Berwick M. UV or not UV: metals are the answer. Cancer Epidemiol Biomarkers Prev 2008;17(2):268–70.
41. Wolff T, Tai E, Miller T. Screening for skin cancer: an update of the evidence for the U.S. Preventive Services Task Force. Ann Intern Med 2009;150(3):194–8.
42. Fears TR, Guerry D, Pfeiffer RM, et al. Identifying individuals at high risk of melanoma: a practical predictor of absolute risk. J Clin Oncol 2006;24(22):3590–6.
43. Ford D, Bliss JM, Swerdlow AJ, et al. Risk of cutaneous melanoma associated with a family history of the disease. The International Melanoma Analysis Group (IMAGE). Int J Cancer 1995;62(4):377–81.
44. Rutter JL, Bromley CM, Goldstein AM, et al. Heterogeneity of risk for melanoma and pancreatic and digestive malignancies: a melanoma case-control study. Cancer 2004;101(12):2809–16.
45. Goldstein AM, Chan M, Harland M, et al. Features associated with germline CDKN2A mutations: a GenoMEL study of melanoma-prone families from three continents. J Med Genet 2007;44(2):99–106.

46. Bishop DT, Demenais F, Goldstein AM, et al. Geographical variation in the penetrance of CDKN2A mutations for melanoma. J Natl Cancer Inst 2002;94(12): 894–903.
47. Begg CB, Orlow I, Hummer AJ, et al. Lifetime risk of melanoma in CDKN2A mutation carriers in a population-based sample. J Natl Cancer Inst 2005;97(20): 1507–15.
48. Goldstein AM, Chan M, Harland M, et al. High-risk melanoma susceptibility genes and pancreatic cancer, neural system tumors, and uveal melanoma across GenoMEL. Cancer Res 2006;66(20):9818–28.
49. Goldstein AM. Familial melanoma, pancreatic cancer and germline CDKN2A mutations. Hum Mutat 2004;23(6):630.
50. Gerstenblith MR, Goldstein AM, Fargnoli MC, et al. Comprehensive evaluation of allele frequency differences of MC1R variants across populations. Hum Mutat 2007;28(5):495–505.
51. Raimondi S, Sera F, Gandini S, et al. MC1R variants, melanoma and red hair color phenotype: a meta-analysis. Int J Cancer 2008;122(12):2753–60.
52. Landi MT, Bauer J, Pfeiffer RM, et al. MC1R germline variants confer risk for BRAF-mutant melanoma. Science 2006;313(5786):521–2.
53. Fargnoli MC, Pike K, Pfeiffer RM, et al. MC1R variants increase risk of melanomas harboring BRAF mutations. J Invest Dermatol 2008;128(10):2485–90.
54. Landi MT, Kanetsky PA, Tsang S, et al. MC1R, ASIP, and DNA repair in sporadic and familial melanoma in a Mediterranean population. J Natl Cancer Inst 2005; 97(13):998–1007.
55. Goldstein AM, Landi MT, Tsang S, et al. Association of MC1R variants and risk of melanoma in melanoma-prone families with CDKN2A mutations. Cancer Epidemiol Biomarkers Prev 2005;14(9):2208–12.
56. Goldstein AM, Chaudru V, Ghiorzo P, et al. Cutaneous phenotype and MC1R variants as modifying factors for the development of melanoma in CDKN2A G101W mutation carriers from 4 countries. Int J Cancer 2007;121(4):825–31.
57. Zuo L, Weger J, Yang Q, et al. Germline mutations in the p16INK4a binding domain of CDK4 in familial melanoma. Nat Genet 1996;12(1):97–9.
58. Brown KM, Macgregor S, Montgomery GW, et al. Common sequence variants on 20q11.22 confer melanoma susceptibility. Nat Genet 2008;40(7):838–40.
59. Sulem P, Gudbjartsson DF, Stacey SN, et al. Genetic determinants of hair, eye and skin pigmentation in Europeans. Nat Genet 2007;39(12):1443–52.
60. Sulem P, Gudbjartsson DF, Stacey SN, et al. Two newly identified genetic determinants of pigmentation in Europeans. Nat Genet 2008;40(7):835–7.
61. Gudbjartsson DF, Sulem P, Stacey SN, et al. ASIP and TYR pigmentation variants associate with cutaneous melanoma and basal cell carcinoma. Nat Genet 2008; 40(7):886–91.

Applications of Genomics in Melanoma Oncogene Discovery

Michael F. Berger, PhD[a], Levi A. Garraway, MD, PhD[a,b,c],*

KEYWORDS

- Melanoma • Oncogene • DNA sequencing • Microarrays
- Gene amplification • Targeted therapy

The notion of cancer as a genetic disease is, by now, well established.[1] The accumulation of genomic mutations and epigenetic changes that dysregulate genes controlling key hallmarks of malignancy[2] (proliferation, survival, invasion, and so forth) is considered to be the main cause of cancer. The last decade has seen the discovery of mutations in many genes driving the progression of a host of different cancers. These include activating mutations in growth-promoting oncogenes, inactivating mutations in growth-inhibiting tumor-suppressor genes, and alterations to stability genes. Collectively, somatic base pair mutations have been identified in almost 10% of genes in human cancers, although only a subset of these are believed to be driver events.[3] Ongoing efforts to elucidate these genes and their roles in promoting the growth of different tumor types constitute a major component of molecular cancer research.

Melanoma, a malignant tumor of melanocytes, is responsible for 80% of all deaths from skin cancer. An estimated 62,000 new melanoma cases were diagnosed in the United States in 2008.[4] The poor prognosis of advanced melanoma and the relative ineffectiveness of conventional therapies for patients with metastatic disease underscore a dire need for improved therapeutic agents. Recent discoveries of recurrent mutations in the melanoma genome have provided an improved understanding of the biology of melanoma genesis and progression as well as an opportunity for the development of new classes of targeted drugs. In this review, the discoveries of

This work was supported by Grant No. DP2OD002750 (NIH), the Burroughs-Wellcome Fund, and the Starr Cancer Consortium.

[a] The Broad Institute of MIT and Harvard, 7 Cambridge Center, Cambridge, MA 02142, USA
[b] Department of Medical Oncology, Dana-Farber Cancer Institute, 44 Binney Street, D1542, Boston, MA 02115, USA
[c] Center for Cancer Genome Discovery, Dana-Farber Cancer Institute, 44 Binney Street, D1542, Boston, MA 02115, USA
* Corresponding author. Department of Medical Oncology, Dana-Farber Cancer Institute, 44 Binney Street, D1542, Boston, MA 02115.
E-mail address: levi_garraway@dfci.harvard.edu (L.A. Garraway).

several critical melanoma oncogenes are described and the role played by genomic technologies is highlighted. Our goal is not to provide a comprehensive list of all genetic alterations observed in melanoma, but to illustrate through melanoma onco-gene discovery how genomic analysis can lead to a better understanding of tumor biology and novel therapeutic avenues. The article concludes with a discussion of emerging "omic" technologies and how these might lead to the discovery of additional oncogenes that indicate a path to improved prognosis and treatment of patients suffering from this deadly malignancy.

MELANOMA ONCOGENES

Genetic mutations involving numerous genes have been linked to melanoma genesis and progression. These genes encompass many signaling pathways, including the receptor tyrosine kinase (RTK), phosphatidylinositol-3-kinase (PI(3)K), retinoblastoma (RB), p53, Wnt, and NF-kB pathways. The supporting evidence implicating these oncogenes in melanoma ranges from positional cloning studies in familial melanoma to elevated frequencies of mutation or amplification in patient cohorts, to functional studies in vitro and in vivo. Five well-studied melanoma oncogenes and their contribu-tions to overall morbidity are considered (**Table 1**). Each of these genes was identified by a different approach, highlighting alternate strategies for melanoma oncogene discovery and emphasizing the expanding importance of technology and integrative genomic analysis.

NRAS

One of the first genes shown to be specifically mutated in melanoma was *NRAS*, a gene encoding a member of the RAS family of small GTP-binding proteins. The RAS proteins lie at the top of the RAS/RAF/MEK/ERK MAP kinase pathway, which activates a large number of growth-promoting genes in response to signals trans-mitted from growth factors and cytokines. Regulation of RAS signaling is achieved by alternating between active (GTP-bound) and inactive (GDP-bound) forms of the RAS protein. The prototypic members of the RAS family, HRAS and KRAS, were orig-inally discovered as the transforming oncoproteins in Harvey and Kirsten murine sarcoma viruses.[5] Human cellular versions of the *HRAS* and *KRAS* genes were subse-quently identified, and single nucleotide mutations were shown to confer transforming capabilities on these genes on transfection into the mouse embryonic fibroblast NIH

Table 1
Summary of exemplary melanoma oncogenes

Gene	Function	Alteration	Prevalence	Discovery Method
NRAS	Growth, proliferation	Mutation	15%–30%	Transformation assay, genotyping
BRAF	Proliferation, survival	Mutation	50%–70%	Systematic DNA sequencing
MITF	Lineage survival	Amplification	10%–20%	Copy number and gene expression profiling
NEDD9	Invasion, metastasis	Amplification	36%	Copy number profiling and evolutionary conservation
KIT	Proliferation, survival	Mutation, amplification	2%–5%	DNA sequencing

3T3 cell line.[6–8] *NRAS* was later discovered as the transforming gene of a neuroblastoma cell line, and sequence analysis revealed considerable homology with *HRAS* and *KRAS*.[9,10] Mutations converting all 3 genes to active oncogenes nearly always occur in residues 12, 13, or 61 of the protein.[11] These mutations impair the GTPase catalytic activity of RAS, resulting in a constitutively GTP-bound and activated state. Altogether, approximately 20% to 30% of human tumors carry a mutation in one of the *RAS* genes.

NRAS was first shown to be mutated in melanoma in the mid-1980s when 2 studies demonstrated that *NRAS* DNA isolated from 4 human melanoma cell lines was sufficient to transform NIH 3T3 cells.[12,13] Subsequent sequencing and genotyping efforts revealed that *NRAS* is mutated in 15% to 30% of melanomas, more than 10 times more frequently than *HRAS* or *KRAS*.[14–18] Notably, the mutations occur most often at residue 61. The spatial distribution of *NRAS*-mutated tumors on the skin and their proclivity for dipyrimidine mutations suggest a possible correlation with UV exposure.[14,17] Transgenic mice with oncogenic NRAS targeted to the melanocytic compartment show hyperpigmented skin and develop cutaneous metastasizing melanoma.[19] In addition to its role in tumor formation, mutant *RAS* is also critical for tumor maintenance.[20] Knockdown of mutant *NRAS* (but not wild-type *NRAS*) by RNA interference reduces the viability of melanoma cell lines, suggesting a possible therapeutic avenue in patients whose tumors harbor this mutation.[21] However, the development of small molecules that target RAS proteins directly has proved exceedingly difficult.

As stated earlier, RAS operates in the MAP kinase pathway. This pathway is hyperactivated in up to 90% of human melanomas.[22] This underscores the contribution of *NRAS* mutations to the development of melanoma but also indicates the involvement of other genes in the pathway, discussed later. At the same time, RAS-activating mutations can influence the phosphoinositide-3-OH kinase (PI(3)K) pathway. The specificity of mutations in melanoma for *NRAS* compared with *HRAS* and *KRAS* is notable considering that all 3 isoforms are expressed in primary melanomas and melanoma-derived short-term cultures,[23,24] and that *HRAS* and *KRAS* are mutated in a variety of other human cancers. For example, *KRAS* mutations are found in 15% to 20% of lung cancers, approximately 30% of colorectal cancers, and up to 90% of pancreatic adenocarcinomas.[11] *HRAS* mutations have been detected in Spitz nevi, yet they rarely occur in malignant melanoma.[25] Comparisons of the transformation efficiencies of different RAS isoforms suggest that the activity of different isoforms may depend on the cellular context.[26]

In summary, the recurrence and high transforming potential of oncogenic *NRAS* mutations in human melanomas demonstrate the critical role of this gene and its downstream effector mechanisms in melanoma genesis and maintenance. As with many other classic oncogenes described in cancer, the original discovery and validation of *NRAS* as a melanoma oncogene required a laborious series of low-throughput experiments spanning many years and multiple research groups. The following examples illustrate how recent melanoma oncogene discoveries have emerged from powerful systematic approaches enabled by the massive technology revolution that accompanied the genomic era.

BRAF

BRAF, a serine-threonine kinase, lies downstream of RAS in the MAP kinase signaling pathway (**Fig. 1**). BRAF induces MEK to phosphorylate ERK, which enhances cell growth and proliferation. In 2002, as part of a large-scale DNA sequencing effort to identify mutant oncogenes in the MAP kinase pathway, Davies and colleagues[27] discovered highly recurrent oncogenic BRAF mutations in melanoma through systematic resequencing across 545 cancer cell lines. The *BRAF* gene was observed to be mutated in 20 of 34 (59%) melanoma cell lines and an additional 18 of 24 (75%) patient-derived primary melanomas and short-term cultures, compared with an over-all mutation frequency of 8% in all cancers. (After melanoma, *BRAF* was mutated in 15% of colon cancers, 11% of gliomas, and 10% of ovarian cancers, considering cell lines and primary tumors.) Notably, greater than 90% of the *BRAF* mutations in melanoma involved a single substitution of valine to glutamic acid in the kinase domain (V600E).[27] Subsequent studies have confirmed the specificity for V600E mutations and established the overall frequency of *BRAF* mutations at 50% to 70% in cutaneous melanomas.[28-32] Unlike the mutation patterns observed in *NRAS*, the T → A transversion associated with the V600E mutation is not suggestive of UV-induced DNA damage, although there is an apparent association between this mutation and intermittent exposure to sun.[31] Surprisingly, the V600E mutation was also observed in 39 of 44 (89%) benign melanocytic nevi, suggesting that mutation of *BRAF* represents an early event in melanocytic neoplasia but one that is insufficient by itself for tumorigenesis.[29] However, mutant *BRAF* does seem to induce transformation of NIH 3T3 cells and murine melanocytes and allow them to grow as tumors in nude mice, clearly implicating it as an oncogene.[27,33-35]

As noted earlier, the oncogenic potential of BRAF lies in its ability to phosphorylate MEK, leading to ERK activation and cell proliferation (**Fig. 1**). The kinase activity of BRAF is normally regulated by the phosphorylation of 2 amino acids, T599 and S602, which disrupts the interaction between the activation segment and P loop and causes a conformational change to the active state.[36] The V600E mutant mimics these phosphorylation events by inserting a negatively charged residue in the activation segment, resulting in constitutively active BRAF.[27,34] The absence of comparable mutations from *ARAF* and *CRAF* (paralogs of *BRAF* that also function in MAP kinase

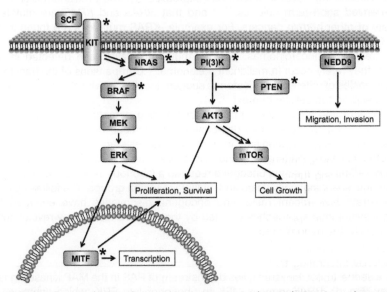

Fig. 1. Cell signaling pathways that undergo oncogenic dysregulation in melanoma. The receptor tyrosine kinase-driven MAP kinase and PI(3)K pathways are featured. Genes mutated in melanoma are marked with an asterisk. These include *KIT, NRAS, BRAF, MITF, PI(3)K, PTEN, AKT3,* and *NEDD9*.

signaling) is likely due to the further requirement of phosphorylation of an additional regulatory region (N region) in the kinase domain of these proteins. Unlike ARAF and CRAF, the N region of BRAF is constitutively phosphorylated such that BRAF is primed for activation.[33] Recent studies have identified several genes functioning downstream of BRAF in melanoma, including critical cell cycle regulators, tumor maintenance enzymes, and microphthalmia-associated transcription factor (MITF, discussed later).[37] These findings underscore the key role of BRAF in melanoma genesis and progression.

Depletion of oncogenic BRAF (but not ARAF or CRAF) by RNA interference in cultured human melanoma cells and mouse xenograft models has been shown to inhibit proliferation and induce apoptosis.[38,39] This suggests an essential role for the MAP kinase pathway in tumor maintenance. Consequently, inhibitors of BRAF and MEK are of considerable interest as potential targeted therapies for melanomas harboring BRAF mutations. To this end, several BRAF inhibitors (such as BAY 43-9006 and CHIR-265) and MEK inhibitors (such as PD0325901 and AZD6244) are currently in various stages of development or clinical trials.[37] One well-studied MEK inhibitor, CI-1040, clearly inhibits proliferation and soft-agar colony formation in vitro and causes rapid regression of BRAF mutant xenografts in mouse.[40] Given the additional role of RAS in MAP kinase signaling, it would stand to reason that MEK inhibition would produce a similar effect in NRAS mutant cells. However, human melanoma cell lines with BRAF mutations proved to be demonstrably more sensitive to CI-1040 and the related (but more potent) MEK inhibitor PD0325901 than did many NRAS mutant melanoma cell lines.[41] This suggests that activation of additional pathways by RAS, such as the PI(3)K/PTEN pathway, decreases the dependence of melanoma cells on MEK. Consistent with this, NRAS and BRAF mutations, as well as NRAS and PTEN mutations, are mutually exclusive in melanoma due to their shared pathway membership, whereas BRAF and PTEN mutations are coincident in up to 20% of melanomas.[42] BRAF and PTEN operate in different pathways downstream of RAS, such that separate mutations are required to activate both pathways. It thus remains uncertain as to why BRAF would be mutated so much more frequently than NRAS in melanoma.

Microphthalmia-Associated Transcription Factor

In addition to nucleotide substitutions, DNA copy number alterations are frequently observed in cancer. More than just passive reflections of the genomic instability of cancer, such amplifications and deletions often function as driver events in tumorigenesis by altering the expression levels of important genes regulating cell growth, survival, and so forth. Changes in DNA copy number are readily profiled at high resolution by hybridizing tumor genomic DNA to microarrays comprised of oligonucleotides spanning the entire human genome.[43] As an illustration of the use of recurrent chromosomal aberrations to identify a novel melanoma oncogene, Garraway and colleagues[44] profiled genomic copy gains and losses in the NCI-60 cancer cell line collection using high-density single nucleotide polymorphism (SNP) microarrays and observed a focal amplification at 3p14-3p13 shared among 6 out of 8 melanoma cell lines. By integrating these copy number data with gene expression signatures for this cell line collection, the investigators identified only 1 highly expressed gene located within the amplified region. The product of this gene, microphthalmia-associated transcription factor (MITF), was already known to be a master regulator of the melanocyte lineage and a sensitive marker for melanoma diagnosis.[45,46] However, this integrative genomics approach provided the first evidence that MITF is an oncogene in human melanoma and the target of a specific somatic alteration in this malignancy.

Detailed characterization of this locus by fluorescence in situ hybridization (FISH) established the frequency of *MITF* amplification in melanomas at 10% to 20%, with a higher incidence among advanced tumors and an associated decrease in survival of 5 years.[44] *MITF* amplifications are coincident with mutations in *BRAF*. Growth of NCI-60 cell lines harboring *MITF* amplification was inhibited following RNAi-mediated knockdown of MITF or introduction of dominant-negative MITF.[44] In an apparent contradiction, high levels of MITF also seem to reduce tumorigenicity and promote melanocyte differentiation, perhaps by transcriptionally activating p16INK4A and p21, 2 cyclin-dependent kinase inhibitors.[37] Tight regulation of MITF levels may therefore be necessary for maximal proliferation.

As a master regulator of melanocyte development and differentiation, MITF represents an emerging class of lineage-survival oncogenes.[47] Unlike oncogenic *NRAS* and *BRAF*, which acquire new and tumor-specific cellular functions through nucleotide mutations, *MITF* becomes oncogenic by way of deregulation, affecting survival mechanisms that are also present in the normal melanocyte lineage. It is well established that wild-type MITF is essential for lineage survival and that deficiency of MITF results in the absence (or loss) of melanocytes during development.[48] The same survival mechanisms that govern melanocyte proliferation and development may subsequently persist or become deregulated during tumor progression. Additional lineage-survival oncogenes have been implicated in other cancers for which normal lineage programs become aberrantly regulated. For example, the androgen receptor (*AR*) and thyroid transcription factor 1 (*TITF1*) are targeted by genetic alterations in carcinomas of the prostate and lung, respectively.[49,50] Like *MITF*, these genes encode transcription factors that are essential master regulators during development for their particular lineage, but whose functions provide key tumor survival roles in prostate and lung adenocarcinoma. These observations emphasize the importance of lineage in providing a context for additional oncogenic alterations and help to explain why certain mutations occur at different frequencies in discrete tumor types.

NEDD9

The identification of *MITF* within a locus of recurrent amplification in cancer was enabled by the integration of copy number and gene expression data. Subsequently, Kim and colleagues[51] used a related integrative genomics approach that incorporated evolutionary conservation to implicate *NEDD9* as a melanoma metastasis gene from within a broad gain of chromosome 6p. Amplification of 6p had been previously associated with 36% of human metastatic, but not primary, melanomas.[52] However, the shared amplified region spans more that 35 megabases, making recognition of the underlying driver gene(s) nearly impossible by analysis of copy number data alone. Using high-resolution microarray comparative genome hybridization, Kim and colleagues identified a recurrent focal amplification associated with metastatic potential in a genetically engineered inducible mouse model of melanoma. By performing a cross-species comparison between the mouse and human genomes, the investigators dramatically narrowed the minimal region of overlap to an 850-kilobase region on human chromosome 6p24-25. Further integration with expression data revealed *NEDD9* (*n*eural precursor cell *e*xpressed, *d*evelopmentally *d*own-regulated 9) as the only resident gene that was overexpressed compared with nontransformed primary melanocyte cultures. Accordingly, *NEDD9* is amplified in 36% of human metastatic melanomas and overexpressed at mRNA and protein levels in approximately 50%.

NEDD9 protein expression was shown to be up-regulated in a manner correlated with tumor progression.[51]

Functional studies provided further support of *NEDD9* as a melanoma gene important for invasion and metastasis.[51] Knockdown of *NEDD9* by RNAi reduced the number of distal metastases in vivo and limited cellular proliferation and invasion in vitro. In addition, gain-of-function studies demonstrated that overexpression of *NEDD9* enhances the metastatic potential of primary melanocytes and nonmetastatic melanoma cells. This increased invasiveness is conferred by a functional and physical interaction between NEDD9 and focal adhesion kinase (FAK) at the cell periphery. These results demonstrate the usefulness of genome-wide cross-species comparisons for oncogene discovery; in particular, the integration of genomic data from a mouse model and human tumors led to the identification of *NEDD9*. Genetically engineered mouse models also enabled the design of appropriate functional assays and suggested the genetic context in which these assays would be most informative.

KIT

As discussed earlier, *NRAS* and *BRAF* mutations represent common mechanisms of up-regulating the MAP kinase pathway in melanoma. In particular, *BRAF* mutations are prevalent in cutaneous melanomas without chronic sun-induced damage, whereas they almost never occur in melanomas of the palms and soles (acral melanomas), mucosal membranes (mucosal melanomas), and occur less frequently on skin with chronic sun-induced damage (CSD melanomas). In an attempt to discover oncogenic mutations in melanomas with wild-type *NRAS* and *BRAF*, Curtin and colleagues[53] identified a shared region of amplification at 4q12 using comparative genomic hybridization (CGH) to microarrays. This amplicon was specific to the acral and mucosal melanoma subtypes where *BRAF* mutations are rare, and it contained an attractive candidate oncogene, *KIT*. *KIT* encodes a receptor tyrosine kinase (RTK) for the stem cell factor (SCF) ligand and functions as an upstream activator of the MAP kinase signaling pathway (**Fig. 1**). Like *MITF*, *KIT* is an essential gene for melanocyte survival and development,[54] although its expression is usually lost during cutaneous melanoma progression. Resequencing of *KIT* in melanomas with amplification of 4q12 revealed mutations in 3 of 7 cases. More extensive tumor sequencing confirmed that although they may occur in only 2% to 5% of all melanomas,[55,56] *KIT* mutations are much more prevalent in acral (12%–23%), mucosal (16%–25%), and CSD (8%–20%) melanomas.[53,57] Just as many additional cases exhibit amplifications without observed sequence mutations.[53]

The *KIT* mutations that have been observed in melanoma nearly always occur in exon 11, which is similar to the spectrum of activating *KIT* mutations in patients with gastrointestinal stromal tumors (GISTs).[58] GISTs have been successfully treated by the KIT inhibitor, imatinib mesylate.[59] (Imatinib, or Gleevec, also targets the BCR-ABL tyrosine kinase produced by the Philadelphia chromosome in chronic myelogenous leukemia [CML] and leads to response in more than 95% of cases.[60]) GIST patients whose tumors express an exon 11 mutant KIT protein exhibit an 84% partial response rate to imatinib.[58] These results have prompted multiple phase II clinical trials of imatinib in patients with metastatic melanoma. Results are inconclusive to date, but at least 2 melanoma patients with activating *KIT* mutations in exon 11 have demonstrated a marked response to imatinib treatment.[61,62] These results illustrate the emerging need for systematic cancer mutation profiling before enrolling patients in clinical trials for targeted agents, and suggest an immediate benefit of profiling melanoma patients for *KIT* mutations. The results also anticipate a scenario that may ultimately typify personalized cancer medicine, in which a drug used to treat one type of cancer can be applied in a new cancer based on a shared genetic mechanism.

Additional Oncogenes

The genes described earlier account for only a fraction of the altered loci observed in melanoma. Oncogenes and tumor suppressor genes in many critical pathways have been implicated from a variety of experimental systems. The MAP kinase signaling pathway is commonly altered as shown by mutations in *NRAS*, *BRAF*, and *KIT*, but *NRAS* and receptor tyrosine kinases also contribute to the PI(3)K pathway. Oncogenic signaling through PI(3)K leads to the activation of AKT, a prominent downstream oncogenic effector in many tumor types. The AKT3 isoform is highly expressed in neural crest-derived cells such as melanocytes, and *AKT3* has been found to undergo chromosomal copy gains or overexpression in up to 60% of melanomas.[63] Recently, activating point mutations in *AKT3* have also been described in melanoma.[64] Hyperactivation of the PI(3)K/AKT pathway arises from a variety of additional perturbations including activating PI(3)K mutations in 3% of metastatic melanomas,[65] and deletions or loss-of-function mutations in *PTEN* in 40% of melanoma cell lines.[66,67] The p16/RB pathway is another common target of melanoma genomic alterations; lesions affecting this pathway enable cells to avoid senescence and acquire extended proliferative potential. Germline mutations in the cyclin-dependent kinase inhibitor p16 (encoded by *CDKN2A*), and in the cyclin-dependent kinase *CDK4*, preventing binding by p16, are common in familial melanoma.[68–71] *CDKN2A* also encodes p14/ARF in an alternate reading frame, which serves to inhibit the p53 antagonist MDM2. Likewise, *p53* is lost or mutated in 10% to 20% of melanomas.[72,73] Finally, the Wnt pathway can provide additional proliferative and survival signals in melanoma through loss of adenomatous polyposis coli (*APC*)[74] or mutation of b-catenin (*CTNNB1*).[75,76] The complex interplay among these pathways warrants further study to determine their total contribution to melanoma genesis and progression.

MELANOMA ONCOGENES AND PERSONALIZED MEDICINE

The completion of the human genome project marked the beginning of the genomic era in biology. However, for this knowledge to truly transform medicine, accessible and affordable technologies are needed that can probe the genomes of many individuals to understand the genetic basis of disease and, ultimately, to stratify cancer patients in the clinical arena for optimal therapy. For cancer in particular, the ability to profile the genetic makeup of a patient's tumor can indicate which pathways are activated, thus enabling the prediction of disease outcome and the most appropriate course of treatment. The discovery of critical oncogenes, even if mutated in only a small percentage of tumors, can provide new putative targets for drugs tailored for specific patient subpopulations. DNA sequencing, copy number measurements, and gene expression profiling have already led to the identification of many key genes underlying melanoma progression. As described earlier, these technologies are likely to turn up many new candidate genes in the coming years and shed light on the dependencies operant among these genes and pathways in cancer subtypes defined by genomic or other molecular criteria (**Table 2**). Further, the emergence of next-generation DNA sequencing technologies is expected to dramatically accelerate the search for genes and the movement toward personalized medicine.

Table 2
Genomic technologies for oncogene discovery

Genomic Approach	Type of Tumor Data
SNP microarrays, comparative genomic hybridization (CGH)	Chromosomal copy number Loss of heterozygosity
Gene expression microarrays	Gene expression profiles miRNA profiles
Sanger DNA sequencing	Point mutations Small insertions and deletions
Mutation profiling	Known or "druggable" mutations
Next-generation DNA sequencing	Point mutations Small insertions and deletions Chromosomal rearrangements, translocations Chromosomal copy number DNA methylation (with bisulfite treatment) Epigenetics (with chromatin immunoprecipitation)
RNAi screening	Essential genes Suppressor genes

Discovery of Additional Oncogenes

Despite the success of previous oncogene discovery efforts, a large part of the genetic basis of melanoma remains uncharacterized. As discussed earlier, the MAP kinase pathway is hyperactivated in 90% of melanomas.[22] This is frequently the result of *BRAF* mutations, but *NRAS* and *KIT* are often mutated as well. However, many melanomas harbor wild-type sequences for all 3 genes, suggesting that additional mutations may perturb this pathway. (The recent discovery of *FGFR1* mutations in 2 melanoma lines with wild-type *BRAF* and *NRAS* may indicate a possible alternate mechanism for MAP kinase activation.[23]) Further, perturbations to this pathway alone are not sufficient to drive melanoma progression. *BRAF* is mutated in 50% to 70% of malignant melanomas, and it is also mutated in as many as 90% of benign melanocytic nevi.[29] *MITF* overexpression and *BRAF* mutations together are sufficient to transform primary human melanocytes (in the context of deficient p53 and p16/RB pathways), but only about 15% of *BRAF* mutated melanomas also exhibit *MITF* amplification.[44] Undoubtedly, additional melanoma oncogenes in many other pathways await discovery.

Large-scale, systematic DNA sequencing and copy number profiling efforts will aid the search for new oncogenes. Several groups have used large-scale Sanger sequencing to identify novel mutations in other tumor types. Greenman and colleagues[77] sequenced the coding exons of 518 protein kinase genes in 210 diverse human cancers and found evidence for high-frequency driver mutations in more than 100 genes. A separate, multi-institutional study identified 26 genes significantly mutated in a single tumor type on sequencing 623 genes in 188 lung adenocarcinoma samples.[78] Vogelstein, Velculescu, Kinzler, and colleagues have sequenced the coding exons of approximately 20,000 genes in breast, colorectal, and pancreatic cancers, as well as glioblastoma multiforme, albeit in small discovery cohorts, which may have constrained the statistical power.[79–82] Genome-wide copy number profiling across many samples can also reveal regions of shared copy gain or loss, leading to the discovery of novel lineage-specific oncogenes and tumor suppressors.[50] To provide an organizational and scientific framework for systematically mapping genetic abnormalities that lead to cancer, the US National Cancer Institute and National Human Genome Research Institute established The Cancer Genome Atlas (TCGA) initiative.[83] By integrating genomic data generated by multiple scientific teams using different platforms, including DNA sequence, gene expression, copy number alterations, and DNA methylation, TCGA will lead to the identification of genes and pathways significantly altered in different cancers.[84] Although the pilot stage of TCGA only includes glioblastoma, lung cancer, and ovarian cancer, it will serve as a model for similar large-scale efforts to comprehensively catalog and characterize the genomic changes involved in melanoma.

Most of the DNA mutations discussed to this point involve somatic changes that accumulate over the lifetime of an individual tumor. However, allelic variants of certain genes can be transmitted through the germline and result in an inherited predisposition to developing melanoma. Much remains to be understood about this heritable component of melanoma. Genetic linkage studies have demonstrated that rare mutations in *CDKN2A* on 9p21 segregate with melanoma susceptibility in large melanoma-prone families.[68,69] More common physical characteristics, such as fair complexion and red hair, are also often accompanied by an increased risk of melanoma. To identify the common genetic variants underlying susceptibility to melanoma in large populations, genome-wide association studies will be particularly useful. Genome-wide association studies involve simultaneously genotyping hundreds of thousands of genetic polymorphisms in large sets of cases and controls. One recent study identified a susceptibility locus for melanoma on chromosome 20q11 by pooling 2,019 cases and 2,105 controls.[85] Additional genetic loci known to affect hair, eye, and skin pigmentation in Europeans show clear associations with cutaneous melanoma and basal cell carcinoma.[86] Further studies using additional populations and larger cohorts will likely narrow these loci and reveal novel associations with melanoma susceptibility genes.

Further Characterization of Genetic Lesions

Even as more oncogenic mutations in melanoma become known, the precise mechanisms by which existing mutations confer tumorigenicity remain poorly understood. In vitro transformation assays monitoring proliferation, pathway activation, and anchorage-independent growth have been informative, yet these assays must be performed in the appropriate genetic background. For certain types of mutations, the underlying oncogene may not always be apparent. Amplifications and deletions typically encompass many genes. To narrow down regions of copy gain or loss, additional genomic information can be incorporated. The examples of MITF and NEDD9 discussed earlier demonstrate how gene expression and evolutionary conservation can be successfully used to pinpoint the driver oncogene within a broader locus. However, many additional significant regions of copy number alteration remain uncharacterized. For example, a recent study identified 27 significant copy gains and losses across 101 melanoma cell lines and short-term cultures using high-density SNP arrays.[23]

An additional strategy for the functional characterization of commonly amplified regions involves systematic gene knockdown by RNA interference. Although many regions harbor attractive candidate oncogenes, all constituent genes can be examined through systematic RNAi screens. For instance, one would expect RNAi knockdown of an oncogene to result in decreased proliferation of all cell lines harboring an amplification of that locus. Similarly, restoring the expression of a tumor suppressor gene that has been deleted should produce a similar antiproliferative effect.

The high prevalence of particular mutations in melanoma underscores the critical roles played by the associated pathways. However, no single mutation is sufficient to lead to malignant melanoma. The interdependence among various mutations affecting different pathways needs to be further examined. From the distribution of mutations in *NRAS*, *BRAF*, and *PTEN*, it is clear that the MAP kinase pathway and the PI(3)K/PTEN pathway are often simultaneously targeted. The context dependence of oncogenic mutations can be explored by RNAi screens in multiple cell lines with different genetic backgrounds.[87] Additional genes whose knockdown reduces proliferation in some, but not all, cell lines can be linked to common alterations through supervised analysis. The temporal order in which mutations occur can also be deduced from their distribution. *BRAF* is mutated in approximately 90% of benign melanocytic nevi, whereas *MITF* amplification is restricted to malignant melanoma.[29,44] This suggests that *BRAF* mutations occur early during melanoma progression, perhaps predisposing cells to hyperproliferation following additional genetic alterations.

Next-Generation Technologies for Oncogene Discovery

Looking forward, the discovery of new oncogenes in melanoma and other tumors will largely come about from genome-scale DNA sequencing efforts. Until recently, large-scale DNA sequencing in cancer has been conducted entirely by traditional capillary-based Sanger sequencing methods.[77–82,84] New technologies have now emerged that promise to dramatically reduce the cost and increase the throughput of DNA sequencing.[88] These massively parallel, next-generation, sequencing platforms involve the clonal amplification of millions of individual template molecules without the need for multiwell plates and large quantities of costly reagents. The short sequence readouts (ranging from 20 to 50 to a few hundred bases) that are generated can be mapped onto the reference human genome, and the nucleotide identity at each position is determined by counting discrete readouts. This results in increased sensitivity for detecting rare sequence variants, which is especially important in cancer; confounding factors such as stromal contamination and genetic heterogeneity are common.[89] The first whole-genome sequence of a cancer patient's tumor was recently completed using massively parallel sequencing.[90] In this study, 33-fold coverage was obtained for an acute myeloid leukemia genome, and 14-fold coverage was obtained for a normal skin sample from the patient, leading to the discovery and validation of several novel somatic mutations. For the purposes of oncogene discovery, it is currently more economical to sequence only protein-coding regions rather than sequence across the entire genome. Several groups have developed exon capture methods for targeted resequencing to overcome the cost limitations of parallel polymerase chain reactions.[91,92] Consequently, it will soon be feasible to sequence all human exons (or a subset thereof) in hundreds of tumors at reasonable cost.

The value of next-generation DNA sequencing technologies in cancer is not limited to genome sequencing applications. Microarray-based assays can be adapted to use DNA sequencing as a readout, providing more sensitivity and a greater dynamic range. For instance, gene expression levels can be monitored by counting the number of sequence readouts arising from different cDNAs. In doing so, novel transcription events and alternatively spliced isoforms can be readily identified.[93,94] To demonstrate its usefulness for cancer, Sugarbaker and colleagues[95] used next-generation sequencing of cDNA to characterize RNA mutations and gene expression levels in malignant mesotheliomas. In addition to expression, DNA methylation patterns can be evaluated in different samples using reduced representation bisulfite sequencing.[96] Chromatin modifications and transcription factor binding can be analyzed by DNA sequencing following chromatin immunoprecipitation (ChIP-Seq).[97,98] Copy number alterations can be identified in tumors at high resolution from low-coverage shotgun sequencing of genomic DNA.[99] It is likely that integrative genomic characterization efforts such as The Cancer Genome Atlas will soon deal predominantly (if not exclusively) in various forms of DNA sequence data.

Targeted Therapies and Personalized Medicine

Ultimately, the key cancer-associated mutations uncovered through these discovery efforts can serve as important clinical biomarkers for the diagnosis and prognosis of melanoma, the prediction of a patient's response to a particular treatment, and the development of novel rational therapeutics targeting specific subsets of patients. With regard to mutations as prognostic biomarkers, Curtin and colleagues[100] used genome-wide copy number measurements and *BRAF* and *NRAS* mutational status to classify 126 melanomas into 4 clinically distinct groups with 70% percent accuracy. In addition, as discussed earlier, *MITF* amplification in melanoma correlates with a 5-year decrease in survival.[44] Global gene expression patterns have also revealed discernible subclasses of cutaneous melanoma.[101] The FDA has recently approved several anticancer drugs that specifically target the products of mutated genes in other malignancies. These include imatinib (*BCR-ABL* translocation in CML, *KIT* mutation in GIST),[59,60] trastuzumab (*ERBB2* amplification in breast cancer),[102] and gefitinib and erlotinib (*EGFR* mutation in non–small cell lung cancer).[103–105] Imatinib represents a potential therapy for malignant melanomas harboring *KIT* mutations, as shown by the marked response of at least 2 patients to imatinib treatment.[61,62] Given the large number of melanomas with activating mutations in the MAP kinase pathway (*NRAS* and *BRAF*), multiple RAF and MEK inhibitors are currently being developed and investigated in clinical trials.[106]

The usefulness of these genetic biomarkers for the development and administration of targeted therapies hinges on being able to profile patients for mutations in an efficient, cost-effective manner. Although this goal has not yet been attempted categorically, recent advances suggest that there is room for optimism. Thomas and colleagues[107] described a mass spectrometry-based strategy whereby they genotyped more than 200 high-frequency cancer-associated mutations in 1,000 human tumors. Using this platform, termed OncoMap, the investigators discovered that certain mutations commonly associated with particular cancers were also present at lower frequencies in many other cancers. This reinforced the notion that existing targeted treatments such as imatinib may be applied to additional cancers with shared genetic lesions. In its current embodiment, OncoMap relies on the observation that a small number of recurrent base pair mutations accounts for most somatic events known to drive tumor progression. However, extending this strategy to next-generation sequencing of whole exons will enable the rapid profiling of all mutations—both base pair mutations and copy number alterations—in cancer-associated genes. The ability to interrogate large panels of tumors will have a large impact on the discovery of targeted therapies, as pharmacologic data from drug screens can be correlated with the mutational status of the associated tumor-derived cell lines.[23,108] It will also enable efficient patient stratification for clinical trial design. Such an approach, if applied universally, can transform patient care through improved diagnosis and prognosis in the movement toward personalized medicine.

SUMMARY

The identification of melanoma oncogenes, such as *NRAS*, *BRAF*, *MITF*, *NEDD9*, and *KIT*, have led to an improved understanding of the biology of melanoma. These discoveries have come about from a variety of genomic approaches, including systematic DNA sequencing, chromosomal copy number profiling, gene expression profiling, evolutionary conservation analysis, and RNA interference. Despite these initial successes, the genetic basis of melanoma progression remains largely uncharacterized. It is clear that additional knowledge will come from the use of improved genomic technologies with increased throughput and sensitivity for mutation detection and discovery, as well as analyses that integrate these diverse data types. These technologies (and the biologic insight gained from their deployment) hold great promise for the development of improved diagnostics and targeted therapies, and carry the potential to dramatically transform patient care.

REFERENCES

1. Vogelstein B, Kinzler KW. Cancer genes and the pathways they control. Nat Med 2004;10(8):789–99.
2. Hanahan D, Weinberg RA. The hallmarks of cancer. Cell 2000;100(1):57–70.
3. Futreal PA, Coin L, Marshall M, et al. A census of human cancer genes. Nat Rev Cancer 2004;4(3):177–83.
4. American Cancer Society. Cancer facts and figures: 2008. Atlanta (GA): American Cancer Society; 2008.
5. Shih TY, Papageorge AG, Stokes PE, et al. Guanine nucleotide-binding and autophosphorylating activities associated with the p21src protein of Harvey murine sarcoma virus. Nature 1980;287(5784):686–91.
6. Parada LF, Tabin CJ, Shih C, et al. Human EJ bladder carcinoma oncogene is homologue of Harvey sarcoma virus ras gene. Nature 1982;297(5866):474–8.
7. Santos E, Tronick SR, Aaronson SA, et al. T24 human bladder carcinoma oncogene is an activated form of the normal human homologue of BALB- and Harvey-MSV transforming genes. Nature 1982;298(5872):343–7.
8. Der CJ, Krontiris TG, Cooper GM. Transforming genes of human bladder and lung carcinoma cell lines are homologous to the ras genes of Harvey and Kirsten sarcoma viruses. Proc Natl Acad Sci U S A 1982;79(11):3637–40.
9. Shimizu K, Goldfarb M, Suard Y, et al. Three human transforming genes are related to the viral ras oncogenes. Proc Natl Acad Sci U S A 1983;80(8):2112–6.
10. Taparowsky E, Shimizu K, Goldfarb M, et al. Structure and activation of the human N-ras gene. Cell 1983;34(2):581–6.
11. Bos JL. ras oncogenes in human cancer: a review. Cancer Res 1989;49(17):4682–9.
12. Albino AP, Le Strange R, Oliff AI, et al. Transforming ras genes from human melanoma: a manifestation of tumour heterogeneity? Nature 1984;308(5954):69–72.
13. Padua RA, Barrass NC, Currie GA. Activation of N-ras in a human melanoma cell line. Mol Cell Biol 1985;5(3):582–5.
14. van 't Veer LJ, Burgering BM, Versteeg R, et al. N-ras mutations in human cutaneous melanoma from sun-exposed body sites. Mol Cell Biol 1989;9(7):3114–6.
15. Albino AP, Nanus DM, Mentle IR, et al. Analysis of ras oncogenes in malignant melanoma and precursor lesions: correlation of point mutations with differentiation phenotype. Oncogene 1989;4(11):1363–74.
16. Jafari M, Papp T, Kirchner S, et al. Analysis of ras mutations in human melanocytic lesions: activation of the ras gene seems to be associated with the nodular

type of human malignant melanoma. J Cancer Res Clin Oncol 1995;121(1): 23–30.

17. van Elsas A, Zerp SF, van der Flier S, et al. Relevance of ultraviolet-induced N-ras oncogene point mutations in development of primary human cutaneous melanoma. Am J Pathol 1996;149(3):883–93.

18. Demunter A, Stas M, Degreef H, et al. Analysis of N- and K-ras mutations in the distinctive tumor progression phases of melanoma. J Invest Dermatol 2001; 117(6):1483–9.

19. Ackermann J, Frutschi M, Kaloulis K, et al. Metastasizing melanoma formation caused by expression of activated N-RasQ61K on an INK4a-deficient background. Cancer Res 2005;65(10):4005–11.

20. Chin L, Tam A, Pomerantz J, et al. Essential role for oncogenic Ras in tumour maintenance. Nature 1999;400(6743):468–72.

21. Eskandarpour M, Kiaii S, Zhu C, et al. Suppression of oncogenic NRAS by RNA interference induces apoptosis of human melanoma cells. Int J Cancer 2005; 115(1):65–73.

22. Cohen C, Zavala-Pompa A, Sequeira JH, et al. Mitogen-actived protein kinase activation is an early event in melanoma progression. Clin Cancer Res 2002; 8(12):3728–33.

23. Lin WM, Baker AC, Beroukhim R, et al. Modeling genomic diversity and tumor dependency in malignant melanoma. Cancer Res 2008;68(3):664–73.

24. Winnepenninckx V, Lazar V, Michiels S, et al. Gene expression profiling of primary cutaneous melanoma and clinical outcome. J Natl Cancer Inst 2006; 98(7):472–82.

25. Bastian BC, LeBoit PE, Pinkel D. Mutations and copy number increase of HRAS in Spitz nevi with distinctive histopathological features. Am J Pathol 2000;157(3): 967–72.

26. Whitwam T, Vanbrocklin MW, Russo ME, et al. Differential oncogenic potential of activated RAS isoforms in melanocytes. Oncogene 2007;26(31):4563–70.

27. Davies H, Bignell GR, Cox C, et al. Mutations of the BRAF gene in human cancer. Nature 2002;417(6892):949–54.

28. Brose MS, Volpe P, Feldman M, et al. BRAF and RAS mutations in human lung cancer and melanoma. Cancer Res 2002;62(23):6997–7000.

29. Pollock PM, Harper UL, Hansen KS, et al. High frequency of BRAF mutations in nevi. Nat Genet 2003;33(1):19–20.

30. Gorden A, Osman I, Gai W, et al. Analysis of BRAF and N-RAS mutations in metastatic melanoma tissues. Cancer Res 2003;63(14):3955–7.

31. Maldonado JL, Fridlyand J, Patel H, et al. Determinants of BRAF mutations in primary melanomas. J Natl Cancer Inst 2003;95(24):1878–90.

32. Shinozaki M, Fujimoto A, Morton DL, et al. Incidence of BRAF oncogene mutation and clinical relevance for primary cutaneous melanomas. Clin Cancer Res 2004;10(5):1753–7.

33. Garnett MJ, Marais R. Guilty as charged: B-RAF is a human oncogene. Cancer Cell 2004;6(4):313–9.

34. Wan PT, Garnett MJ, Roe SM, et al. Mechanism of activation of the RAF-ERK signaling pathway by oncogenic mutations of B-RAF. Cell 2004;116(6): 855–67.

35. Wellbrock C, Ogilvie L, Hedley D, et al. V599EB-RAF is an oncogene in melanocytes. Cancer Res 2004;64(7):2338–42.

36. Zhang BH, Guan KL. Activation of B-Raf kinase requires phosphorylation of the conserved residues Thr598 and Ser601. EMBO J 2000;19(20):5429–39.

37. Gray-Schopfer V, Wellbrock C, Marais R. Melanoma biology and new targeted therapy. Nature 2007;445(7130):851–7.
38. Hingorani SR, Jacobetz MA, Robertson GP, et al. Suppression of BRAF(V599E) in human melanoma abrogates transformation. Cancer Res 2003;63(17): 5198–202.
39. Hoeflich KP, Gray DC, Eby MT, et al. Oncogenic BRAF is required for tumor growth and maintenance in melanoma models. Cancer Res 2006;66(2): 999–1006.
40. Collisson EA, De A, Suzuki H, et al. Treatment of metastatic melanoma with an orally available inhibitor of the Ras-Raf-MAPK cascade. Cancer Res 2003; 63(18):5669–73.
41. Solit DB, Garraway LA, Pratilas CA, et al. BRAF mutation predicts sensitivity to MEK inhibition. Nature 2006;439(7074):358–62.
42. Tsao H, Goel V, Wu H, et al. Genetic interaction between NRAS and BRAF mutations and PTEN/MMAC1 inactivation in melanoma. J Invest Dermatol 2004; 122(2):337–41.
43. Hoheisel JD. Microarray technology: beyond transcript profiling and genotype analysis. Nat Rev Genet 2006;7(3):200–10.
44. Garraway LA, Widlund HR, Rubin MA, et al. Integrative genomic analyses identify MITF as a lineage survival oncogene amplified in malignant melanoma. Nature 2005;436(7047):117–22.
45. King R, Weilbaecher KN, McGill G, et al. Microphthalmia transcription factor. A sensitive and specific melanocyte marker for MelanomaDiagnosis. Am J Pathol 1999;155(3):731–8.
46. Levy C, Khaled M, Fisher DE. MITF: master regulator of melanocyte development and melanoma oncogene. Trends Mol Med 2006;12(9):406–14.
47. Garraway LA, Sellers WR. Lineage dependency and lineage-survival oncogenes in human cancer. Nat Rev Cancer 2006;6(8):593–602.
48. Chin L, Garraway LA, Fisher DE. Malignant melanoma: genetics and therapeutics in the genomic era. Genes Dev 2006;20(16):2149–82.
49. Heinlein CA, Chang C. Androgen receptor in prostate cancer. Endocr Rev 2004; 25(2):276–308.
50. Weir BA, Woo MS, Getz G, et al. Characterizing the cancer genome in lung adenocarcinoma. Nature 2007;450(7171):893–8.
51. Kim M, Gans JD, Nogueira C, et al. Comparative oncogenomics identifies NEDD9 as a melanoma metastasis gene. Cell 2006;125(7):1269–81.
52. Bastian BC, LeBoit PE, Hamm H, et al. Chromosomal gains and losses in primary cutaneous melanomas detected by comparative genomic hybridization. Cancer Res 1998;58(10):2170–5.
53. Curtin JA, Busam K, Pinkel D, et al. Somatic activation of KIT in distinct subtypes of melanoma. J Clin Oncol 2006;24(26):4340–6.
54. Geissler EN, Ryan MA, Housman DE. The dominant-white spotting (W) locus of the mouse encodes the c-kit proto-oncogene. Cell 1988;55(1):185–92.
55. Willmore-Payne C, Holden JA, Tripp S, et al. Human malignant melanoma: detection of BRAF- and c-kit-activating mutations by high-resolution amplicon melting analysis. Hum Pathol 2005;36(5):486–93.
56. Willmore-Payne C, Holden JA, Hirschowitz S, et al. BRAF and c-kit gene copy number in mutation-positive malignant melanoma. Hum Pathol 2006;37(5): 520–7.
57. Beadling C, Jacobson-Dunlop E, Hodi FS, et al. KIT gene mutations and copy number in melanoma subtypes. Clin Cancer Res 2008;14(21):6821–8.

58. Heinrich MC, Corless CL, Demetri GD, et al. Kinase mutations and imatinib response in patients with metastatic gastrointestinal stromal tumor. J Clin Oncol 2003;21(23):4342–9.
59. Demetri GD, von Mehren M, Blanke CD, et al. Efficacy and safety of imatinib mesylate in advanced gastrointestinal stromal tumors. N Engl J Med 2002;347(7):472–80.
60. Kantarjian H, Sawyers C, Hochhaus A, et al. Hematologic and cytogenetic responses to imatinib mesylate in chronic myelogenous leukemia. N Engl J Med 2002;346(9):645–52.
61. Kim KB, Eton O, Davis DW, et al. Phase II trial of imatinib mesylate in patients with metastatic melanoma. Br J Cancer 2008;99(5):734–40.
62. Hodi FS, Friedlander P, Corless CL, et al. Major response to imatinib mesylate in KIT-mutated melanoma. J Clin Oncol 2008;26(12):2046–51.
63. Stahl JM, Sharma A, Cheung M, et al. Deregulated Akt3 activity promotes development of malignant melanoma. Cancer Res 2004;64(19):7002–10.
64. Davies MA, Stemke-Hale K, Tellez C, et al. A novel AKT3 mutation in melanoma tumours and cell lines. Br J Cancer 2008;99(8):1265–8.
65. Omholt K, Krockel D, Ringborg U, et al. Mutations of PIK3CA are rare in cutaneous melanoma. Melanoma Res 2006;16(2):197–200.
66. Wu H, Goel V, Haluska FG. PTEN signaling pathways in melanoma. Oncogene 2003;22(20):3113–22.
67. Guldberg P, thor Straten P, Birck A, et al. Disruption of the MMAC1/PTEN gene by deletion or mutation is a frequent event in malignant melanoma. Cancer Res 1997;57(17):3660–3.
68. Hussussian CJ, Struewing JP, Goldstein AM, et al. Germline p16 mutations in familial melanoma. Nat Genet 1994;8(1):15–21.
69. Kamb A, Shattuck-Eidens D, Eeles R, et al. Analysis of the p16 gene (CDKN2) as a candidate for the chromosome 9p melanoma susceptibility locus. Nat Genet 1994;8(1):23–6.
70. Wolfel T, Hauer M, Schneider J, et al. A p16INK4a-insensitive CDK4 mutant targeted by cytolytic T lymphocytes in a human melanoma. Science 1995;269(5228):1281–4.
71. Zuo L, Weger J, Yang Q, et al. Germline mutations in the p16INK4a binding domain of CDK4 in familial melanoma. Nat Genet 1996;12(1):97–9.
72. Straume O, Akslen LA. Alterations and prognostic significance of p16 and p53 protein expression in subgroups of cutaneous melanoma. Int J Cancer 1997;74(5):535–9.
73. Ragnarsson-Olding BK, Karsberg S, Platz A, et al. Mutations in the TP53 gene in human malignant melanomas derived from sun-exposed skin and unexposed mucosal membranes. Melanoma Res 2002;12(5):453–63.
74. Worm J, Christensen C, Gronbaek K, et al. Genetic and epigenetic alterations of the APC gene in malignant melanoma. Oncogene 2004;23(30):5215–26.
75. Omholt K, Platz A, Ringborg U, et al. Cytoplasmic and nuclear accumulation of beta-catenin is rarely caused by CTNNB1 exon 3 mutations in cutaneous malignant melanoma. Int J Cancer 2001;92(6):839–42.
76. Rubinfeld B, Robbins P, El-Gamil M, et al. Stabilization of beta-catenin by genetic defects in melanoma cell lines. Science 1997;275(5307):1790–2.
77. Greenman C, Stephens P, Smith R, et al. Patterns of somatic mutation in human cancer genomes. Nature 2007;446(7132):153–8.
78. Ding L, Getz G, Wheeler DA, et al. Somatic mutations affect key pathways in lung adenocarcinoma. Nature 2008;455(7216):1069–75.

79. Jones S, Zhang X, Parsons DW, et al. Core signaling pathways in human pancreatic cancers revealed by global genomic analyses. Science 2008;321(5897): 1801–6.

80. Parsons DW, Jones S, Zhang X, et al. An integrated genomic analysis of human glioblastoma multiforme. Science 2008;321(5897):1807–12.

81. Sjoblom T, Jones S, Wood LD, et al. The consensus coding sequences of human breast and colorectal cancers. Science 2006;314(5797):268–74.

82. Wood LD, Parsons DW, Jones S, et al. The genomic landscapes of human breast and colorectal cancers. Science 2007;318(5853):1108–13.

83. Collins FS, Barker AD. Mapping the cancer genome. Pinpointing the genes involved in cancer will help chart a new course across the complex landscape of human malignancies. Sci Am 2007;296(3):50–7.

84. The Cancer Genome Atlas Research Network. Comprehensive genomic characterization defines human glioblastoma genes and core pathways. Nature 2008; 455(7216):1061–8.

85. Brown KM, Macgregor S, Montgomery GW, et al. Common sequence variants on 20q11.22 confer melanoma susceptibility. Nat Genet 2008;40(7):838–40.

86. Gudbjartsson DF, Sulem P, Stacey SN, et al. ASIP and TYR pigmentation variants associate with cutaneous melanoma and basal cell carcinoma. Nat Genet 2008; 40(7):886–91.

87. Luo B, Cheung HW, Subramanian A, et al. Highly parallel identification of essential genes in cancer cells. Proc Natl Acad Sci U S A 2008;105(51):20380–5.

88. Shendure J, Ji H. Next-generation DNA sequencing. Nat Biotechnol 2008; 26(10):1135–45.

89. Thomas RK, Nickerson E, Simons JF, et al. Sensitive mutation detection in heterogeneous cancer specimens by massively parallel picoliter reactor sequencing. Nat Med 2006;12(7):852–5.

90. Ley TJ, Mardis ER, Ding L, et al. DNA sequencing of a cytogenetically normal acute myeloid leukaemia genome. Nature 2008;456(7218):66–72.

91. Hodges E, Xuan Z, Balija V, et al. Genome-wide in situ exon capture for selective resequencing. Nat Genet 2007;39(12):1522–7.

92. Olson M. Enrichment of super-sized resequencing targets from the human genome. Nat Methods 2007;4(11):891–2.

93. Sultan M, Schulz MH, Richard H, et al. A global view of gene activity and alternative splicing by deep sequencing of the human transcriptome. Science 2008; 321(5891):956–60.

94. Wang ET, Sandberg R, Luo S, et al. Alternative isoform regulation in human tissue transcriptomes. Nature 2008;456(7221):470–6.

95. Sugarbaker DJ, Richards WG, Gordon GJ, et al. Transcriptome sequencing of malignant pleural mesothelioma tumors. Proc Natl Acad Sci U S A 2008; 105(9):3521–6.

96. Meissner A, Mikkelsen TS, Gu H, et al. Genome-scale DNA methylation maps of pluripotent and differentiated cells. Nature 2008;454(7205):766–70.

97. Mikkelsen TS, Ku M, Jaffe DB, et al. Genome-wide maps of chromatin state in pluripotent and lineage-committed cells. Nature 2007;448(7153):553–60.

98. Johnson DS, Mortazavi A, Myers RM, et al. Genome-wide mapping of in vivo protein-DNA interactions. Science 2007;316(5830):1497–502.

99. Chiang DY, Getz G, Jaffe DB, et al. High-resolution mapping of copy-number alterations with massively parallel sequencing. Nat Methods 2008;6:99–103.

100. Curtin JA, Fridlyand J, Kageshita T, et al. Distinct sets of genetic alterations in melanoma. N Engl J Med 2005;353(20):2135–47.

101. Bittner M, Meltzer P, Chen Y, et al. Molecular classification of cutaneous malignant melanoma by gene expression profiling. Nature 2000;406(6795):536–40.
102. Slamon DJ, Leyland-Jones B, Shak S, et al. Use of chemotherapy plus a monoclonal antibody against HER2 for metastatic breast cancer that overexpresses HER2. N Engl J Med 2001;344(11):783–92.
103. Lynch TJ, Bell DW, Sordella R, et al. Activating mutations in the epidermal growth factor receptor underlying responsiveness of non-small-cell lung cancer to gefitinib. N Engl J Med 2004;350(21):2129–39.
104. Paez JG, Janne PA, Lee JC, et al. EGFR mutations in lung cancer: correlation with clinical response to gefitinib therapy. Science 2004;304(5676):1497–500.
105. Pao W, Miller V, Zakowski M, et al. EGF receptor gene mutations are common in lung cancers from "never smokers" and are associated with sensitivity of tumors to gefitinib and erlotinib. Proc Natl Acad Sci U S A 2004;101(36):13306–11.
106. Adjei AA, Cohen RB, Franklin W, et al. Phase I pharmacokinetic and pharmacodynamic study of the oral, small-molecule mitogen-activated protein kinase kinase 1/2 inhibitor AZD6244 (ARRY-142886) in patients with advanced cancers. J Clin Oncol 2008;26(13):2139–46.
107. Thomas RK, Baker AC, Debiasi RM, et al. High-throughput oncogene mutation profiling in human cancer. Nat Genet 2007;39(3):347–51.
108. McDermott U, Sharma SV, Dowell L, et al. Identification of genotype-correlated sensitivity to selective kinase inhibitors by using high-throughput tumor cell line profiling. Proc Natl Acad Sci U S A 2007;104(50):19936–41.

Melanoma Genetics: An Update on Risk-Associated Genes

Durga Udayakumar, PhD[a], Hensin Tsao, MD, PhD[b,c],*

KEYWORDS

• Genetics • Melanoma • *CDKN2A* • Polymorphism
• Germline mutations

The notion that melanoma has a genetic component was posited by William Norris in some of the earliest descriptions of the disease.[1] The general practitioner noted that some cases of "melanosis" (ie, melanoma) were associated with a family history. These observations lay largely fallow until Clark[2] and Lynch[3] independently described the "B-K mole" and familial atypical mole-melanoma syndromes, respectively. Through these reports, the hereditary nature of melanoma was formally codified along with the atypical mole phenotype in a subset of melanoma-prone families.

With the advances in linkage analysis that occurred through the 1980s and early 1990s, much attention was trained on high-risk, high-penetrance loci that were associated with familial malignancies. In 1994, germline mutations in *CDKN2A* were first demonstrated in a subset of melanoma-prone kindreds;[4] a few families lacking *CDKN2A* were later found to harbor heritable alterations in *CDK4*, the target of inhibition for p16.[5] The last 15 years bore witness to the completion of the Human Genome Project and unprecedented gains in the discovery of low-to-medium–risk predisposition alleles. In 2008, a harvest of new lower-risk melanoma loci were uncovered through genome-wide association studies (GWAS), thereby painting a much richer view of melanoma genetics. In this study, we highlight the latest findings related to high- and low-risk alleles predisposing individuals to melanoma.

[a] Department of Dermatology, Wellman Center for Photomedicine, Harvard Medical School, Massachusetts General Hospital, Edwards 211, 50 Blossom Street, Boston, MA 02114, USA
[b] Department of Dermatology, Wellman Center for Photomedicine, Harvard Medical School, Massachusetts General Hospital, Bartlett 622, 48 Blossom Street, Boston, MA 02114, USA
[c] The Melanoma and Pigmented Lesion Center, Massachusetts General Hospital, 50 Staniford Street, Suite 200, Boston, MA 02114, USA
* Corresponding author. Department of Dermatology, Wellman Center for Photomedicine, Harvard Medical School, Massachusetts General Hospital, Bartlett 622, 48 Blossom Street, Boston, MA 02114.
E-mail address: htsao@partners.org (H. Tsao).

Hematol Oncol Clin N Am 23 (2009) 415–429
doi:10.1016/j.hoc.2009.03.011
0889-8588/09/$ – see front matter © 2009 Elsevier Inc. All rights reserved.

hemonc.theclinics.com

RISK ALLELES IN MELANOMA PREDISPOSITION

Like most cancers, risk factors for melanoma include both environmental and genetic components. As shown in **Fig. 1**, variants in genes such as *CDKN2A* confer extraordinary risk but are limited to a small fraction of the general melanoma population. In contrast, alterations at other common phenotype-determining loci (such as those for pigmentation) are quite prevalent but are associated with much lower risk levels for the disease.[6,7] These observations support the emerging adage of "common disease, common variant; rare disease, rare variant." Although the allele-specific risk for variants in high-risk loci is great, the attributable burden for the more common risk alleles is greater at the population level.

HIGH-RISK MELANOMA GENES

A family history of melanoma occurs in about 10% of melanoma patients and confers about a 2-fold increase in melanoma risk.[8] High-risk melanoma alleles often manifest as (1) multiple cases of melanoma in several generations on one side of the lineage, (2) multiple primary melanomas (MPMs) in a given individual, and (3) early onset of disease. Hereditary melanoma is usually considered an autosomal dominant condition consonant with other familial cancer syndromes. Within this category, there are families with an increased occurrence of both melanoma and clinically atypical moles (**Fig. 2**). With the clinical recognition and the systematic collection of B-K mole and FAMMM kindreds worldwide, several groups performed linkage analysis on these families and identified evidence of melanoma-predisposing loci on chromosome 1p36[9] and 9p21.[10] Contemporaneous with this linkage, Serrano and colleagues[11] isolated a cell-cycle regulator, p16, using a yeast two-hybrid technology and proved that the short motif directly bound and inhibited the cyclin-dependent protein kinase 4 (Cdk4). Since p16 (derived from the *CDKN2A* locus) is located on chromosome 9p21 and is functionally related to cell proliferation, it quickly became an attractive candidate for the melanoma locus on chromosome 9. Hussussian and colleagues[4] then demonstrated deleterious germline mutations in *CDKN2A* among a subset of melanoma-prone families, thereby establishing the first molecular correlates for hereditary melanoma.

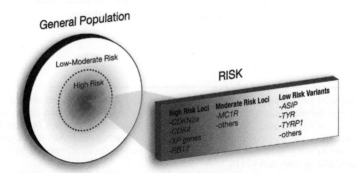

Fig. 1. Melanoma susceptibility loci. The darker-toned region represents the high-risk population; the lighter-toned region represents the low-moderate risk in the general population and their corresponding risk-associated alleles. The prevalence of high-risk alleles is quite low in the general population, although the prevalence of low-moderate risk alleles can be quite high. Overall, common low-risk predisposing alleles probably account for most of the melanoma burden.

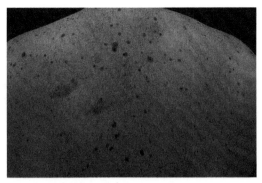

Fig. 2. Patient who has multiple clinically atypical moles.

CDKN2A

Locus

The *CDKN2A* locus is composed of 4 exons and encodes for 2 distinct proteins through alternative splicing: p16/Ink4a and p14/Arf (**Fig. 3**); interestingly, both proteins are potent tumor suppressors with critical roles in cell cycle and apoptosis regulation. P16/Ink4a binds Cdk4, thereby inhibiting the protein kinase from phosphorylating another tumor suppressor, the retinoblastoma (Rb) protein.[12,13] Hyperphosphorylation of Rb leads to the release of the transcription factor E2F1, which, in turn, induces the

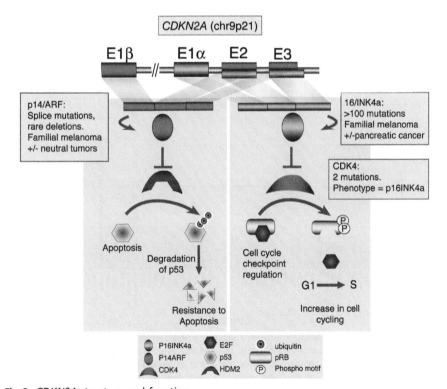

Fig. 3. *CDKN2A* structure and function.

synthesis of S phase genes. Thus, loss of p16/Ink4a encourages melanocytes to negotiate out of G1 arrest and promotes the transition of G1 to S and cell cycling.

On the other hand, p14/Arf is directly involved in p53 regulation.[14] P14/Arf binds to human double minute-2 (HDM2) through N terminal domain and sequesters HDM2 in the nucleolus so it can not interact with p53. Because HDM2 downregulates p53 through accelerated destruction, depletion of HDM2 stabilizes p53.[15–17] Thus, loss of p14/Arf through *CDKN2A* inactivation destabilizes p53. Thus, in tumor cells, *CDKN2A* lesions functionally abrogate both the Rb and p53 pathways through loss of p16/Ink4a and p14/Arf, respectively.[18]

The tumor suppressive effects of *CDKN2A* have been validated through animal models. Mice with targeted deletions of both exons 2 and 3, which inactivate both p16/Ink4a and p19/Arf (the mouse homolog), develop spontaneous tumors at an early age and are highly sensitive to carcinogens.[19] When the *Cdkn2a*-null mice are crossed with mice that carry a melanocyte-specific oncogenic *HRAS*, murine melanomas develop with high penetrance.[20]

Fig. 4 presents the vast array of *CDKN2A* mutations identified in various melanoma families throughout the world.[21] Most mutations appear to involve exons 1(and 2), which then support the argument that p16/Ink4a is preferentially targeted transcript. There are some highly recurrent alterations that result from founder mutations—some of these have eponymic designations—for example, the "Scottish" (p.Met53Ile) and "Leiden" (p.225-243del19) mutations. Changes at the p14/Arf-specific exon 1β are much less commonly detected among melanoma-prone kindreds. Rare deletions and a 16-bp insertion involving exon 1[22,23] have both been reported. More recently, a mutational hotspot at the exon 1 splice site has also been identified.[22] Rare deep intronic mutations of *CDKN2A* have also been described, although these account for very few cases worldwide.[24,25]

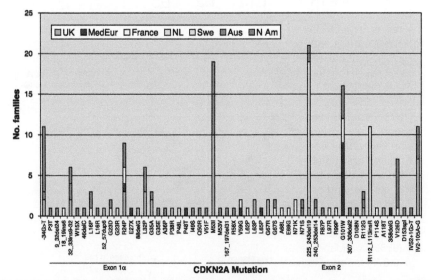

Fig. 4. Distribution of p16/Ink4a mutations along coding sequence. Some highly prevalent mutations are in fact founder mutations (eg, pMet53Ile). (*Reproduced from* Goldstein AM, Chan M, Harland M, et al. High-risk melanoma susceptibility genes and pancreatic cancer, neural system tumors, and uveal melanoma across GenoMEL. Cancer Res 2006;66:9818–28; with permission.)

Phenotypic features

Family history is one of the strongest predictors of germline *CDKN2A* mutation status. In a large study of 385 families worldwide by the international melanoma genetics consortium GenoMEL, 39% of families (n = 150) had mutations, although the frequency of mutations ranged from 20% (32/162) in Australia to 45% (29/65) in North America and 57% (89/157) in Europe.[26] The mutation rate also increases as the number of affected individuals in the family increases, although this is subject to modulation by the ambient melanoma rates. For instance, in pedigrees with 4 affected members, the prevalence of *CDKN2A* mutations is about 70% in low baseline incidence (LBI) regions such as Europe and only 10% in high-baseline incidence (HBI) regions such as Australia. This disparity probably reflects the large number of phenocopies in HBI zones, that is, in HBI regions, there may be clusters of sporadic cases within families by pure statistical chance rather than genetic transmission. Although most initial studies were performed on melanoma-prone families, a recent population-based study found that the prevalence of *CDKN2A* among individuals with a single primary melanoma (SPM) is 1.2%.[27]

Initial reports of smaller case series found that the rate of germline *CDKN2A* mutations among persons with MPMs ranged from 5% to 15%.[28–35] However, many of these cases were from multiplex families and therefore expected to have greater genetic risk. A more unbiased population-based estimate for MPM patients is 2.9%.[27]

The increased incidence of pancreatic cancer among *CDKN2A*-mutation-bearing families[36] is now well established. In the GenoMEL analysis of 385 families, 72% of families with 1 reported patient with pancreatic cancer had mutations (31/43), and 81% of families with 2 patients or more with pancreatic cancer had mutations (13/16). Interestingly, pancreatic cancer was associated with mutations in Europe and North America but not in Australia, raising the possibility of additional environmental risk factors that are still unknown.[26]

Early age of disease onset alone does not appear to be associated with a high *CDKN2A* mutation rate.[29,37–39] However, within high-risk families, a younger age of diagnosis is significantly associated with a higher *CDKN2A* mutation rate.[26] In contrast, individuals with early onset melanoma and MPMs have a much higher rate of *CDKN2A* mutations in LBI regions such as Greece when compared with HBI regions.[40] Taken together, there is now the view that the apparent genetic contribution from germline *CDKN2A* mutagenesis is greatest in regions where ambient melanoma incidences, and thus phenocopy rates, are low. These geographic considerations need to be factored into any clinical evaluation involving melanoma patients.

Niendorf and colleagues[41] recently created a logistic regression model to estimate mutation probability among individuals with specific phenotypic features. Proband age at diagnosis, number of proband primaries, and number of additional family primaries were most closely associated with germline mutations. The estimated probability of the proband being a mutation carrier based on the logistic regression model (MELPREDICT) is given by $e^L/(1 + e^L)$, where L = 1.99+[0.92×(no. of proband primaries)]+[0.74×(no. of additional family primaries)]-[2.11×ln(age)]. As a test of performance, the area under the curve from receiver operator characteristic analyses was 0.881 (95% confidence interval [CI], 0.739–1.000) for the training set and 0.803 (0.729–0.877) for an external validation set.[41]

CDKN2A penetrance

There are two robust estimates of *CDKN2A* mutation penetrance. In the GenoMEL estimate, the overall penetrance was calculated to be 30% by age 50 years and 67% by age 80 years (**Fig. 5**). However, this was also subject to geographic effects.

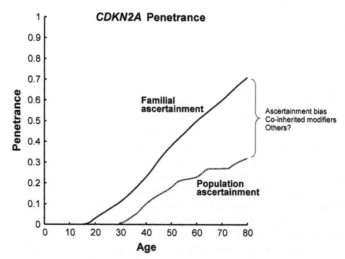

Fig. 5. *CDKN2A* mutation penetrance by familial and population ascertainment.

By age 50 years, penetrance reached 13% in Europe, 50% in the United States, and 32% in Australia; however, by age 80 years, it was 58% in Europe, 76% in the United States, and 91% in Australia.[42] When cases were ascertained through the general melanoma population rather than through families, the *CDKN2A* penetrance appeared to be lower: 14%, 24%, and 28% by ages 50, 70, and 80 years, respectively.[43] Other coinherited factors that elevate genetic risk may in fact contribute to the higher observed penetrance among familial cases. These genetic modifiers may include a host of low-to-medium risk genes. The mere study design of selecting for family history may enrich far more penetrant lesions, and, thus, it is not surprising that the estimates would be higher. Nevertheless, it is reasonable to consider the penetrance estimates as lying within a continuum that is modulated by pedigree structure and environmental input.

Genetic testing for CDKN2A

One controversial area within melanoma genetics is the role of commercial testing for *CDKN2A*.[44] Before any consideration for genetic testing, a formalized and rigorous genetic counseling session is conducted to directly address

1. the information on the specific test
2. the nature of the result (both positive and negative) and its implications
3. risk estimation without genetic testing
4. risk of transmission to children
5. technical accuracy of assay used for testing
6. risks of psychological stress and confidentiality issues
7. risks of genetic discrimination
8. clinical treatment guidelines after testing is not required
9. and insurance coverage of testing fees.

The current commercial test is focused on the coding regions of the p16/Ink4a transcript and does not include *CDK4*, exon 1β of p14/Arf, or deep intronic regions; thus, there will be some mutations that will be missed.

If an affected individual tests positive for a *CDKN2A* mutation, he or she may be at an increased risk to develop a second melanoma compared with the general population, although all melanoma patients are at increased risk of a second melanoma independent of genetic status.[45] This result does provide a family signature so that other family members who subsequently seek genetic testing will in fact have a reference for their results. For the relatives, it is reasonable to assume that a noncarrier will exhibit a lower genetic risk of melanoma than a carrier, although coinherited modifiers may still confer a higher melanoma risk than the general population. Shared exposure risks, such as repeated sun exposure on family vacations, may also play a significant role.

If an unaffected individual in a high-risk family tests positive for a *CDKN2A* mutation, future melanoma risk is estimated by the penetrance. This scenario is less common in practice, since it makes greater logistical sense to also test an affected member of the family to tease out any underlying mutations. If an unaffected individual from the high-risk kindred tests negative for a mutation and no mutation has yet been identified in the family, it is very difficult to draw any genetic or clinical conclusions. Without testing an affected individual or individuals from this family, it is impossible to rule out *CDKN2A* involvement in the kindred. A *CDKN2A* alteration may be present in the family, but the tested individual can be a noncarrier. Alternatively, a mutation in another melanoma-predisposing gene (eg, *CDK4*) that is not identifiable by the test is in fact operating in the kindred. Thus, proper counseling should steer the patient away from a false sense of security if a genetic signature has not been identified in the family. If an affected individual in a family tests negative for a *CDKN2A* mutation, it is still not possible to eliminate the possibility of hereditary melanoma. Because some 50% to 60% of strong melanoma pedigrees do not harbor *CDKN2A* or *CDK4* mutations, other unknown high-risk alleles probably exist and may be transmitted in the family. Lastly, there is no useful information that can be gleaned from an equivocal result, that is, when the impact of the mutation on the protein function cannot be predicted. Until sufficient functional analyses are performed on reported mutations, patients with novel missense mutations should be referred to centers for possible participation in ongoing studies. Furthermore, they should continue to follow stringent sun-protective guidelines.

The clinical utility of *CDKN2A* testing continues to evolve. Theoretical benefits include increased surveillance and earlier detection of lesions in carriers and potential anxiety reduction in noncarriers once identity of a *CDKN2A* mutation has been established. Potential but unproven downsides include oversampling, disruption of family dynamics, and individual distress. It is imperative to stress that because the risk of developing melanoma is not zero even among known noncarriers, abandonment of preventive and surveillance behaviors could negatively impact the individual to a serious extent. As alluded to above, pancreatic cancer risk has also been reported to be increased among some *CDKN2A* families. The absolute risk of pancreatic cancer among carriers has not been rigorously determined. Pancreatic cancer is notoriously difficult to detect at early stages, and currently, there are no data to demonstrate that screening reduces the incidence or mortality from the disease. However, it is not unreasonable that patients with known *CDKN2A* mutations at least consult with a gastroenterologist to discuss pancreatic cancer risk and possible screening strategies. Because of its diagnostic sensitivity and limited invasiveness, endoscopic ultrasound is appealing. One proposed approach for hereditary pancreatic cancer families recommends endoscopic ultrasound examinations beginning 10 years before the diagnosis of the youngest pancreatic cancer patient in the family.[46] Others have endorsed the use of endoscopic ultrasound in conjunction with endoscopic retrograde cholangiopancreatography and serologic marker CA 19-9.[47] More studies are clearly needed before a formalized pancreatic cancer intervention can be recommended.

CDK4

Cell division is tightly controlled by set of cell cycle regulators, which are activated or deactivated at certain checkpoints in the cell cycle, which allows progression through the cycle. Any perturbation in these regulators would contribute to cancer by uncontrolled cell proliferation. A commitment to DNA synthesis during cell cycle is controlled by a set of complexes comprising cyclins and Cdks (see **Fig. 3**). More specifically, Cdk4 or Cdk6 along with cyclin D control passage through the G1 checkpoint of the cell cycle; these Cdks are selectively inhibited by p16/Ink4a. Biochemical data have shown that missense germline mutations in p16/Ink4a impair its ability to inhibit the Cdk complexes. Similarly, Cdk4 mutations that fall within the p16-binding region (ie, Arg24) create oncogenic variants that are resistant to physiologic inhibition by p16/Ink4a.[48,49] Both somatic and germline mutations of Cdk4 have been identified in melanoma cell lines and in families.[5,50] Two recurrent mutations have been described—p.Arg24Cys[5] and p.Arg24His[51]—for a limited number of families worldwide. An analysis by Goldstein and colleagues found that clinical factors were indistinguishable between melanoma case subjects from CDKN2A versus CDK4 families[52] consonant with their epistatic relationship on the Rb pathway.

LOW-TO-MODERATE–RISK SUSCEPTIBILITY GENES

The CDKN2A/CDK4 risk loci appear to be rather selective in that the predominant phenotype is that of cutaneous melanoma (CM). As one approaches the lower risk genes, the phenotype is more related to general pigmentary traits, that is, skin color, hair color, and sun sensitivity. One would expect that many individuals who are predisposed to melanoma are similarly at risk for other cutaneous malignancies including basal cell carcinomas (BCCs).

MC1R

Epidemiologic studies have directly linked pigmentation and melanoma risk.[8] More than 120 genes determine constitutive and facultative pigmentation of the skin (reviewed in[18,53]). One of these, the melanocortin-1-receptor, MC1R, has been recently implicated in melanoma predisposition.

Mc1r is a seven-transmembrane protein that belongs to the family of G-protein–coupled receptors. Upon α-MSH binding, Mc1r activates a G protein, which in turn stimulates adenylate cyclase to increase intracellular cAMP (**Fig. 6**).[54,55] Increased cAMP levels eventually lead to the production of dark eumelanin in preference over the red pheomelanin. Eumelanin confers greater skin pigmentation and protection against exogenous ultraviolet radiation (UVR).

Germline variants of Mc1r are detected in 80% of the individuals with red hair color (RHC) and/or fair skin and who tan poorly, but less than 20% in individuals with brown or black hair and less than 4% of people with good tanning response.[56] Genetic association studies have found that the Mc1r variants p.Asp84Glu, p.Arg151Cys, p.Arg160Trp, and p.Asp294His, defined as "R'" alleles, were strongly associated with the RHC phenotype and, hence, are designated the "R" variants, whereas two other less frequent variants (p.Arg142His and p.Ile155Thr) have also been classified as "R" alleles based on strong familial association with RHC phenotype. The p.Val60-Leu, p.Val92Met, and p.Arg163Gln variants seem to have weaker association with the RHC phenotype and are designated as "r'" alleles.[57] An early study found that Mc1r

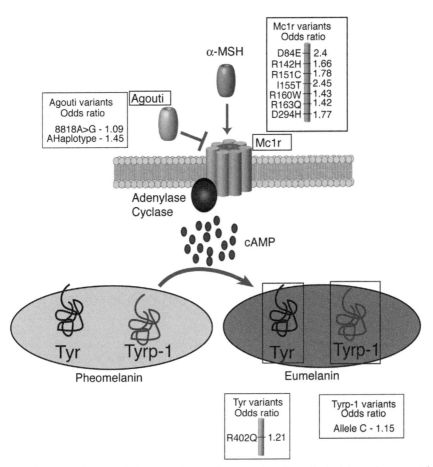

Fig. 6. Biochemical map of pigmentation pathway and loci implicated in melanoma risk. Melanocyte stimulating hormone (MSH) binds to the melanocortin-1-receptor (Mc1r) and stimulates adenylate cyclase (AC) to produced cAMP; agouti protein competitively inhibits this binding. Increased cAMP levels then shift pheomelanin synthesis to eumelanin synthesis. This process is mediated by a large number of melanosomal enzymes including tyrosinase (Tyr) and tyrosinase-related protein-1 (*TYRP1*). The odds ratio represents the risk of melanoma in the patients carrying the indicated gene variants.

variants increased CM risk by 3.9-fold.[56] Another larger study found that, after adjusting for the skin type, a single Mc1r variant confers a 2.7-fold risk, whereas two variants lead to a 3.6-fold risk. The p.Asp84Glu change seems to be associated with the highest risk, with an odds ratio (OR) of 16.1. Some CM risk alleles are not strongly associated with the pigmentary phenotypes, suggesting that *MC1R* alterations may have cancer-related effects outside of hair and skin color.[58] In a recent meta-analysis of Mc1r variants and melanoma risk, all but 2 variants (p.Val60Leu and p.Val92Met) were significantly associated with melanoma risk, with ORs (95% CI) ranging from 1.42 (1.09–1.85) for p.Arg163Gln to 2.45 (1.32–4.55) for p.Ile155Thr.[57] The two common variants—p.Arg151Cys and p.Arg160Trp—account for 7.48% and 4.54%, respectively, of the attributable risk. Overall, the p.Val60Leu and p.Val92Met variants do not appear to be significantly associated with either red hair or melanoma risk; the p.Ile155Thr and p.Arg163Gln variants are associated with melanoma risk but not red hair; and the p.Arg84Glu, p.Arg142His, p.Arg151Cys, p.Arg160Trp, and p.Asp294His variants are associated with both red hair and melanoma (see **Fig. 6**).

In addition to the independent function as a common low-penetrant, low-risk melanoma locus, *MC1R* was also implicated to have a role as a modifier gene in melanoma risk. Among *CDKN2A* mutation carriers, the presence of consensus *MC1R* leads to a penetrance of 50% with a mean onset age of 58.1 years, whereas the presence of an *MC1R* variant increases the penetrance to 84% with a mean onset age of 37.8 years.[59] In this study from Australia, the melanoma risk was largely based on three variants—p.Arg151Cys, p.Arg160Trp, and p.Asp294His. In another study of 395 subjects from 16 American *CDKN2A* families, the presence of multiple Mc1r variants was significantly associated with melanoma, especially among individuals with MPMs. All MPM patients had at least one Mc1r variant, whereas 65% of MPM patients versus only 17% of SPM patients had at least two Mc1r variants. There was a statistically significant decrease in median age at diagnosis as numbers of Mc1r variants increased.[60] Recently, intratumoral Braf mutations were found to be significantly associated with germline Mc1r variants, suggesting that inheritance of these alleles may predispose individuals to develop Braf-driven tumors.[61,62]

Low to Moderate Risk Melanoma Loci—Lessons from Genome-Wide Association Studies

For the previous genes, the population and familial genetics have been tightly linked to proven biologic plausibility. However, recent GWAS have led to several additional melanoma risk loci with suggestive, but unproven, biology. In a survey of 5130 Icelanders, with follow-up analyses in 2116 Icelanders and 1214 Dutch individuals, two coding variants in *TPCN2* were found to be associated with hair color, whereas a variant at the agouti (*ASIP*) locus showed strong association with skin sensitivity to sun, freckling, and red hair—phenotypic features similar to those carrying variants in *MC1R*.[63] In a larger follow-up study of 810 individuals with CM and 36723 non-CM controls from Iceland, 1033 CM cases and 2650 controls from Sweden and 278 CM cases and 1297 controls from Spain, 11 single nucleotide polymorphisms (SNPs) from 8 pigmentation-related loci (*SLC24A4, KITLG*, 6p25.3, *TYR, OCA2, TPCN2, ASIP, TYRP1*) were further tested for melanoma risk effects. A 2-SNP haplotype at the *ASIP* locus was the variant most strongly associated with CM (combined for all 3 CM samples, OR = 1.45; $P = 1.2 \times 10^{-9}$), whereas an additional nonsynonymous coding variant in *TYR* (combined for all 3 samples, OR = 1.21; $P = 2.8 \times 10^{-7}$) and a noncoding SNP at the tyrosinase-related protein 1 (*TYRP1*) locus also associated significantly with melanoma risk (rs1408799; combined for all 3 samples, OR = 1.15; $P = .00043$). A second independent GWAS based in Australia also found evidence of a melanoma risk locus at the *ASIP* locus on chromosome 20q11.[64] The genetic interactions that have emerged from the GWAS appear to be more complicated than thought at first. Interestingly, in the large Icelandic-based GWAS, *MC1R* variants conferred little or no increased risk of CM among the Icelandic population, whereas significant risks for CM were observed in both the Swedish and Spanish cohorts.[63] These findings are consistent with the observation that RHC is not a strong risk factor for CM in Iceland. **Table 1** enumerates the known relationships between the various GWAS loci and their associated pigmentary and cancer phenotypes.

Other Low-Risk Genes

Though inactivating mutations in the *CDKN2A* gene has a very high impact, carriers with rare *CDKN2A* polymorphisms (C500G and C540T) have been associated with

Table 1
GWAS loci and the associated pigmentary and cancer phenotypes

Chromosomal Region/Locus (SNP Region)	Pigmentation Status	Cancer Phenotype
20q11 (Multiple)	Blonde/red hair, green eyes, freckling	Skin sensitivity, CM, BCC
TYR (rs1126809)	Green eyes	Skin sensitivity, CM, BCC
TYR (rs1042602)	Freckling	CM
TYRP1 (rs1408799)	Blonde hair (weak), brown eyes, green eyes (weak)	CM
SLC24A4 (rs12896399)	Blonde hair, green eyes brown eyes (weak)	
KITLG (rs12821256)	Blonde hair	
6p25.3 (rs1540771)	Blonde hair, freckling	Skin sensitivity (weak)
OCA2 (rs1667394)	Blonde hair, green and brown eyes	Skin sensitivity (weak)
OCA2 (rs7495174)	Brown eyes	Skin sensitivity (weak)
TPCN2 (rs35264875, rs3829241)	Blonde hair	
MCIR (RHC, NRHC)	Blonde/red hair, freckling	Skin sensitivity, CM, BCC

Abbreviations: BCC, basal cell carcinoma; CM, cutaneous melanoma; NRHC, non-red hair color variants; RHC, red hair color variants; SNP, singe-nucleotide polymorphism.

the risk of developing melanoma.[65] Another potential risk gene is glutathione S-transferase (*GSTM1 and GSTP1 variants*). Lira and colleagues[66] have shown that the allele *GSTP1*A* is associated with nonmelanoma skin cancer (NMSC) (OR, 1.7), and the *GSTM1* null/null variants have been associated with the risk of developing BCC (OR, 3.1). Analysis of interaction between allelic variants showed significant association between combined *GSTM1* and *CYP1A1* Val462 genotypes (variant of cytochrome P450 debrisoquine hydroxylase locus), where the combined occurrence of these variants showed a higher risk of developing NMSC (OR, 4.5) and also squamous cell carcinoma (SCC) (OR, 6.5).[66] Finally, the vitamin D receptor (*VDR*) has also been implicated in melanoma risk; one of the VDR variants, *Bsm1*, has been shown to confer a higher risk of developing melanoma (OR, 1.3).[67]

UNCOMMON CONDITIONS ASSOCIATED WITH MELANOMA RISK
Hereditary Retinoblastoma

Germline mutations in the *Rb1* gene cause Rb in approximately 85% to 95% of cases, usually bilaterally. The protein product, Rb1, is downstream of the melanoma-related proteins, p16/Ink4a and Cdk4/6. Studies have documented an increased incidence of or mortality from melanoma among survivors of Rb.[68] Given the small number of cases, an accurate relative risk is not possible to estimate. The genetic pathway that links *CDKN2A* and *RB1* provides obvious biologic rationale for the observed melanoma risk.

Xeroderma Pigmentosum

These autosomal recessive conditions result from deficiencies in nucleotide excision repair (NER), the DNA repair process responsible for removing UVR-induced photoadducts. As a consequence, children with xeroderma pigmentation (XP) develop

Table 2
Major known xeroderma pigmentosum genes and thier function

Chromosomal Region	Gene	Function
9q34.1	XPA	Recognizes and binds damaged DNA
2q21	XPB	3'-5' DNA helicase activity
3p25.1	XPC	Initial recognition of DNA damage,and binds single strand DNA
19q13.2	XPD	5'-3' DNA helicase
11p11-12(DDB2 subunit)	XPE	Binds to UV damaged DNA
16p13.3	XPF	Makes DNA incision 5' to the damaged site
13q32-33	XPG	Makes DNA incision 3' to the damaged site

exquisite sun sensitivity at a very early age and cutaneous malignancies decades before their unaffected counterparts.[69,70] There are at least 7 complementation groups that correspond to 7 unique genes that participate in NER. **Table 2** summarizes the major known XP genes and their functions.

XP-C is the most common form of XP, and mutations are associated with an impaired repair of UVR-induced DNA lesions, leading to dramatic increases of UVR-associated skin tumors, predominantly BCC and SCC. Patients with XP have about a 1000-fold increased risk of developing skin cancer with a 600- to 8000-fold elevated risk of melanoma. About 5% to 20% of the patients are eventually diagnosed with CM.[71] Interestingly, in XP, there is a shift away from the more common non–sun-exposed superficial spreading subtype toward a chronic sun-exposed lentigo maligna subtype.

REFERENCES

1. McLead RG, Davis NC, Sober AJ. A history of melanoma: from hunter to clark. In: Balch CM, Houghton A, Sober AJ, et al, editors. Cutaneous melanoma. 4th edition. St. Louis (MO): Quality Medical Publishing Inc; 2003. p. 1–12.
2. Clark WH Jr, Reimer RR, Greene M, et al. Origin of familial malignant melanomas from heritable melanocytic lesions. 'The B-K mole syndrome'. Arch Dermatol 1978;114:732–8.
3. Lynch HT, Frichot BC 3rd, Lynch JF. Familial atypical multiple mole-melanoma syndrome. J Med Genet 1978;15:352–6.
4. Hussussian CJ, Struewing JP, Goldstein AM, et al. Germline p16 mutations in familial melanoma. Nat Genet 1994;8:15–21.
5. Zuo L, Weger J, Yang Q, et al. Germline mutations in the p16INK4a binding domain of CDK4 in familial melanoma. Nat Genet 1996;12:97–9.
6. Bishop JN, Harland M, Bishop DT. The genetics of melanoma. Br J Hosp Med (Lond) 2006;67:299–304.
7. Fargnoli MC, Argenziano G, Zalaudek I, et al. High- and low-penetrance cutaneous melanoma susceptibility genes. Expert Rev Anticancer Ther 2006;6:657–70.
8. Gandini S, Sera F, Cattaruzza MS, et al. Meta-analysis of risk factors for cutaneous melanoma: III. Family history, actinic damage and phenotypic factors. Eur J Cancer 2005;41:2040–59.
9. Bale SJ, Dracopoli NC, Tucker MA, et al. Mapping the gene for hereditary cutaneous malignant melanoma-dysplastic nevus to chromosome 1p. N Engl J Med 1989;320:1367–72.

10. Cannon-Albright LA, Goldgar DE, Meyer LJ, et al. Assignment of a locus for familial melanoma, MLM, to chromosome 9p13-p22. Science 1992;258:1148–52.
11. Serrano M, Hannon GJ, Beach D. A new regulatory motif in cell-cycle control causing specific inhibition of cyclin D/CDK4. Nature 1993;366:704–7.
12. Koh J, Enders GH, Dynlacht BD, et al. Tumour-derived p16 alleles encoding proteins defective in cell-cycle inhibition. Nature 1995;375:506–10.
13. Lukas J, Parry D, Aagaard L, et al. Retinoblastoma-protein-dependent cell-cycle inhibition by the tumour suppressor p16. Nature 1995;375:503–6.
14. Pomerantz J, Schreiber-Agus N, Liegeois NJ, et al. The Ink4a tumor suppressor gene product, p19Arf, interacts with MDM2 and neutralizes MDM2's inhibition of p53. Cell 1998;92:713–23.
15. Kamijo T, Weber JD, Zambetti G, et al. Functional and physical interactions of the ARF tumor suppressor with p53 and Mdm2. Proc Natl Acad Sci U S A 1998;95: 8292–7.
16. Stott FJ, Bates S, James MC, et al. The alternative product from the human CDKN2A locus, p14(ARF), participates in a regulatory feedback loop with p53 and MDM2. EMBO J 1998;17:5001–14.
17. Zhang Y, Xiong Y, Yarbrough WG. ARF promotes MDM2 degradation and stabilizes p53: ARF-INK4a locus deletion impairs both the Rb and p53 tumor suppression pathways. Cell 1998;92:725–34.
18. Lin J, Hocker TL, Singh M, et al. Genetics of melanoma predisposition. Br J Dermatol 2008;159:286–91.
19. Serrano M, Lee H, Chin L, et al. Role of the INK4a locus in tumor suppression and cell mortality. Cell 1996;85:27–37.
20. Chin L, Pomerantz J, Polsky D, et al. Cooperative effects of INK4a and ras in melanoma susceptibility in vivo. Genes Dev 1997;11:2822–34.
21. Goldstein AM, Chan M, Harland M, et al. High-risk melanoma susceptibility genes and pancreatic cancer, neural system tumors, and uveal melanoma across GenoMEL. Cancer Res 2006;66:9818–28.
22. Harland M, Taylor CF, Chambers PA, et al. A mutation hotspot at the p14ARF splice site. Oncogene 2005;24:4604–8.
23. Hewitt C, Lee Wu C, Evans G, et al. Germline mutation of ARF in a melanoma kindred. Hum Mol Genet 2002;11:1273–9.
24. Harland M, Taylor CF, Bass S, et al. Intronic sequence variants of the CDKN2A gene in melanoma pedigrees. Genes Chromosomes Cancer 2005;43:128–36.
25. Harland M, Mistry S, Bishop DT, et al. A deep intronic mutation in CDKN2A is associated with disease in a subset of melanoma pedigrees. Hum Mol Genet 2001;10:2679–86.
26. Goldstein AM, Chan M, Harland M, et al. Features associated with germline CDKN2A mutations: a GenoMEL study of melanoma-prone families from three continents. J Med Genet 2007;44:99–106.
27. Berwick M, Orlow I, Hummer AJ, et al. The prevalence of CDKN2A germ-line mutations and relative risk for cutaneous malignant melanoma: an international population-based study. Cancer Epidemiol Biomarkers Prev 2006;15:1520–5.
28. Berwick M, Orlow I, Mahabir S, et al. Estimating the relative risk of developing melanoma in INK4A carriers. Eur J Cancer Prev 2004;13:65–70.
29. Soufir N, Lacapere JJ, Bertrand G, et al. Germline mutations of the INK4a-ARF gene in patients with suspected genetic predisposition to melanoma. Br J Cancer 2004;90:503–9.
30. Blackwood MA, Holmes R, Synnestvedt M, et al. Multiple primary melanoma revisited. Cancer 2002;94:2248–55.

31. Auroy S, Avril MF, Chompret A, et al. Sporadic multiple primary melanoma cases: CDKN2A germline mutations with a founder effect. Genes Chromosomes Cancer 2001;32:195–202.
32. Hashemi J, Platz A, Ueno T, et al. CDKN2A germ-line mutations in individuals with multiple cutaneous melanomas. Cancer Res 2000;60:6864–7.
33. Ruiz A, Puig S, Malvehy J, et al. CDKN2A mutations in Spanish cutaneous malignant melanoma families and patients with multiple melanomas and other neoplasia. J Med Genet 1999;36:490–3.
34. MacKie RM, Andrew N, Lanyon WG, et al. CDKN2A germline mutations in U.K. patients with familial melanoma and multiple primary melanomas. J Invest Dermatol 1998;111:269–72.
35. Monzon J, Liu L, Brill H, et al. CDKN2A mutations in multiple primary melanomas. N Engl J Med 1998;338:879–87.
36. Goldstein AM, Fraser MC, Struewing JP, et al. Increased risk of pancreatic cancer in melanoma-prone kindreds with p16INK4 mutations. N Engl J Med 1995;333:970–4.
37. Tsao H, Zhang X, Kwitkiwski K, et al. Low prevalence of germline CDKN2A and CDK4 mutations in patients with early-onset melanoma. Arch Dermatol 2000; 136:1118–22.
38. Berg P, Wennberg AM, Tuominen R, et al. Germline CDKN2A mutations are rare in child and adolescent cutaneous melanoma. Melanoma Res 2004;14:251–5.
39. Debniak T, van de Wetering T, Scott R, et al. Low prevalence of CDKN2A/ARF mutations among early-onset cancers of breast, pancreas and malignant melanoma in Poland. Eur J Cancer Prev 2008;17:389–91.
40. Stratigos AJ, Yang G, Dimisianos R, et al. Germline CDKN2A mutations among Greek patients with early-onset and multiple primary cutaneous melanoma. J Invest Dermatol 2006;126:399–401.
41. Niendorf KB, Goggins W, Yang G, et al. MELPREDICT: a logistic regression model to estimate CDKN2A carrier probability. J Med Genet 2006;43:501–6.
42. Bishop DT, Demenais F, Goldstein AM, et al. Geographical variation in the penetrance of CDKN2A mutations for melanoma. J Natl Cancer Inst 2002;94: 894–903.
43. Begg CB, Orlow I, Hummer AJ, et al. Lifetime risk of melanoma in CDKN2A mutation carriers in a population-based sample. J Natl Cancer Inst 2005;97:1507–15.
44. Tsao H, Niendorf K. Genetic testing in hereditary melanoma. J Am Acad Dermatol 2004;51:803–8.
45. Goggins WB, Tsao H. A population-based analysis of risk factors for a second primary cutaneous melanoma among melanoma survivors. Cancer 2003;97: 639–43.
46. Kimmey MB, Bronner MP, Byrd DR, et al. Screening and surveillance for hereditary pancreatic cancer. Gastrointest Endosc 2002;56:S82–6.
47. Parker JF, Florell SR, Alexander A, et al. Pancreatic carcinoma surveillance in patients with familial melanoma. Arch Dermatol 2003;139:1019–25.
48. Ranade K, Hussussian CJ, Sikorski RS, et al. Mutations associated with familial melanoma impair p16INK4 function. Nat Genet 1995;10:114–6.
49. Reymond A, Brent R. p16 proteins from melanoma-prone families are deficient in binding to Cdk4. Oncogene 1995;11:1173–8.
50. Tsao H, Benoit E, Sober AJ, et al. Novel mutations in the p16/CDKN2A binding region of the cyclin-dependent kinase-4 gene. Cancer Res 1998;58:109–13.
51. Soufir N, Avril MF, Chompret A, et al. Prevalence of p16 and CDK4 germline mutations in 48 melanoma-prone families in France. The French Familial Melanoma Study Group. Hum Mol Genet 1998;7:209–16.

52. Goldstein AM, Struewing JP, Chidambaram A, et al. Genotype-phenotype relationships in U.S. melanoma-prone families with CDKN2A and CDK4 mutations. J Natl Cancer Inst 2000;92:1006–10.

53. Rouzaud F, Kadekaro AL, Abdel-Malek ZA, et al. MC1R and the response of melanocytes to ultraviolet radiation. Mutat Res 2005;571:133–52.

54. Garcia-Borron JC, Sanchez-Laorden BL, Jimenez-Cervantes C. Melanocortin-1 receptor structure and functional regulation. Pigment Cell Res 2005;18:393–410.

55. Mas JS, Gerritsen I, Hahmann C, et al. Rate limiting factors in melanocortin 1 receptor signalling through the cAMP pathway. Pigment Cell Res 2003;16:540–7.

56. Valverde P, Healy E, Jackson I, et al. Variants of the melanocyte-stimulating hormone receptor gene are associated with red hair and fair skin in humans. Nat Genet 1995;11:328–30.

57. Raimondi S, Sera F, Gandini S, et al. MC1R variants, melanoma and red hair color phenotype: a meta-analysis. Int J Cancer 2008;122:2753–60.

58. Kennedy C, ter Huurne J, Berkhout M, et al. Melanocortin 1 receptor (MC1R) gene variants are associated with an increased risk for cutaneous melanoma which is largely independent of skin type and hair color. J Invest Dermatol 2001;117:294–300.

59. Box NF, Duffy DL, Chen W, et al. MC1R genotype modifies risk of melanoma in families segregating CDKN2A mutations. Am J Hum Genet 2001;69:765–73.

60. Goldstein AM, Landi MT, Tsang S, et al. Association of MC1R variants and risk of melanoma in melanoma-prone families with CDKN2A mutations. Cancer Epidemiol Biomarkers Prev 2005;14:2208–12.

61. Landi MT, Bauer J, Pfeiffer RM, et al. MC1R germline variants confer risk for BRAF-mutant melanoma. Science 2006;313:521–2.

62. Fargnoli MC, Pike K, Pfeiffer RM, et al. MC1R variants increase risk of melanomas harboring BRAF mutations. J Invest Dermatol 2008;128:2485–90.

63. Sulem P, Gudbjartsson DF, Stacey SN, et al. Two newly identified genetic determinants of pigmentation in Europeans. Nat Genet 2008;40:835–7.

64. Brown KM, Macgregor S, Montgomery GW, et al. Common sequence variants on 20q11.22 confer melanoma susceptibility. Nat Genet 2008;40:838–40.

65. Hayward NK. Genetics of melanoma predisposition. Oncogene 2003;22:3053–62.

66. Lira MG, Provezza L, Malerba G, et al. Glutathione S-transferase and CYP1A1 gene polymorphisms and non-melanoma skin cancer risk in Italian transplanted patients. Exp Dermatol 2006;15:958–65.

67. Mocellin S, Nitti D. Vitamin D receptor polymorphisms and the risk of cutaneous melanoma: a systematic review and meta-analysis. Cancer 2008;113:2398–407.

68. Kleinerman RA, Tucker MA, Tarone RE, et al. Risk of new cancers after radiotherapy in long-term survivors of retinoblastoma: an extended follow-up. J Clin Oncol 2005;23:2272–9.

69. Somoano B, Tsao H. Genodermatoses with cutaneous tumors and internal malignancies. Dermatol Clin 2008;26:69–87, viii.

70. Somoano B, Niendorf KB, Tsao H. Hereditary cancer syndromes of the skin. Clin Dermatol 2005;23:85–106.

71. Kraemer KH, Lee MM, Andrews AD, et al. The role of sunlight and DNA repair in melanoma and nonmelanoma skin cancer. The xeroderma pigmentosum paradigm. Arch Dermatol 1994;130:1018–21.

Tumor Angiogenesis in Melanoma

Alexander G. Marneros, MD, PhD[a,b,*]

KEYWORDS

- Melanoma • Angiogenesis
- Vascular endothelial growth factor
- Bone marrow–derived cells • Antiangiogenesis
- Endothelial cells

PRINCIPLES OF TUMOR ANGIOGENESIS IN MELANOMA
Angiogenic Factors and Endogenous Angiogenesis Inhibitors in Melanoma

Various types of cells in the melanoma microenvironment produce a large number of inhibitors and stimulators of angiogenesis. These cells include tumor cells, tumor-infiltrating inflammatory cells, endothelial cells, or other cells of the tumor stroma. It has been hypothesized that an imbalance between such inhibitors and stimulators of angiogenesis, favoring stimulators, promotes tumor angiogenesis. In this context, it has been proposed that growth of tumor blood vessels could be inhibited by excess of endogenous inhibitors of angiogenesis.[1,2] The observation that some primary tumors are able to inhibit the growth of distant metastases led to the hypothesis that tumors may secret endogenous inhibitors of angiogenesis. This notion has led to the identification of various endogenous angiogenesis inhibitors, including endostatin and angiostatin,[1,2] which are proteolytic fragments of the basement membrane collagen XVIII and plasminogen, respectively. For example, endostatin was shown to suppress tumor angiogenesis and growth of B16F10 melanomas in mice.[1] Other extracellular matrix proteins or their proteolytic derivatives, such as thrombospondins, or fragments of perlecan or collagen IV, were also shown to possess antiangiogenic activity and to inhibit tumor growth in mouse models.[3–5] The concept of an angiogenic switch from a quiescent resident vasculature to an expanding proliferative tumor vasculature, which is required for tumor cells to form expanding solid tumors, was proposed, and endogenous angiogenesis inhibitors were found to inhibit this angiogenic switch in mouse tumor models.[6,7]

In contrast, growth factors that stimulate endothelial cell proliferation and migration, such as vascular endothelial growth factor (VEGF) and fibroblast growth

[a] Cutaneous Biology Research Center, Massachusetts General Hospital, Building 149, 13th Street, Charlestown, MA 02129, USA
[b] Department of Dermatology, Harvard Medical School, Boston, MA, USA
* Cutaneous Biology Research center, Massachusetts General Hospital, Building 149, 13th Street, Charlestown, MA 02129.
E-mail address: alexander_marneros@yahoo.com

Hematol Oncol Clin N Am 23 (2009) 431–446
doi:10.1016/j.hoc.2009.03.007
0889-8588/09/$ – see front matter © 2009 Elsevier Inc. All rights reserved.

hemonc.theclinics.com

factor-2 (FGF-2), promote blood vessel formation. Multiple studies have examined the expression of proangiogenic growth factors and their receptors in melanomas, to assess whether vascular invasion of primary melanomas is predictive for a risk of metastasis. Initial studies led to conflicting results regarding the prognostic value of vascular invasion of melanomas for the risk of metastasis.[8] These initial descriptive studies did not distinguish between blood and lymph vessels in melanomas, due to the lack of specific lymph vessel markers. When such markers became available, detailed analyses of lymph and blood vessels in melanomas were undertaken. For example, it was shown that melanomas overexpressing the lymphangiogenic growth factor, VEGF-C, have increased intratumoral blood and lymph vessels.[9] VEGF-C was found to be expressed in primary cutaneous melanomas.[10] The intratumoral lymph vessels are likely sprouting from the surrounding preexisting lymphatic network, and are not the result of bone marrow–derived endothelial progenitor cell recruitment.[11]

When intratumoral lymph vessels in melanomas that had metastasized to lymph nodes were compared with those in nonmetastatic melanomas, a significant increase in intratumoral lymphatics was observed in metastatic primary melanomas.[12] These findings suggest that the extent of intratumoral lymphatics in primary melanomas may be a prognostic indicator for the risk of lymph node metastasis.

Similarly, in a chemically induced skin carcinogenesis model in transgenic mice overexpressing VEGF-A in the epidermis, sentinel lymph nodes of VEGF-A–expressing skin tumors had increased lymphangiogenesis.[13] Increased lymph vessels were already observed in sentinel lymph nodes before any lymph node metastasis had occurred, a process that may facilitate further metastatic spread along the lymphatics. Lymphangiogenesis was also increased in sentinel lymph nodes in carcinogenesis experiments in transgenic mice overexpressing VEGF-C in the epidermis.[14]

Analysis of the expression of VEGF and its receptors in melanomas showed that VEGF is frequently expressed by melanoma cells, but the prognostic value of this finding is not clear.[8] Some data indicated an increase of VEGF-A and VEGF-C expression in melanomas compared with their expression in benign melanocytic lesions.[15] The presence of VEGF receptors on melanoma cells may suggest an autocrine effect of VEGF.[16] In vitro, melanoma cells expressing VEGF-A and VEGF receptor-2 (VEGFR2) showed an increased ability to invade the extracellular matrix.[17] Other proangiogenic factors were also found to be expressed in melanomas, including FGF-2, interleukin-8 (IL-8), placental growth factor (PlGF), or platelet-derived growth factor (PDGF).[16,18–22]

Recent evidence demonstrates that tumor angiogenesis and metastasis are not only directed by the interactions between tumor cells and stroma cells at the site of the primary tumor, but that cells from the bone marrow are critically involved in promoting tumor angiogenesis and metastasis.

Bone Marrow–Derived Cells Contribute to Tumor Angiogenesis: the Role of Myeloid Cells

Distinct populations of bone marrow–derived cells contribute to tumor angiogenesis. Endothelial progenitor cells (EPCs) incorporate into the vessel wall, and pericyte progenitor cells (PPCs) surround endothelial cell linings. In the early stages of tumor angiogenesis, secretion of matrix metalloproteinase-9 (MMP9) by tumor-infiltrating neutrophils results in an increase in VEGF-VEGFR interactions and activation of tumor angiogenesis.[23,24] Similarly, bone marrow–derived dendritic cell precursors have been shown to integrate into the tumor vasculature and promote tumor growth.[25]

Myeloid progenitor cell populations, including Gr1$^+$CD11b$^+$ cells, have been shown to differentiate into endothelial-like cells that are able to incorporate into the vessel wall.[26] These myeloid immune suppressor cells promote tumor growth through a mechanism that depends on high MMP9 expression by these cells, resulting in an increase of matrix-bound VEGF release from the tumor tissue.[26] When these cells were coinjected with tumor cells in mice, increased vascular density and maturation were observed, associated with less tumor cell hypoxia and necrotic tumor areas.[26] MMP9 seems to be essential in this process. In addition to releasing matrix-bound VEGF in tumors and thereby promoting angiogenesis, MMP9 derived from Gr1$^+$CD11b$^+$ cells releases soluble Kit ligand (sKitL) in the bone marrow, thereby mobilizing hematopoietic and endothelial progenitor cells.[26,27] It has previously been shown that MMP9-mediated release of sKitL leads endothelial and hematopoietic progenitor cells in the bone marrow to enter a proliferative niche, in which sKitL recruits c-Kit$^+$ stem and progenitor cells.[27] Furthermore, in tumor mouse models MMP9 was shown to be important for the production and tumor infiltration of Gr1$^+$CD11b$^+$ cells.[26]

Refractoriness to antiangiogenic treatment with an anti-VEGF antibody in tumor-bearing mice was shown to be mediated by Gr1$^+$CD11b$^+$ myeloid cells that infiltrated the tumor tissue.[28] An increased antitumor effect was noticed in this study when a combination of antibodies that target VEGF and Gr1$^+$CD11b$^+$ myeloid cells was administered. The refractoriness to anti-VEGF treatments differed between the various tumor types studied. For example, B16F1 melanomas responded well to anti-VEGF treatment, with an observed reduction in tumor growth of more than 70%, whereas Lewis lung carcinoma growth was inhibited by only about 30%. The investigators demonstrated that when mixing nonrefractory B16F1 melanoma cells with bone marrow–derived myeloid cells that were primed in mice bearing refractory tumors, such as Lewis lung carcinomas, these B16F1 melanomas acquired anti-VEGF resistance.[28] Experiments with conditioned media from these different tumors revealed that recruitment of Gr1$^+$CD11b$^+$ myeloid cells was increased for tumors that exhibit anti-VEGF treatment refractoriness. Therefore, the role of these myeloid cells in promoting tumor growth and tumor angiogenesis differs significantly between various tumors, and their specific contribution to tumor angiogenesis in patients with melanomas remains to be determined.

It has been speculated that the combination of antiangiogenic treatments with cytotoxic agents may also enhance antitumor effects to some extent through ablation of myeloid cells that may mediate anti-VEGF refractoriness. How these myeloid cells lead to anti-VEGF refractoriness in some tumors is not entirely clear at this point, but a recently identified component of this mechanism may be Bv8.

Bv8 (also called prokinectin-2) has a high similarity with endocrine gland–derived VEGF (EG-VEGF). It binds to G-protein–coupled receptors, which are also expressed by hematopoietic stem cells.[29] Bv8 is expressed in the bone marrow and promotes hematopoietic stem cell mobilization. Tumor-bearing mice showed an up-regulation of Bv8 expression in Gr1$^+$CD11b$^+$ cells, and Bv8 expression was shown to be up-regulated by granulocyte–colony stimulating factor (G-CSF). Thus, tumor or tumor stroma cell–derived G-CSF is likely to increase mobilization of Gr1$^+$CD11b$^+$ cells. Bv8 was shown to promote tumor angiogenesis, whereas treatment with anti-Bv8 antibodies inhibited tumor growth and tumor angiogenesis associated with a reduction in tumoral Gr1$^+$CD11b$^+$ cells and mobilization of these cells from the bone marrow.[28] Treatment with a combination of antibodies against Bv8 and VEGF inhibited tumor growth, even in tumors that were refractory to anti-VEGF treatment.[28] In addition, anti-Bv8 antibodies increased the antitumor effects of cytotoxic agents.

Hematopoietic Progenitor Cells in Tumor Angiogenesis

A population of CXCR4+VEGFR1+ hematopoietic progenitor cells, designated as "hemangiocytes," has also been shown to contribute to angiogenesis.[30] Various factors, in particular sKitL and thrombopoietin, induced release of stroma-derived factor-1 (SDF-1) from platelets, which mobilized CXCR4+VEGFR1+ hemangiocytes to sites of angiogenesis.[30] These findings emphasize the importance of platelets as regulators of angiogenesis. It has been shown that platelets are able to actively secret pro- and antiangiogenic factors. Thrombin stimulation can induce the release of VEGF from platelets, thereby promoting neovascularization at sites of injury.[31] Some evidence suggests that proangiogenic factors and antiangiogenic factors are present in distinct α-granules in platelets, and can be released selectively through distinct mechanisms.[32] An antiangiogenic effect of platelets may be mediated by the release of antiangiogenic endostatin or thrombospondin. For example, thrombospondin release from platelets resulted in significant antiangiogenic activity and in an inhibition of thrombopoiesis.[33] In contrast, platelets are also able to sequester proangiogenic factors, such as tumor-derived VEGF.[34]

The mobilization of the hemangiocytes from the bone marrow and their contribution to angiogenesis is an example of the complex interplay between tumor cells, peritumoral blood vessels, and bone marrow cells. Secretion of VEGF and SDF-1 activates CXCR4+VEGFR1+ cells in the bone marrow and induces MMP9 release, which results in sKitL release. In turn, these cells are mobilized from the bone marrow into the circulation and home to the tumor vascular bed, in part through SDF-1 secretion by tumor cells. These bone marrow–derived cells can release MMP9 and promote tumor growth, possibly by the release of matrix-bound VEGF.[35]

As bone marrow–derived cells home toward SDF-1 secreting cells, it can be speculated that bone marrow–derived chemokines may also attract tumor cells to the bone marrow, explaining the high rate of bone marrow infiltration of certain tumors. The chemoattractant SDF-1 has been shown to be expressed by specialized bone marrow endothelial cells that also express E-selectin. These specialized endothelial cells in the bone marrow can be a site for tumor cell homing and thus provide a microenvironment for metastatic spread to the bone marrow.[36] These specialized vascular structures in the bone marrow were also the site of entry of circulating hematopoietic progenitor cells and lymphocytes, suggesting that tumor cells may use a physiologic mechanism for cellular entry in the bone marrow by way of specialized vascular structures.

For example, breast cancer commonly metastasizes to the bone. Breast cancer cells were shown to express the chemokine receptors, CXCR4 and CCR7. Their respective ligands, SDF-1 (CXCL12) and CCL21, were found to have their highest levels of expression at tissue sites that are the first destinations for breast cancer metastasis, including the bone marrow.[37] When the chemokine receptor profile was investigated in melanoma cell lines, it became apparent that, in addition to CXCR4 and CCR7, the chemokine receptor CCR10 was found to be expressed at high levels by melanoma cells. Melanoma often shows a similar pattern of metastatic spread as some breast cancers, but it also commonly metastasizes to the skin. Consistent with this clinical experience, the ligand for CCR10, namely CCL27 (CTACK), is specifically expressed in the skin, supporting the hypothesis that chemokines play important roles in directing sites of metastasis.[37] Treatment of mice with neutralizing antibodies against endogenous CCL27 blocked the growth of CCR10-expressing melanoma cells in skin.[38] Furthermore, lymphatic endothelium secretes CCL21, and may thus stimulate melanoma metastasis through mobilization of CCR7-expressing melanoma cells.[39,40]

Endothelial Progenitor Cells in Tumor Angiogenesis

The extent to which EPCs incorporate into the tumor vasculature and promote angiogenesis has been a subject of controversy, with significant differences in the reported contributions of EPCs to tumor vasculature in different studies. Some of these differences may be related to the use of different types of tumors in these experiments, and whether tumor vessels were examined at an early or late phase of tumor growth. A study involving bone marrow transplant patients who received donor cells from individuals of the opposite sex and who developed cancers at a later stage, used sex chromosome-specific fluorescence in situ hybridization probes to identify tumor endothelium derived from bone marrow cells. Less than 5% of tumor endothelial cells in cancers were derived from bone marrow cells in this study.[41] In contrast, a recent study in mice using syngeneic melanomas and other tumors, reported no endothelial progenitor cell incorporation into the tumor vessel endothelial cell lining, but instead found recruitment of bone marrow–derived cells to the perivascular area of tumor vessels.[42]

Strong evidence for a role of circulating EPCs in tumor angiogenesis came from a recent study in a mouse lung metastasis model. Bone marrow–derived EPCs were shown to promote progression of micrometastases to macrometastases in this model, associated with increased tumor angiogenesis.[43] This angiogenic switch was mediated by the transcription factor Id1. The expression of Id1was found to be increased specifically in EPCs in the bone marrow after tumor challenge.[43] Suppression of this transcription factor in EPCs inhibited tumor angiogenesis and metastatic progression in this mouse model, suggesting a critical role for EPCs in metastatic progression of cancers through promoting angiogenesis. It has been suggested that Id1 is important for the mobilization and recruitment of EPCs to tumors. Although only a minority of the endothelial cells that are incorporated into the tumor vasculature were derived from EPCs in this model, it is likely that these cells also stimulate proliferation of other endothelial cells in the tumor microenvironment through secretion of proangiogenic factors.[43]

Using an antibody against the monomeric vascular endothelial (VE)–cadherin, present on EPCs but not on mature endothelial cells, tumor angiogenesis was significantly reduced, accompanied by a reduction of EPCs within tumors.[44] In this study, EPCs were defined by cell surface expression of VE-cadherin, VEGFR2, endoglin, prominin I/AC133, and low expression of CD31. The investigators showed differentiation of these EPCs into ECs that luminally incorporated into tumor vessels. A contribution of EPCs to tumor angiogenesis was particularly apparent in the early stages of tumor vascularization, whereas endothelial cells from preexisting vessels diluted the pool of EPCs in tumor vessels at later stages.

The term EPCs has been used for different cell populations in the recent literature, and cells from the monocyte lineage with similarities to endothelial cells, as well as other hematopoietic cells, may have been described as EPCs.[45] The lack of a uniform and specific marker for EPCs has made it difficult to determine the role of EPCs versus other endothelial cell–like progenitor cells in tumor angiogenesis with certainty.

In earlier studies, it was shown that mice mutant for Id transcription factors (Id1$^{-/+}$ Id3$^{-/-}$) showed significantly reduced tumor angiogenesis.[46] However, tumor angiogenesis was restored after transplantation of bone marrow obtained from wild-type mice. This effect was mediated through recruitment of VEGF-responsive hematopoietic cells and circulating EPCs.[47] In addition to VEGFR2$^+$ EPCs, VEGFR1$^+$ bone marrow–derived hematopoietic cells contributed to tumor angiogenesis and were incorporated into the perivascular space of tumor vessels in this study.[47] VEGF was shown to be critical for the mobilization of hematopoietic stem cells and EPCs from the bone marrow.[48]

The recruitment of these different bone marrow–derived cell populations during angiogenesis is likely to be the result of a concerted effort between tumor cells, endothelial cells, but also perivascular myofibroblasts or other stromal cells. For example, VEGF, which can recruit bone marrow–derived circulating myeloid cells to the site of angiogenesis, has been shown to induce SDF-1 expression in activated perivascular myofibroblasts. SDF-1, in turn, may promote incorporation of these circulating myeloid cells into the perivascular space, which then secrete proangiogenic factors that stimulate endothelial cell proliferation or EPC incorporation.[49]

Pericytes and Mesenchymal Stem Cells in Tumor Angiogenesis

Vessel maturation depends on the proper assembly of pericytes that cover endothelial cells. VEGF and PDGF act in concert to regulate this interaction between endothelial cells and pericytes. Endothelial cell–derived PDGF has been shown to stimulate pericytes to express proangiogenic factors. It has recently been demonstrated that VEGF can inhibit vessel maturation if present with PDGF at pericytes. VEGF/PDGF can induce the formation of a receptor complex between VEGFR2 and PDGFR-β, suppressing PDGF signaling in pericytes and ablating pericyte coverage, thereby destabilizing the vessels.[50] Fibrosarcomas expressing VEGF were shown to develop an immature vasculature with little pericyte coverage, whereas fibrosarcomas lacking VEGF expression had mature blood vessels with extensive pericyte coverage.[50] Therefore, anti-VEGF therapy in cancer patients may stimulate tumor vessel maturation. Consistent with these findings, vessels in tumors lacking myeloid-derived VEGF had increased pericyte coverage with morphologic signs of vessel normalization.[51] This effect was associated with reduced tumor hypoxia and tumor cell death, resulting in accelerated tumor progression. Notably, loss of myeloid cell–derived VEGF also led to an increased susceptibility of tumors to chemotherapeutic cytotoxicity. Thus, myeloid cell–derived VEGF may inhibit tumor progression, rather than promote it. Total tumoral VEGF levels were unaltered in mice lacking myeloid cell–derived VEGF, and therefore the functions of myeloid cell–derived VEGF for the tumor vasculature cannot be replaced by tumor cell–derived VEGF.[51]

Whereas vessel stabilization was associated in this study with accelerated tumor progression, this finding does not necessarily argue for therapeutic approaches that target the tumoral pericytes. It is possible that, although pericyte coverage of tumor vessels may stabilize vessels and thereby stimulate primary tumor growth, it may at the same time reduce the likelihood of tumor cell invasion into the vessel and subsequent metastatic spread. Genetic ablation of pericytes in PDGF-β mutant mice was associated with increased metastases in a fibrosarcoma tumor model in these mice.[52] Therefore, pericyte-mediated stabilization of the tumoral blood vessel wall may limit metastasis.

In another study, PDGFR-β–expressing perivascular cells in tumor vessels were in part recruited from the bone marrow and led to vessel stabilization. Ablation of PDGFR-β signaling led to loss of these perivascular cells with subsequent endothelial cell apoptosis.[53]

It is possible that pericytes in tumors have more complex roles beyond their effects on vessel stabilization. In the normal vasculature of multiple tissues, it has recently been shown that pericytes have characteristics of mesenchymal stem cells, in that they are able to differentiate into muscle cells, chondrocytes, osteocytes, and adipocytes, and show clonal proliferation.[54] Furthermore, they were shown to express markers that have been associated with mesenchymal stem cells. Therefore, pericytes may serve as progenitor cells during tissue regeneration. These findings raise the question whether pericytes in tumors can also act like mesenchymal stem cells.

When bone marrow–derived human mesenchymal stem cells were mixed with breast carcinoma cells, which have only weak metastatic potential in tumor xenograft assays, the rate of metastasis increased greatly.[55] This increase in metastasis was shown to involve a paracrine mechanism between the breast cancer cells and the mesenchymal stem cells involving the chemokine, CCL5 (RANTES), expressed by mesenchymal stem cells. These findings raise the question whether tumor vessel pericytes could increase the metastatic potential of some types of tumor cells through a direct paracrine effect, rather than inhibit metastasis through blocking tumor cell invasion into the vessel wall as seen in the fibrosarcoma model.[52] Alternatively, the observed prometastatic effect of mesenchymal stem cells in the breast cancer model may, at least in part, be mediated through tumor vessel stabilization. CCL5 has been shown to attract macrophages and endothelial cells to sites of tumor formation, thereby stimulating tumor angiogenesis.[56] It will be important to determine whether tumor vessel pericytes have mesenchymal stem cell–like characteristics similar to those described for pericytes in normal tissues and whether they promote or inhibit tumor metastasis.

It is also not clear if tumor cells attract mesenchymal stem cells in a paracrine fashion, or if the evolving blood vessels supplying the tumor cells secrete chemokines that attract mesenchymal stem cells to integrate into the tumor vessel wall and stabilize these vessels. Endothelial cells were shown to attract pericyte precursor cells and promote their perivascular incorporation and differentiation into mature pericytes.[53] This cell population was partly derived from bone marrow hematopoietic stem cells.

Bone marrow–derived cells expressing pericyte markers (like NG2) localized to blood vessels in a subcutaneous B16F1 melanoma tumor model.[57] In this study, the investigators demonstrated that the major contribution of bone marrow–derived cells to the tumor vasculature was in forming perivascular cells. These findings make the distinction between bone marrow–derived mesenchymal stem cells and pericytes difficult. It has been shown that bone marrow–derived mesenchymal stem cells incorporated in a perivascular location when injected into gliomas and expressed pericyte markers, such as neuron-glia 2 (NG2), PDGFR-β, or α-smooth muscle actin.[58] Similarly, when bone marrow–derived mesenchymal stem cells were coinjected with melanoma cells in mouse xenograft studies, these stem cells engrafted into the tumor stroma.[59] Systemic administration of mesenchymal stem cells showed that these cells engrafted preferentially into the stroma of tumors (melanomas in this case). Furthermore, adenoviral transfection of mesenchymal stem cells with interferon-β and subsequent intravenous administration of these cells, resulted in tumor engraftment and inhibition of tumor growth.[59] Such an effect was not observed when cells were implanted at a distant subcutaneous site.

Thus, it may be possible to use mesenchymal stem cells as delivery systems for antitumor agents. Similarly, IFN-α–expressing mesenchymal stem cells inhibited tumor growth in a lung metastasis model of melanoma after intravenous injection of B16F10 melanoma cells into mice.[60] This model was also used to show inhibition of melanoma metastasis with mesenchymal stem cells stably transfected with IL-12.[61]

Bone Marrow–Derived Cells and the "Premetastatic Niche"

It is becoming increasingly clear that bone marrow–derived cells have essential functions in promoting tumor angiogenesis and tumor growth. It has recently been shown that some tumors are able to stimulate the growth of distant indolent tumors. Osteopontin secretion by these tumors was shown to be necessary for this effect.[62] The concept that a primary tumor stimulates the growth of distant tumors is contrary to the concept of a primary tumor secreting antiangiogenic factors that suppress distant tumors, such as reported for endostatin.[1] The tumor-promoting effect of osteopontin was dependent on activation of bone marrow–derived cells, more specifically hematopoietic stem cells expressing the osteopontin receptors CD44 and α4-integrin, eventually resulting in an increase in mobilization and incorporation of bone marrow–derived cells into the tumor that is being stimulated to grow. In human cancers, high levels of osteopontin in the blood have been reported as a poor prognostic marker and are associated with an increased rate of metastasis. An increase in osteopontin levels has also been reported to be a poor prognostic marker in patients with melanoma, and to be significantly predictive of melanoma sentinel lymph node metastasis.[63]

Recent findings have provided evidence for a further mechanism through which a primary tumor promotes metastasis, namely in establishing a "premetastatic niche" as a supporting environment to which metastatic cells home. Following this hypothesis, primary tumor cells secrete factors that support the formation of a premetastatic niche at a distant site, for example in the lung. Bone marrow–derived hematopoietic precursor cells that express VEGFR1 and VLA-4 (integrin α4β1) were shown to home to such tumor-specific premetastatic niches and form cellular clusters before the arrival of tumor cells, to establish a supporting environment for metastatic cells. Bone marrow–derived cells clustered in tissues that are common sites of melanoma metastasis before arrival of tumor cells in tumor mouse models using B16 melanoma cells.[64] In addition, primary tumors secrete factors that increase fibronectin expression in resident fibroblasts in these niches to which the bone marrow-derived hematopoietic precursor cells can home by binding of VLA-4 to fibronectin.[64] Conditioned media from different tumors with distinct metastatic profiles were shown to induce fibronectin expression at distinct peripheral sites. These findings provide compelling evidence for an important role of hematopoietic bone marrow–derived cells in metastasis. Thus, tumor cells not only interact with tumoral stroma cells in a paracrine fashion and through direct cell-cell interactions but also in an endocrine manner, activating cells in the bone marrow and at distant sites.

Tumor-derived VEGF, TGF-β, and TNF-α were shown to induce expression of S100A8 and S100A9, both being proinflammatory chemokines, in the premetastatic niche in the lung.[65] These chemokines promoted the homing of Mac1$^+$ myeloid cells to this niche and tumor cell invasion. S100A8 and S100A9 increased levels of serum amyloid A3 (SAA3) at these premetastatic sites.[66] SAA3, in turn, stimulates its own secretion by a positive feedback mechanism that involves Toll-like receptor-4 (TLR4), and leads to activation of NF-κB signaling in macrophages. Therefore, the microenvironment created at these premetastatic niches by tumor cells has been compared with an inflammation-like state that favors tumor cell invasion and metastasis.[67] Blocking this pathway, which involves SAA3 and TLR4, may provide a new therapeutic approach to inhibit metastasis in the lung.

These findings reveal extensive communications between the primary tumor site, the bone marrow, and the sites of future metastasis, involving factors that act locally and systemically. Therefore, a model of "niche-to-niche" migration of cells has been put forward as a multidirectional system between the bone marrow, the tumor, and the peripheral premetastatic niche (**Fig. 1**).[68]

Cancer-Associated Fibroblasts and Tumor Angiogenesis

Cancer-associated fibroblasts (CAFs), with features of myofibroblasts, have been shown in a breast cancer xenograft model to stimulate tumor growth through secretion

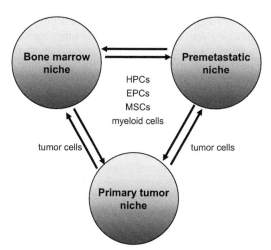

Fig. 1. Model of "niche-to-niche" migration of cells as a multidirectional system between the bone marrow, the tumor, and the "premetastatic niche." Hematopoietic progenitor cells (HPCs), EPCs, MSCs, and myeloid cells are essential in promoting tumor angiogenesis and metastasis. Factors derived from cells from the primary tumor niche prepare resident cells in the "premetastatic niche" to provide a supportive environment for tumor cells.

of SDF-1.[69] This factor promotes tumor cell growth directly through effects on cancer cells, and indirectly by recruiting EPCs and thereby stimulating tumor angiogenesis.[69] CAFs may represent a heterogenous population of cells with similar features. They may be "activated" resident fibroblasts that stimulate tumor cell growth locally. Alternatively, these cells may be actively recruited to the site of tumor growth from a pool of circulating progenitor cells, or these cells may be derived from perivascular cells with characteristics of mesenchymal stem cells, which also express pericyte markers.

Although it seems that a large number of different cell populations contribute to the tumor cell microenvironment, it remains to be determined if some cell populations that are categorized as distinct subsets of cells, may actually be cells of similar origin and function. For example, pericytes, stromal myofibroblasts, and mesenchymal stem cells may have similar functions regarding the stimulation of tumor growth.

ANTIANGIOGENESIS TREATMENTS IN PATIENTS WITH MELANOMA

Various experimental treatment approaches have been conducted that target critical steps in melanoma tumor angiogenesis. For example, a synthetic molecule that inhibits binding of VEGF to its receptor VEGFR2 was able to reduce B16F10 melanoma growth in mice.[70] As VEGF and VEGFR2 expression have been reported in melanoma cells, and therefore an autocrine VEGF-growth promoting effect has been proposed, melanoma cells were treated with the anti-VEGF antibody bevacizumab. Consistent with an autocrine effect of VEGF in melanoma cells, bevacizumab inhibited growth of VEGFR2-expressing melanoma cells.[71] Inhibition of melanoma cell survival was enhanced when combining bevacizumab with rapamycin in these experiments.

The anti-VEGF antibody bevacizumab has Food and Drug Administration approval for certain types of breast cancer, non–small cell lung cancer, and metastatic colorectal cancer. Multiple clinical trials, currently in phase I or II, are being conducted with bevacizumab, either alone or in combination with other medications, in patients with metastatic melanoma (**Table 1**). The experience of anti-VEGF treatments in melanoma mouse models suggests that antiangiogenesis treatments are likely to be more successful if combined with cytotoxic agents or other forms of antitumor treatment. Clinical reports have also shown that bevacizumab alone may be effective in reducing tumor angiogenesis and melanoma growth initially, but tumor recurrence has been observed despite continued administration of bevacizumab.[72] Thus, combination treatment approaches are currently being investigated in several clinical trials.

Some chemotherapeutic agents, commonly used in the treatment of patients with melanoma, have also been shown to have direct antiangiogenic effects. For example, the methylating agent temozolomide has been shown to inhibit endothelial cell proliferation and angiogenesis.[73] In contrast, dacarbazine, commonly used in chemotherapy for metastatic melanoma, was shown to increase the expression of the proangiogenic factors VEGF and IL-8 in melanoma cell lines.[74] Such findings further support the concept of combining antiangiogenic therapies with cytotoxic agents in the treatment of melanoma. For example, a clinical study, currently in phase II, treats melanoma patients with bevacizumab, dacarbazine, and IFN-α. However, a recent clinical pilot study did not provide evidence that IFN-α2b in combination with bevacizumab alone was of clinical benefit.[75]

Other clinical studies have combined bevacizumab with sorafenib tosylate, or added oxaliplatin to this combination as a triple therapy (**Table 1**). A phase II study

Table 1
Selected clinical trials involving antiangiogenesis agents in patients with metastatic melanoma

Trial ID	Trial Phase	Treatment
NCT00111007	Phase III	Sorafenib + paclitaxel + carboplatin versus placebo + paclitaxel + carboplatin
NCT00304200	Phase I/II	Temozolomide + sunitinib
NCT00349206	Phase I/II	Sorafenib + temsirolimus
NCT00538005	Phase I/II	Sorafenib + bevacizumab + oxiplatin
NCT00496223	Phase I/II	Sunitinib + dacarbazine
NCT00527657	Phase I/II	Temozolomide + lomustine + thalidomide
NCT00811759	Phase I/II	Sorafenib + temozolomide
NCT00026221	Phase II	Bevacizumab with or without low- or high-dose IFN-α
NCT00139360	Phase II	Bevacizumab monotherapy
NCT00281957	Phase II	Sorafenib + temsirolimus or tipifarnib
NCT00308607	Phase II	Bevacizumab + dacarbazine + IFN-α
NCT00387751	Phase II	Bevacizumab + sorafenib
NCT00397982	Phase II	Temsirolimus + bevacizumab
NCT00450255	Phase II	VEGF-trap
NCT00462423	Phase II	Bevacizumab + paclitaxel
NCT00483301	Phase II	Sorafenib + paclitaxel + carboplatin
NCT00568048	Phase II	Temozolomide + bevacizumab
NCT00602576	Phase II	Temozolomide + sorafenib
NCT00631618	Phase II	Sunitinib
NCT00130442	Phase II	Heparanase inhibitor (PI-88) + dacarbazine
NCT00304525	Phase I	CHIR-265 (Raf kinase and VEGFR2 inhibitor)
NCT00790010	Phase I	Bevacizumab + ipilimumab

Data from the National Cancer Institute. December, 2008.

treats patients with metastatic melanoma with bevacizumab and temsirolimus. Paclitaxel is also being combined with bevacizumab in patients with metastatic melanoma. A clinical trial, currently in phase I, treats patients who have stage III or IV melanoma with the combination treatment of bevacizumab and ipilimumab (MDX-010). Ipilimumab is an antibody that targets cytotoxic T lymphocyte antigen-4 (CTLA-4), thereby stimulating T cell responses, possibly through enhancing NY-ESO-1 antigen-specific immune responses in melanoma patients.[76]

However, it is critical to take potential adverse effects into account when proposing antiangiogenic treatment regimens, and particularly if combined with other anticancer medications. For example, in a recent study, the treatment of patients with melanoma brain metastases with the antiangiogenic thalidomide and temozolomide resulted in a high rate of severe thromboembolic events, with no objective responses to the treatment in these patients.[77] Similarly, bevacizumab treatment in combination with chemotherapy increased the risk of arterial thromboembolic events compared with chemotherapy alone.[78]

Multi-kinase inhibitors are being tested on melanoma patients in multiple clinical trials, either alone or in combination with other treatments. Sunitinib is one such multi-kinase inhibitor that inhibits VEGF receptors (VEGFR-1, -2, and -3), PDGF receptors (PDGFR-α and -β), KIT receptor tyrosine kinase, fms-related tyrosine kinase 3 (FLT3), and other targets. Therefore, sunitinib may, at least in part, lead to tumor inhibition through an antiangiogenic effect. A current clinical study combines sunitinib treatment with temozolomide. Another study uses sunitinib specifically in metastatic melanomas with KIT mutations.

Sorafenib, another multi-kinase inhibitor used in clinical melanoma studies, targets VEGF receptor signaling and Raf kinases.[79] It is currently used in a phase III trial with paclitaxel and carboplatin in patients with metastatic melanoma. Current phase II studies include combination treatments of sorafenib with temozolomide or dacarbazine.[80]

SUMMARY

A large number of clinical studies are currently being conducted to assess the effects of angiogenesis inhibitors in the treatment of patients with metastatic melanoma. It has become increasingly clear that a therapeutic approach that combines angiogenesis inhibitors with cytotoxic agents or other treatment modalities is more likely to result in a clinical benefit for patients rather than antiangiogenesis treatments alone. However, a targeted treatment approach with antiangiogenic agents needs to be based on an in-depth understanding of the complex mechanisms involved in melanoma tumor angiogenesis. For example, the antitumor effects of myeloid cell–derived VEGF raise the question whether broad anti-VEGF therapy is indeed a promising therapeutic approach. The increasing knowledge about the various cell types and factors involved in tumor angiogenesis is likely to result in the development of novel and much more specific angiogenesis inhibitors that may target specific subsets of cells or factors involved.

REFERENCES

1. O'Reilly MS, Boehm T, Shing Y, et al. Endostatin: an endogenous inhibitor of angiogenesis and tumor growth. Cell 1997;88:277–85.
2. O'Reilly MS, Holmgren L, Shing Y, et al. Angiostatin: a novel angiogenesis inhibitor that mediates the suppression of metastases by a Lewis lung carcinoma. Cell 1994;79:315–28.

3. Miao WM, Seng WL, Duquette M, et al. Thrombospondin-1 type 1 repeat recombinant proteins inhibit tumor growth through transforming growth factor-beta-dependent and -independent mechanisms. Cancer Res 2001;61:7830–9.
4. Streit M, Stephen AE, Hawighorst T, et al. Systemic inhibition of tumor growth and angiogenesis by thrombospondin-2 using cell-based antiangiogenic gene therapy. Cancer Res 2002;62:2004–12.
5. Marneros AG, Olsen BR. The role of collagen-derived proteolytic fragments in angiogenesis. Matrix Biol 2001;20:337–45.
6. Bergers G, Javaherian K, Lo KM, et al. Effects of angiogenesis inhibitors on multistage carcinogenesis in mice. Science 1999;284:808–12.
7. Hanahan D, Folkman J. Patterns and emerging mechanisms of the angiogenic switch during tumorigenesis. Cell 1996;86:353–64.
8. Streit M, Detmar M. Angiogenesis, lymphangiogenesis, and melanoma metastasis. Oncogene 2003;22:3172–9.
9. Skobe M, Hamberg LM, Hawighorst T, et al. Concurrent induction of lymphangiogenesis, angiogenesis, and macrophage recruitment by vascular endothelial growth factor-C in melanoma. Am J Pathol 2001;159:893–903.
10. Salven P, Lymboussaki A, Heikkila P, et al. Vascular endothelial growth factors VEGF-B and VEGF-C are expressed in human tumors. Am J Pathol 1998;153:103–8.
11. He Y, Rajantie I, Ilmonen M, et al. Preexisting lymphatic endothelium but not endothelial progenitor cells are essential for tumor lymphangiogenesis and lymphatic metastasis. Cancer Res 2004;64:3737–40.
12. Dadras SS, Paul T, Bertoncini J, et al. Tumor lymphangiogenesis: a novel prognostic indicator for cutaneous melanoma metastasis and survival. Am J Pathol 2003;162:1951–60.
13. Hirakawa S, Kodama S, Kunstfeld R, et al. VEGF-A induces tumor and sentinel lymph node lymphangiogenesis and promotes lymphatic metastasis. J Exp Med 2005;201:1089–99.
14. Hirakawa S, Brown LF, Kodama S, et al. VEGF-C-induced lymphangiogenesis in sentinel lymph nodes promotes tumor metastasis to distant sites. Blood 2007;109:1010–7.
15. Brychtova S, Bezdekova M, Brychta T, et al. The role of vascular endothelial growth factors and their receptors in malignant melanomas. Neoplasma 2008;55:273–9.
16. Lacal PM, Failla CM, Pagani E, et al. Human melanoma cells secrete and respond to placenta growth factor and vascular endothelial growth factor. J Invest Dermatol 2000;115:1000–7.
17. Lacal PM, Ruffini F, Pagani E, et al. An autocrine loop directed by the vascular endothelial growth factor promotes invasiveness of human melanoma cells. Int J Oncol 2005;27:1625–32.
18. Reed JA, McNutt NS, Albino AP. Differential expression of basic fibroblast growth factor (bFGF) in melanocytic lesions demonstrated by in situ hybridization. Implications for tumor progression. Am J Pathol 1994;144:329–36.
19. Giehl KA, Nagele U, Volkenandt M, et al. Protein expression of melanocyte growth factors (bFGF, SCF) and their receptors (FGFR-1, c-kit) in nevi and melanoma. J Cutan Pathol 2007;34:7–14.
20. Nurnberg W, Tobias D, Otto F, et al. Expression of interleukin-8 detected by in situ hybridization correlates with worse prognosis in primary cutaneous melanoma. J Pathol 1999;189:546–51.
21. Barnhill RL, Xiao M, Graves D, et al. Expression of platelet-derived growth factor (PDGF)-A, PDGF-B and the PDGF-alpha receptor, but not the PDGF-beta receptor, in human malignant melanoma in vivo. Br J Dermatol 1996;135:898–904.

22. Westermark B, Johnsson A, Paulsson Y, et al. Human melanoma cell lines of primary and metastatic origin express the genes encoding the chains of platelet-derived growth factor (PDGF) and produce a PDGF-like growth factor. Proc Natl Acad Sci U S A 1986;83:7197–200.

23. Nozawa H, Chiu C, Hanahan D. Infiltrating neutrophils mediate the initial angiogenic switch in a mouse model of multistage carcinogenesis. Proc Natl Acad Sci U S A 2006;103:12493–8.

24. Ardi VC, Kupriyanova TA, Deryugina EI, et al. Human neutrophils uniquely release TIMP-free MMP-9 to provide a potent catalytic stimulator of angiogenesis. Proc Natl Acad Sci U S A 2007;104:20262–7.

25. Conejo-Garcia JR, Benencia F, Courreges MC, et al. Tumor-infiltrating dendritic cell precursors recruited by a beta-defensin contribute to vasculogenesis under the influence of Vegf-A. Nat Med 2004;10:950–8.

26. Yang L, DeBusk LM, Fukuda K, et al. Expansion of myeloid immune suppressor Gr+CD11b+ cells in tumor-bearing host directly promotes tumor angiogenesis. Cancer Cell 2004;6:409–21.

27. Heissig B, Hattori K, Dias S, et al. Recruitment of stem and progenitor cells from the bone marrow niche requires MMP-9 mediated release of kit-ligand. Cell 2002; 109:625–37.

28. Shojaei F, Wu X, Malik AK, et al. Tumor refractoriness to anti-VEGF treatment is mediated by CD11b+Gr1+ myeloid cells. Nat Biotechnol 2007;25:911–20.

29. LeCouter J, Zlot C, Tejada M, et al. Bv8 and endocrine gland-derived vascular endothelial growth factor stimulate hematopoiesis and hematopoietic cell mobilization. Proc Natl Acad Sci U S A 2004;101:16813–8.

30. Jin DK, Shido K, Kopp HG, et al. Cytokine-mediated deployment of SDF-1 induces revascularization through recruitment of CXCR4+ hemangiocytes. Nat Med 2006;12:557–67.

31. Mohle R, Green D, Moore MA, et al. Constitutive production and thrombin-induced release of vascular endothelial growth factor by human megakaryocytes and platelets. Proc Natl Acad Sci U S A 1997;94:663–8.

32. Italiano JE Jr, Richardson JL, Patel-Hett S, et al. Angiogenesis is regulated by a novel mechanism: pro- and antiangiogenic proteins are organized into separate platelet alpha granules and differentially released. Blood 2008;111:1227–33.

33. Kopp HG, Hooper AT, Broekman MJ, et al. Thrombospondins deployed by thrombopoietic cells determine angiogenic switch and extent of revascularization. J Clin Invest 2006;116:3277–91.

34. Klement GL, Yip TT, Cassiola F, et al. Platelets actively sequester angiogenesis regulators. Blood 2008.

35. Du R, Lu KV, Petritsch C, et al. HIF1alpha induces the recruitment of bone marrow-derived vascular modulatory cells to regulate tumor angiogenesis and invasion. Cancer Cell 2008;13:206–20.

36. Sipkins DA, Wei X, Wu JW, et al. In vivo imaging of specialized bone marrow endothelial microdomains for tumour engraftment. Nature 2005;435:969–73.

37. Muller A, Homey B, Soto H, et al. Involvement of chemokine receptors in breast cancer metastasis. Nature 2001;410:50–6.

38. Murakami T, Cardones AR, Finkelstein SE, et al. Immune evasion by murine melanoma mediated through CC chemokine receptor-10. J Exp Med 2003; 198:1337–47.

39. Gunn MD, Tangemann K, Tam C, et al. A chemokine expressed in lymphoid high endothelial venules promotes the adhesion and chemotaxis of naive T lymphocytes. Proc Natl Acad Sci U S A 1998;95:258–63.

40. Saeki H, Moore AM, Brown MJ, et al. Cutting edge: secondary lymphoid-tissue chemokine (SLC) and CC chemokine receptor 7 (CCR7) participate in the emigration pathway of mature dendritic cells from the skin to regional lymph nodes. J Immunol 1999;162:2472–5.
41. Peters BA, Diaz LA, Polyak K, et al. Contribution of bone marrow-derived endothelial cells to human tumor vasculature. Nat Med 2005;11:261–2.
42. Purhonen S, Palm J, Rossi D, et al. Bone marrow-derived circulating endothelial precursors do not contribute to vascular endothelium and are not needed for tumor growth. Proc Natl Acad Sci U S A 2008;105:6620–5.
43. Gao D, Nolan DJ, Mellick AS, et al. Endothelial progenitor cells control the angiogenic switch in mouse lung metastasis. Science 2008;319:195–8.
44. Nolan DJ, Ciarrocchi A, Mellick AS, et al. Bone marrow-derived endothelial progenitor cells are a major determinant of nascent tumor neovascularization. Genes Dev 2007;21:1546–58.
45. Hirschi KK, Ingram DA, Yoder MC. Assessing identity, phenotype, and fate of endothelial progenitor cells. Arterioscler Thromb Vasc Biol 2008;28:1584–95.
46. Lyden D, Young AZ, Zagzag D, et al. Id1 and Id3 are required for neurogenesis, angiogenesis and vascularization of tumour xenografts. Nature 1999;401: 670–7.
47. Lyden D, Hattori K, Dias S, et al. Impaired recruitment of bone-marrow-derived endothelial and hematopoietic precursor cells blocks tumor angiogenesis and growth. Nat Med 2001;7:1194–201.
48. Hattori K, Dias S, Heissig B, et al. Vascular endothelial growth factor and angiopoietin-1 stimulate postnatal hematopoiesis by recruitment of vasculogenic and hematopoietic stem cells. J Exp Med 2001;193:1005–14.
49. Grunewald M, Avraham I, Dor Y, et al. VEGF-induced adult neovascularization: recruitment, retention, and role of accessory cells. Cell 2006;124:175–89.
50. Greenberg JI, Shields DJ, Barillas SG, et al. A role for VEGF as a negative regulator of pericyte function and vessel maturation. Nature 2008;456:809–13.
51. Stockmann C, Doedens A, Weidemann A, et al. Deletion of vascular endothelial growth factor in myeloid cells accelerates tumorigenesis. Nature 2008;456:814–8.
52. Xian X, Hakansson J, Stahlberg A, et al. Pericytes limit tumor cell metastasis. J Clin Invest 2006;116:642–51.
53. Song S, Ewald AJ, Stallcup W, et al. PDGFRbeta+ perivascular progenitor cells in tumours regulate pericyte differentiation and vascular survival. Nat Cell Biol 2005; 7:870–9.
54. Crisan M, Yap S, Casteilla L, et al. A perivascular origin for mesenchymal stem cells in multiple human organs. Cell Stem Cell 2008;3:301–13.
55. Karnoub AE, Dash AB, Vo AP, et al. Mesenchymal stem cells within tumour stroma promote breast cancer metastasis. Nature 2007;449:557–63.
56. Hillyer P, Male D. Expression of chemokines on the surface of different human endothelia. Immunol Cell Biol 2005;83:375–82.
57. Rajantie I, Ilmonen M, Alminaite A, et al. Adult bone marrow-derived cells recruited during angiogenesis comprise precursors for periendothelial vascular mural cells. Blood 2004;104:2084–6.
58. Bexell D, Gunnarsson S, Tormin A, et al. Bone marrow multipotent mesenchymal stroma cells act as pericyte-like migratory vehicles in experimental gliomas. Mol Ther 2009;17(1):183–90.
59. Studeny M, Marini FC, Champlin RE, et al. Bone marrow-derived mesenchymal stem cells as vehicles for interferon-beta delivery into tumors. Cancer Res 2002;62:3603–8.

60. Ren C, Kumar S, Chanda D, et al. Therapeutic potential of mesenchymal stem cells producing interferon-alpha in a mouse melanoma lung metastasis model. Stem Cells 2008;26:2332–8.
61. Elzaouk L, Moelling K, Pavlovic J. Anti-tumor activity of mesenchymal stem cells producing IL-12 in a mouse melanoma model. Exp Dermatol 2006;15: 865–74.
62. McAllister SS, Gifford AM, Greiner AL, et al. Systemic endocrine instigation of indolent tumor growth requires osteopontin. Cell 2008;133:994–1005.
63. Rangel J, Nosrati M, Torabian S, et al. Osteopontin as a molecular prognostic marker for melanoma. Cancer 2008;112:144–50.
64. Kaplan RN, Riba RD, Zacharoulis S, et al. VEGFR1-positive haematopoietic bone marrow progenitors initiate the pre-metastatic niche. Nature 2005;438:820–7.
65. Hiratsuka S, Watanabe A, Aburatani H, et al. Tumour-mediated upregulation of chemoattractants and recruitment of myeloid cells predetermines lung metastasis. Nat Cell Biol 2006;8:1369–75.
66. Hiratsuka S, Watanabe A, Sakurai Y, et al. The S100A8-serum amyloid A3-TLR4 paracrine cascade establishes a pre-metastatic phase. Nat Cell Biol 2008;10: 1349–55.
67. Peinado H, Rafii S, Lyden D. Inflammation joins the "niche". Cancer Cell 2008;14: 347–9.
68. Wels J, Kaplan RN, Rafii S, et al. Migratory neighbors and distant invaders: tumor-associated niche cells. Genes Dev 2008;22:559–74.
69. Orimo A, Gupta PB, Sgroi DC, et al. Stromal fibroblasts present in invasive human breast carcinomas promote tumor growth and angiogenesis through elevated SDF-1/CXCL12 secretion. Cell 2005;121:335–48.
70. Sun J, Blaskovich MA, Jain RK, et al. Blocking angiogenesis and tumorigenesis with GFA-116, a synthetic molecule that inhibits binding of vascular endothelial growth factor to its receptor. Cancer Res 2004;64:3586–92.
71. Molhoek KR, Griesemann H, Shu J, et al. Human melanoma cytolysis by combined inhibition of mammalian target of rapamycin and vascular endothelial growth factor/vascular endothelial growth factor receptor-2. Cancer Res 2008;68: 4392–7.
72. Jaissle GB, Ulmer A, Henke-Fahle S, et al. Suppression of melanoma-associated neoangiogenesis by bevacizumab. Arch Dermatol 2008;144:525–7.
73. Kurzen H, Schmitt S, Naher H, et al. Inhibition of angiogenesis by non-toxic doses of temozolomide. Anticancer Drugs 2003;14:515–22.
74. Lev DC, Ruiz M, Mills L, et al. Dacarbazine causes transcriptional up-regulation of interleukin 8 and vascular endothelial growth factor in melanoma cells: a possible escape mechanism from chemotherapy. Mol Cancer Ther 2003;2:753–63.
75. Varker KA, Biber JE, Kefauver C, et al. A randomized phase 2 trial of bevacizumab with or without daily low-dose interferon alfa-2b in metastatic malignant melanoma. Ann Surg Oncol 2007;14:2367–76.
76. Yuan J, Gnjatic S, Li H, et al. CTLA-4 blockade enhances polyfunctional NY-ESO-1 specific T cell responses in metastatic melanoma patients with clinical benefit. Proc Natl Acad Sci U S A 2008;105(51):20410–5.
77. Krown SE, Niedzwiecki D, Hwu WJ, et al. Phase II study of temozolomide and thalidomide in patients with metastatic melanoma in the brain: high rate of thromboembolic events (CALGB 500102). Cancer 2006;107:1883–90.
78. Scappaticci FA, Skillings JR, Holden SN, et al. Arterial thromboembolic events in patients with metastatic carcinoma treated with chemotherapy and bevacizumab. J Natl Cancer Inst 2007;99:1232–9.

79. Egberts F, Kahler KC, Livingstone E, et al. Metastatic melanoma: scientific ratio-
    nale for sorafenib treatment and clinical results. Onkologie 2008;31:398–403.
80. McDermott DF, Sosman JA, Gonzalez R, et al. Double-blind randomized phase II
    study of the combination of sorafenib and dacarbazine in patients with advanced
    melanoma: a report from the 11715 Study Group. J Clin Oncol 2008;26:2178–85.

Transcriptional Regulation in Melanoma

Devarati Mitra[a], David E. Fisher, MD, PhD[b],*

KEYWORDS

- Melanoma • Transcriptional regulation
- Microphthalmia-associated transcription factor
- Therapeutic opportunities in melanoma • Melanocyte survival

THE SIGNIFICANCE OF TRANSCRIPTIONAL REGULATION IN MELANOMA

With the 10 year survival of metastatic melanoma being only 14%, it is clear that we have much to learn about the mechanisms of disease.[1] As with many cancers, it is known that the fundamental defects of melanoma cells involve the dysregulation of melanocyte proliferation and death pathways. One common way the cell changes the activity of such pathways is by altering gene expression, which can perhaps best be understood by studying the similarities and differences of transcriptional regulation in normal melanocytes and transformed melanoma cells.

In general, normal human melanocytes have at least three important programs of transcriptional regulation: (1) differentiation from neural crest precursors; (2) pigment production; and (3) cell survival with potential for proliferation. In melanoma, these normal transcriptional programs become altered such that early developmental genes can become re-expressed or overexpressed, pigment production may be downregulated, and proliferation/survival signals become a dominant force. A key, recurring player in this discussion is microphthalmia-associated transcription factor (MITF), master regulator of melanocyte development, function, and survival.[2,3] In this review, each of these three transcriptional programs are examined and their significance is evaluated in the context of melanoma biology.

This work was supported by grants from NIH and the Melanoma Research Alliance. DEF is a Distinguished Clinical Scholar of the Doris Duke Medical Foundation.
[a] Biology and Biomedical Sciences Program, Cutaneous Biology Research Center, Massachusetts General Hospital, Harvard Medical School, Building 149, 13th Street, Charlestown, MA 02129, USA
[b] Department of Dermatology, Cutaneous Biology Research Center, Melanoma Program in Medical Oncology, Massachusetts General Hospital, Harvard Medical School, Building 149, 13th Street, Charlestown, MA 02129, USA
* Corresponding author.
E-mail address: dfisher3@partners.org (D.E. Fisher).

MELANOCYTE DEVELOPMENT

Melanocytes are pigment-producing cells derived from neural crest progenitors that undergo a complex process of fate specification, proliferation, migration, and differentiation before they arrive at one of several possible final destinations, including the epidermis, hair follicle, eye, cochlea, and meninges.[4] The highest density of melanocytes can be found in the epidermis and hair follicles where melanin, a pigmented polymer stored in melanosomes, is transferred to neighboring keratinocytes to protect the skin against damage from reactive oxygen species and UV radiation.[5] Multiple signaling pathways are critical for this process of melanocyte development and are also frequently dysregulated in melanoma (**Fig. 1**).

Notch is an early signaling receptor that functions to maintain the undifferentiated state of melanoblasts (melanocyte precursors in the neural crest). Studies in zebrafish have suggested that Notch binding to its ligand, Delta, is important to prevent differentiation of cells in the neural crest toward a neuronal cell fate.[6] In melanocytes, the intracellular domain of activated Notch is cleaved by γ-secretase and translocated to the nucleus where association with the transcription factor RBP-J generates a transactivation complex that acts to turn on target genes such as Hes-1, a transcriptional repressor that is important for promoting survival, blocking apoptosis, and preventing further differentiation of melanoblasts in the neural crest and melanocyte stem cells located at the hair follicle bulb.[7,8]

Recent studies have shown that Notch1 expression is elevated in many melanomas relative to normal melanocytes and benign nevi.[9,10] Additional studies supporting the

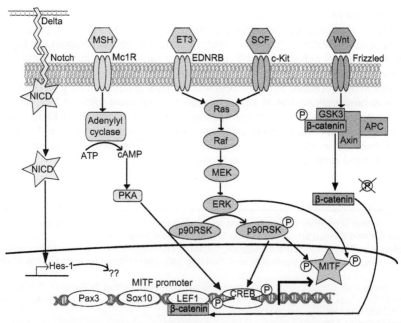

Fig. 1. Multiple melanocyte signaling pathways converge with transcription or activation of MITF, master regulator of melanocyte development, function, and survival. Several of these pathways particularly important in melanocyte development and potentially dysregulated in melanoma include Notch/Delta, Mc1R/MSH, endothelin receptor B/endothelin 3, c-Kit/SCF, and Frizzled/Wnt.

functional relevance of this observation have suggested the importance of Notch1 activation for β-catenin and mitogen-activated protein kinase (MAPK)-mediated melanoma progression.[11,12] Overall, however, studies on the role of Notch in melanoma are still at the early stages.

Wnt signaling is one of the more studied pathways important for determining melanocyte fate from neural crest precursors. The Wnt ligand binds cell surface receptors of the Frizzled family, ultimately blocking β-catenin degradation and allowing its translocation to the nucleus where it serves as a coactivator to T cell factor (TCF)/lymphocyte enhancing factor (LEF) and is recruited to activate transcription of target genes.[13] Wnt signaling is first evident in the neural crest of mice at embryonic day 7.5, at which point β-catenin increases differentiation of neural crest cells to the melanocyte lineage (at the expense of neurons and glia).[14] This process of Wnt-induced melanogenesis was subsequently found to be dependent on MITF as a downstream target.[15,16] MITF also interacts directly with LEF1 to turn on expression of certain MITF target genes, as well as expression of MITF itself.[17–19]

The Wnt pathway is likely to be important in melanoma although the exact mechanism is not yet completely understood. Initially, after a large panel of melanoma cell lines were examined, it was believed that Wnt pathway mutations were common in melanoma, but later it was found that few primary melanomas had β-catenin mutations.[20,21] However, given that one third of primary melanomas have aberrant nuclear localization of β-catenin, the pathway is still likely to be improperly regulated in disease.[21] In vitro, at least, β-catenin is known to induce melanoma growth in a manner that is dependent on downstream target MITF.[22]

Binding of stem cell factor (SCF) to its receptor c-Kit is another early developmental signal for melanocytes. c-Kit is first expressed in the neural crest of mice at E9.5–10.5 and is involved in promoting survival, proliferation, and migration of committed melanocyte progenitors.[23] Further supporting the importance of c-Kit signaling in vivo is the fact that inactivating mutations of c-Kit produce piebaldism, a rare autosomal dominant disorder of melanocyte development, characterized by a congenital white forelock and multiple symmetric hypopigmented patches of hair and skin.[24] The c-Kit signaling pathway has been shown to trigger MAPK-mediated phosphorylation of MITF, which recruits the p300 coactivator to MITF, and ubiquitination and degradation of MITF.[25–27] Recently, an important role for c-Kit in melanoma has been identified, specifically for melanomas arising on acral (palms/soles), mucosal, or chronically sun-damaged cutaneous surfaces.[28] Initial clinical results suggest that Kit-mutated melanomas are susceptible to Kit-targeted kinase inhibitors in patients.[29,30] This clinical finding represents a key advance in melanoma therapeutics, not only because of the opportunity to improve outcomes in a specific patient subgroup, but also in demonstrating the broader concept that rational targeted therapeutics may indeed trigger dramatic clinical responses—even in melanoma.

Sox10 and Pax3 are additional developmental transcription factors that can work together to produce melanogenesis. Both act as transcriptional activators of MITF, which subsequently turns on pigment production.[31,32] Sox10-mediated regulation of MITF requires cooperativity with cAMP regulatory element-binding protein (CREB), suggesting a mechanism of tissue restricted control of MITF expression.[33] Pax3 is expressed in committed but incompletely differentiated melanoblasts and acts to initiate melanogenesis while preventing terminal differentiation. One particularly elegant mechanism by which this is made possible is the simultaneous transcriptional activation of MITF expression and competition with MITF for dopachrome tautomerase (DCT) enhancer occupancy.[32] The potential importance of these transcriptional activators in melanoma is suggested by the fact that Pax3 was found to be improperly expressed in 77% of 35 primary melanomas.[34]

Another signaling pathway known to be important to melanocyte development is endothelin-3 binding to endothelin receptor B, increasing intracellular cAMP levels and activating the MAPK pathway. This ligand-receptor interaction is essential for the development of normal epidermal melanocytes as shown by the fact that mice carrying mutations in either endothelin-3 or its receptor show gross pigment defects resulting from a significant reduction in the number of melanocyte progenitors in the neural crest.[35–37] It has also been suggested that this pathway is important to melanoma development because endothelin receptor B is overexpressed in cutaneous melanoma.[38] More recently, Van Raamsdonk and colleagues identified activating mutations in the G protein adapter, GNAQ, in ~50% of ocular melanomas and blue nevi.[39] GNAQ is believed to participate in endothelin signaling, suggesting that these melanomas may exhibit constitutive endothelin-like signaling as a key oncogenic event.

MITF is a common player in many of these early developmental pathways.[40] Melanoblast precursors evident at E9.5–10.5 are characterized by their state of expressing MITF and c-Kit while being DCT negative. Without MITF, precursor melanoblasts can be identified but will die before further differentiation.[41]

MICROPHTHALMIA-ASSOCIATED TRANSCRIPTION FACTOR
Early Gene Characterization

The first mouse with a pigment defect attributed to loss of melanocytes rather than defective pigmentation in viable melanocytes was identified in 1942. This mouse had been treated with x-ray irradiation and was found to have small eyes in homozygotes (giving it the name *microphthalmia*) as well as white spotted coat color in heterozygotes.[42] On further examination, in homozygous mutant form, these mice were found to have developmental defects in osteoclasts and mast cells with decreased numbers of a variety of immune cells, including natural killer cells, basophils, macrophages, and B cells.[43]

The gene responsible for the *mi* mouse phenotype was found to be a relative of *myc* in the basic helix-loop-helix leucine zipper (HLH-LZ) family, in which the basic domain is responsible for DNA binding and the HLH-LZ domain is important for homodimerization or heterodimerization with related proteins, TFE3 or TFEB.[44,45] Shortly after the *mi* gene was identified, its function was characterized as being a transcription factor responsible for melanocyte development by binding E-box elements in promoter sequences of target genes.[45] In the following years, 24 spontaneous and induced mouse mutations in the newly characterized MITF gene were identified, each producing one of a variety of defects, from problems with DNA binding to an inability to fully dimerize to dysregulated expression, all of which produce phenotypic pigmentation abnormalities.[46]

The significance of MITF for human pigmentation was confirmed by the realization that MITF mutations were a cause of Waardenburg syndrome (WS), an autosomal dominant disorder that affects 1:40,000 people and manifests itself with sensorineural deafness and pigmentation defects caused by the absence of melanocytes from the skin, hair, eyes, and stria vascularis of the cochlea.[47] There are four broad categories of WS, defined clinically by the presence or absence of associated symptoms (**Table 1**). Each subtype has a defect in a key pathway for melanocyte development. WS1 (associated with dystopia canthorum) and WS3 (associated with limb abnormalities) were found to be the result of Pax3 mutations, whereas WS4 (associated with

Table 1
Human auditory-pigmentation defects resulting from melanocyte loss

Type	Inheritance	Geno Type	Pheno Type	Comments
WS1	AD (homozygotes more severe)	PAX3 mutation	Dystopia canthorum, congenital sensorineural hearing loss, abnormal iris pigmentation, white forelock (may have patchy hypopigmented skin and premature hair	Dystopia canthorum is characterized by fusion of inner eyelids, displaced inferior lachrymal ducts, longer than normal interpupillary distance
WS2	AD (homozygotes more severe)	WS2a=MITF, other WS2=Slug	No dystopia canthorum but otherwise the same features as WS1	Catch-all type including auditory-pigmentation syndromes not belonging elsewhere
WS3: Klein-Waardenburg syndrome	AD mostly sporadic	PAX3 mutation	Same as WS1 + hypoplasia of limb muscles and elbow/finger contractures	More severe variant of WS1 (also affects nonmelanocyte neural crest lineages)
WS4: Shah-Waardenburg syndrome	Mostly AR	Heterogeneous (eg, Sox10, ET1 and EDNRB mutations)	Same as WS1 + Hirschsprung's disease (megacolon)	Enteric ganglia abnormalities from other affected neural crest lineages
Tietz-Smith syndrome	AR (in the case of MITF mutation)	Possibly heterogenous but includes MITF mutation	Sensorineural hearing loss + uniform dilution of pigmentation	More severe variant of WS2 (unlike others, nonpatchy hypopigmentation)

Waardenburg syndrome is a genetic disease characterized by the loss of melanocytes leading to abnormalities of pigmentation and hearing, among other variable phenotypic characteristics. There are five major classes of WS, each of which results from various lesions in genes important for normal melanocyte development, and potentially important in the initiation or progression of melanoma.
Abbreviations: AD, autosomal dominant; AR, autosomal recessive.

megacolon) was found to be the result of endothelin ligand or receptor mutations.[48–50] WS2, characterized by a white forelock and auditory defects, has a subtype called WS2a that is associated with MITF mutation.[51,52] A variant of this disease, Tietz syndrome, which manifests with more severe deafness and pigmentation abnormalities, was subsequently found to be the result of a dominant negative allele of MITF.[53] In addition, deletion of SLUG has also been suggested as an alternative cause of WS2[54] The various genetic causes of Waardenburg syndrome represent a remarkable example of epistasis in a human condition, with multiple upstream regulators of MITF (such as Sox10 and Pax3) producing overlapping phenotypic abnormalities, relative to mutations within the coding region of MITF itself.[55]

The MITF gene in humans consists of a 200-kb region at chromosome 3p12.3–14.1 and is conserved across all vertebrate species with similar genes described in *Caenorhabditis elegans*, *Drosophila melanogaster*, *Xenopus laevis*, and other invertebrate species. The gene has at least 9 known promoters and multiple, different first exons with 7 conserved downstream exons across all isoforms.[56] Many isoforms are broadly expressed; the most 3' promoter and first exon are unique to isoform M-MITF, which is believed to be selectively expressed in melanocytes.[2,3,57,58] The gene also has an internal splice variant that produces transcripts with or without 18 additional nucleotides in exon 6a. The splice form containing the resulting extra 6 amino acids has a slightly higher E-box binding affinity than its shorter variant.[45]

Overall, MITF is a unique, important transcription factor involved in all aspects of melanocyte survival and function. Overexpression of the protein was reported to single-handedly change terminally differentiated fibroblasts to cells with significant melanocytic characteristics.[59] The effect of MITF on melanocytes varies depending on a variety of factors, including the degree of expression. Without MITF, melanocytes will die early in development (as shown by WS2 and numerous animal models). There is considerable evidence that varied levels of MITF expression may favor melanocytic quiescence versus differentiation versus proliferation versus senescence, although details of these relationships remain to be worked out.

Microphthalmia-Associated Transcription Factor Target Genes

To better understand the ability of MITF to act as a fine-tuned modulator of melanocyte survival and phenotype, it is helpful to examine the transcription factor's target genes. As noted previously, MITF binds the E-box recognition sequence in gene promoters.[45] Among the various E-box sequence elements (which fit the consensus CANNTG), a sequence termed the *M-box* has been identified at multiple MITF-regulated promoters and is characterized by a flanking thymidine or adenosine (TCATGTG, CATGTGA or TCATGTGA).[60] The general classes of MITF target genes include melanocyte-specific lineage and pigmentation factors, as well as survival and proliferation factors (**Fig. 2**).

MITF is critical for melanocyte function as the key factor that turns on expression of a large program of genes responsible for the synthesis of the components of the pigment production pathway. The best understood pathway of this type involves the tanning response. Specifically, UV radiation produces p53-dependent proopiomelanocorticotrophin (POMC) expression in neighboring keratinocytes of the epidermis.[61] POMC is subsequently cleaved to produce α-melanocyte-stimulating hormone (α-MSH) which is released to bind Mc1R on the surface of melanocytes. Mc1R signaling activates adenylate cyclase, increasing intracellular cAMP levels, and activating CREB, which is then able to turn on MITF expression and ultimately increase skin pigmentation.[26] The specific components of this pigmentation program directly activated downstream of MITF include tyrosinase (the rate-limiting enzyme in

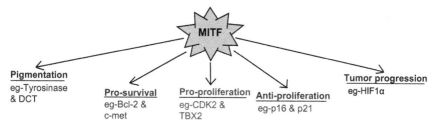

Fig. 2. Transcriptional targets of MITF activate a variety of normal and malignant melanocyte functions, including pigmentation, survival, proliferation, cell cycle arrest, and melanoma progression.

melanin synthesis), other pigment pathway enzymes such as tyrosinase-related protein 1 (TYRP1) and TYRP2 (better known as dopachrome tautomerase or DCT), RAB27 (involved in actin-mediated melanosome distribution to melanocyte dendritic tips), and Mc1R itself.[2,57,62,63]

MITF target genes important in melanocyte proliferation and survival include those that promote survival and block apoptosis, stimulate proliferation, and inhibit cell cycle progression. These 2 latter functions, in particular, can be in direct antagonism to each other, but it is likely that there are as yet unknown mechanisms by which the relative level of MITF expression can promote either a pro-proliferative or pro-differentiation program.

Bcl2 is an MITF target responsible for maintaining melanocyte survival. The relationship between Bcl2 and MITF was first suggested after it was found that, although Bcl2 and MITF homozygous mutant mice have coat pigmentation abnormalities resulting from melanocyte death, both heterozygote mice have essentially normal pigmentation.[46,64,65] However, when compound heterozygotes of MITF and Bcl2 were generated, these mice exhibited significant premature depigmentation.[65] It was subsequently shown that MITF directly binds the Bcl2 promoter and regulates endogenous Bcl2 levels in melanocytes. Epistasis experiments also showed that Bcl2 is downstream of MITF, as its overexpression can partially rescue dominant negative MITF-induced apoptosis in melanoma cell lines.[66]

MITF also activates other pro-survival pathways, including upregulating the transcription of c-met, a growth factor receptor; when its ligand, hepatocyte growth factor (HGF), is overexpressed, it is able to protect melanocytes and melanoma cells from apoptosis.[67,68] c-met signaling also feeds back to MITF by activating phosphorylation of MITF, which subsequently stimulates its proteosome-mediated degradation.[67]

In addition to these pro-survival pathways, MITF promotes expression of genes that actively stimulate proliferation. Specifically, CDK2 has been found to be an MITF target gene that is able to play a role in stimulating melanocyte proliferation. Although CDK2 is a ubiquitously expressed cell cycle kinase, the melanocyte-specific regulation of CDK2 expression by MITF came to light because of the genomic location of the *CDK2* gene. The promoter region of *CDK2* physically overlaps genomically with the *silver* gene, which encodes a melanosomal pigmentation factor.[69] A consensus MITF binding element was identified within intron 1 of *CDK2* (in the 5' upstream region of *silver*), to which MITF binds in melanocytes and melanoma cells. This element seems to be essential for *CDK2* gene expression in melanocytes, but not other cell lineages (which lack MITF).[69] Presumably due in some fashion to this lineage-specific expression of CDK2, MITF binding intron 1 of *CDK2* was found to be essential to survival of melanoma cells (although apparently less essential in other cell types).

Without CDK2, cells undergo G1 arrest but MITF is able to bind the *CDK2* promoter and increase expression of this cyclin-dependent kinase, allowing cell cycle progression. Experiments supporting a functional relationship between MITF and CDK2 showed that CDK2 overexpression could rescue colony formation of melanoma cell lines after MITF depletion.[69]

TBX2 is another MITF target gene with pro-proliferative properties.[70] This transcription factor was found to be overexpressed in at least 6 melanoma cell lines and was found to associate with HDAC1. These investigators also proposed a hypothesis by which TBX2's interaction with HDAC1 maintains low p21 levels, preventing cell cycle arrest.[71]

In contrast to these pro-survival/proliferation target genes, there is also evidence to support the role of MITF in the induction of cell cycle arrest by way of activation of cyclin-dependent kinase inhibitors such as $p16^{INK4a}$ and $p21^{Cip}$. The induction of cell cycle arrest by a factor that (in other contexts) is associated with cell cycle progression may seem paradoxic. However, it is increasingly clear that MITF can function as an oncogene in certain cellular contexts, but as a differentiation factor in others. Presumably, cell cycle arrest occurs in the setting of cellular differentiation. Moreover, the fidelity of CDK-inhibitors (such as p16 or p21) may even help to determine whether MITF can induce cell cycle arrest versus proliferation. In 3T3 fibroblasts, ectopic MITF was found to bind the p21 promoter and cooperate with the tumor suppressor Rb1 to potentiate expression of this cell cycle inhibitor.[72] $p16^{INK4a}$ is known to be a tumor suppressor gene frequently mutated in melanoma.[73–75] Expression of $p16^{INK4a}$ triggers hypophosphorylation of Rb, thereby causing cell cycle arrest. In addition to inducing G1 arrest, the activation of this tumor suppressor was found to be necessary for efficient melanocyte differentiation.[73] This observation suggests that $p16^{INK4a}$ could be a functionally significant downstream effector of MITF, which could help to determine if a melanocyte will continue to proliferate or differentiate to a more senescent phenotype.

In contrast to MITF's ability to promote cell cycle arrest by increasing p21 or p16 expression, there is also some evidence to suggest that MITF decreases activity of p27, a third cdk inhibitor. The proposed mechanism involves MITF increasing Dia1 levels (a Rho effector with a role in actin polymerization), which also increases intracellular Skp2, a regulator of cdk inhibitor p27.[76] As p27 and MITF levels are inversely correlated, a hypothesis has emerged that, under certain unknown conditions, MITF may be preventing cell cycle arrest.

Other MITF target genes also likely contribute to the importance of this transcription factor in melanoma progression beyond initial oncogenesis. For example, MITF also activates the transcription of HIF1α, which stimulates increased production of VEGF, which has known angiogenic properties.[77]

Melastatin (also known as TRPM1) is another MITF target gene the expression of which has been tightly correlated with MITF expression.[78] The precise function of TRPM1 is unknown, although it is believed to be structurally related to the TRP family of Ca channel proteins. The expression of melastatin was originally thought to be lost during progression of melanoma, and this loss of expression in cutaneous melanoma may serve as a marker of aggressive (poorer) prognosis.[79] The melastatin/TRPM1 promoter contains multiple MITF binding sites and seems to be robustly regulated by MITF transcriptional activity.

Regulation of Microphthalmia-Associated Transcription Factor Activity

Given MITF's complex and varied activity, it is understandable that the transcription factor is regulated at many levels from expression to posttranslational modification to cofactor binding. The best understood regulation of expression occurs downstream of UV-induced α-MSH signaling, as discussed previously, but there are many other mechanisms of transcriptional regulation.[26] The M-promoter of MITF in melanocytes carries CREB, LEF1, Sox10, and Pax3 binding sites, all of which activate transcription of this key transcription factor. CREB binding is a known downstream effect of α-MSH, whereas LEF1, Sox10, and Pax3 are all known developmental signals that act to increase MITF expression during melanocyte fate specification and migration.

More recently, oncogenic Braf[V600E] was found to be a transcriptional regulator of MITF in the context of melanoma.[80] The mechanism of this effect was proposed to involve Braf[V600E] inducing the expression of BRN2, a transcription factor normally not expressed in melanocytes but known to be present in neuronal precursors.[81] In three Braf[V600E] melanoma cell lines, MITF expression was found to be dependent on BRN2, which was found by chromatin immunoprecipitation to bind the MITF promoter. Because BRN2 is not expressed in normal melanocytes, the investigators proposed that Braf does not normally regulate MITF expression, but in the context of constitutively active Braf, BRN2 becomes expressed and able to increase MITF levels.[80] Given that activated Braf is also known to produce hyperactivated ERK, which activates MITF but induces induces proteosome-mediated MITF degradation, this BRN2-mediated mechanism could play a role in maintaining sufficient MITF levels to prevent cell cycle arrest or apoptosis.

Recent evidence suggests that MITF is subject to microRNA-mediated regulation. Specifically, miR137 is able to target the 3′ untranslated region of MITF and downregulate its mRNA levels.[82]

There is also preliminary data to suggest that PPARγ and Onecut-2 may play a role in regulating MITF expression levels. Specifically, it was observed that PPARγ activation produces a transient increase in MITF followed by growth arrest and increased pigment gene expression with spindle morphology.[83] However, the mechanism or significance of this activity remains to be determined. Onecut-2, a homeodomain transcription factor known to be expressed in melanocytes also seems able to stimulate MITF expression but in vivo data on its role in melanocyte development, function, or oncogenesis remains unclear.[84]

MITF is also regulated by various post-translational modifications including phosphorylation, sumoylation, and cleavage (**Fig. 3**). The best understood mechanism of phosphorylation occurs downstream of MAPK activation (eg, after SCF binds its cell

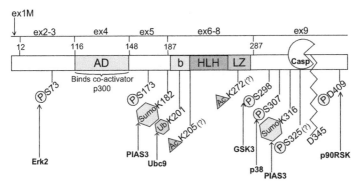

Fig. 3. MITF is subject to many post-translational modifications that regulate its activity. Such modifications include phosphorylation, acetylation, sumoylation, ubiquitination, and caspase-mediated cleavage.

surface receptor c-Kit) whereby MEK1 dual phosphorylates ERK, which is then able to phosphorylate MITF at Ser73.[25] Once phosphorylated at this site, MITF recruits coactivator p300 which upregulates MITF's ability to activate transcription of its target genes, such as tyrosinase.[26] Phosphorylation at Ser73 also results in a built-in subsequent downregulation of MITF activity by stimulating proteosome-mediated MITF degradation. p90-RSK is also able to phosphorylate MITF at Ser409 downstream of c-Kit signaling, resulting in improved proteosome-mediated degradation of MITF.[27]

MITF can be phosphorylated at Ser298 by GSK3β, which enhances MITF binding its target genes. The functional significance of this modification has been confirmed by the fact that this residue has been found to be mutated in a subset of patients with WS2.[85]

Sumoylation is another post-translational modification that regulates MITF activity. PIAS3 is a ubiquitin E3-ligase that was first identified from a yeast 2-hybrid screen as being a repressor of MITF.[86] Subsequently, PIAS3's E3 ligase function was identified as being able to sumoylate MITF at Lys182 or Lys316 thereby repressing MITF-mediated transcription of target genes with more than 1 MITF binding site. However, because sumoylation was found to have no effect on MITF dimerization, DNA binding, stability, or localization, the mechanism by which this repression occurs remains unknown.[87]

There is also evidence that in response to cell surface death signals, such as TRAIL, MITF cleavage at Asp345 by caspases 3, 6, and 7 produces a C-terminal fragment that is pro-apoptotic to melanoma cells.[88] However, the role of this cleavage independent of external death signals is not yet known.

Multiple cofactors play a role in regulating MITF activity. CBP/p300 has been found to bind 18 amino acids upstream of MITF's DNA binding domain and the investigators who recognized that observation have hypothesized that CBP binding may play a role in the dynamic regulation of MITF by differential CBP phosphorylation during the cell cycle.[89]

As noted in the previous discussion of MITF's ability to regulate p21^{Cip}, Rb1 is also a potential MITF cofactor that may help to activate p21^{Cip} expression to regulate cell cycle progression.[72] LEF1 is another MITF cofactor noted previously to be a downstream effector of Wnt signaling in melanocyte development.[17,18]

SWI/SNF chromatin remodeling enzymes also act as important partners for MITF activity but without the need to interact directly with the transcription factor. Chromatin remodeling by SWI/SNF seems to be necessary for expression of some MITF target genes, such as tyrosinase and TYRP1. However, not all MITF target genes seem to need SWI/SNF as shown by the fact that dominant negative components of the SWI/SNF complex have no effect on expression of certain MITF target genes.[90] This implies that MITF may use distinct chromatin-related mechanisms to control expression of separate classes of target genes.

Microphthalmia-Associated Transcription Factor in Melanoma

As shown by MITF's potentially contradictory actions on survival, proliferation, and cell cycle arrest, MITF's role in melanoma is likely complex and varies depending on a variety of conditions, such as relative MITF expression level. MITF itself is a likely lineage survival oncogene amplified in 10% to 15% of melanomas that produce elevated and dysregulated expression. These melanomas are believed to be more aggressive and amplification is associated with poorer prognosis. In addition, overexpression of MITF in conjunction with expression of the most common activating Braf mutation found in melanoma (V600E), can transform human melanocytes (engineered to overexpress hTERT and inactivate the Rb and p53 pathways) to produce growth factor–independent growth and anchorage-independent colony growth in soft agar.[91] In another study, elevated MITF levels were found to counteract Braf^{V600E}'s ability to stimulate melanocyte proliferation. Without additional MITF, this study found that Braf^{V600E} overactivated the MAPK pathway, producing hyperphosphorylated ERK, which is able to phosphorylate MITF for its activation and subsequent proteosome-mediated degradation. Coinciding with these biochemical observations, melanocytes expressing Braf^{V600E} alone were observed to have decreased dendricity and pigmentation, and highly expressing MITF in these same cells returned the normal differentiated melanocyte phenotype.[92]

DIAGNOSIS AND PROGNOSIS

MITF is a well-established melanocyte lineage marker that can be used for melanoma diagnosis. A study from 1999 showed that in 76 consecutive primary human melanoma surgical specimens, 100% were positive for MITF with a nuclear staining pattern. The unique value of MITF as a melanoma marker was confirmed by the fact that staining identified 8/8 amelanotic melanomas as well as melanomas that were negative for other commonly used markers such as HMB-45 or S-100.[93]

Typically, MITF staining in melanocytic lesions has not distinguished between benign and malignant lesions. Because MITF expression tends to be variable across melanomas, it is difficult to draw universal conclusions about the potential for malignancy in a particular melanocytic lesion based on MITF.[2] Analyses of particular subsets of melanoma patients have begun to examine if MITF staining can at least under some circumstances provide any prognostic information. One study used a multivariate analysis to look at MITF expression in intermediate-thickness cutaneous malignant melanoma and found an inverse correlation between degree of MITF expression and overall survival.[94]

Studies on the expression of melastatin (a target gene of MITF, described earlier) have shown significant promise as a prognostic marker. Downregulation of melastatin correlates with increased tumor thickness, increased potential for metastasis, and overall poorer outcomes.[79,95] A prospective study to evaluate melastatin in melanoma patients is currently underway.

MITF gene amplification has also been found to be a prognostic marker for patient survival. One study found that 23% of 104 melanoma patients had more than four copies of MITF, whereas 60% had more than 3 copies. Such amplifications were associated with reduced disease-specific survival time.[96]

Although MITF plays a central role in melanocyte and melanoma biology, it is clear that control of melanoma prognosis is a complex and multivariate process. One study approached this problem by examining microarray expression data for 86 melanomas and defined cohort profiles with differing metastatic potential. These investigators defined a "proliferative" cohort of melanomas with high MITF expression in addition to expression of traditional melanocytic pigmentation genes and neural crest-related factors. This cohort tended to manifest low invasive potential and growth was inhibited by TGF-β treatment. In contrast to this group of melanomas, these investigators also defined an *invasive* cohort with low MITF and pigmentation gene expression that had a lower proliferative rate but increased motility and resistance to TGF-β-mediated growth inhibition.[97] Analyses such as these may help to discriminate distinct classes of melanomas, and may also help to identify different stages of melanoma progression.

FUTURE THERAPEUTIC OPPORTUNITIES

Continuing to improve our understanding of transcriptional regulation in melanoma is likely to provide new opportunities for therapeutic intervention against a disease for which there are insufficient treatment options. Small-molecule chemists are beginning to challenge the current consensus that transcription factors are themselves not ideal drug targets. Understanding the upstream regulatory pathways of transcriptional activators and repressors as well as crucial transcriptional target genes may help to provide options for more traditional drug targets.

An example of a therapeutic approach that targets MITF expression is the recent description of histone deacetylase inhibitors (HDACi), which were found to potently silence expression of the melanocyte-specific MITF promoter.[98] The mechanism of this transcriptional repression seemed to involve downregulation of SOX10, an essential transcriptional regulator of MITF. Although HDACi drugs have numerous effects, there was evidence to support at least a portion of the lethal effect being caused by MITF, because expression of MITF from an exogenous promoter was able to partially rescue HDACi toxicity. Systemic HDACi treatment was also growth suppressive against a human melanoma when tested in a mouse xenograft model.[98] Hopefully, additional targeted therapies will emerge that suppress MITF expression, and might be combined with other agents in a fashion that produces non–cross-reactive toxicity to normal cells/tissues, while focusing toxicity on MITF and melanoma cells.

One area of potential melanoma therapy could involve targeting the pathways important in normal melanocyte development that are commonly dysregulated in oncogenesis. Wnt inhibitors are one class of small molecule that is currently receiving much attention in the field of gastrointestinal cancers.[99] Although general enthusiasm for the Wnt pathway in melanoma has declined since it was realized that only a few primary melanomas have β-catenin mutations, it is nonetheless true that one third of primary melanomas exhibit aberrant nuclear localization of β-catenin, suggesting that this pathway is still activated in melanoma and may be a useful drug target.

Similarly, although it has not yet been established conclusively that overactive Notch signaling plays an important role in the maintenance or progression of melanomas, if this pathway is functionally validated, there are already γ-secretase inhibitors capable of downregulating Notch signaling that could subsequently be tested in melanoma patients.[100]

Another class of potentially effective drug targets in melanoma could include those upstream of MITF activation. Specifically, given that >60% of primary melanomas have an activating mutation in Braf, there is much current excitement about targeted Braf inhibitors in early clinical trials.[101] Although kinase inhibitors such as these are not directly suppressing MITF, it is likely that synergistic opportunities may exist to combine BRAF/MAPK targeted approaches with MITF-pathway inhibition—perhaps with the latter providing lineage specificity and thus enhancing the therapeutic index.

Similarly, recent evidence has shown that suppression of mutated/activated c-Kit in mucosal/acral melanomas (with major clinical efficacy) is likely to operate through an intersection with MITF-controlled pathways in the cell. It will be important to better understand the mechanism of cancer cell death in such imatinib-treated Kit-mutant melanomas, because this may reveal opportunities for enhancing treatment efficacy, for example, using additional drug combinations. In addition, it will be important to determine the efficacy of different Kit-targeted small-molecule kinase inhibitors.

MITF target genes important for maintaining melanocyte survival or proliferation could also be melanoma drug targets. c-met is one such well-characterized growth factor receptor for which several small-molecule inhibitors are already available.[102] Although such inhibitors have not yet been used in melanoma, clinical trials of met inhibition are currently being conducted on clear cell sarcoma, a soft tissue sarcoma with melanocytic differentiation that results from dysregulated expression of MITF.[103] The MIT family of human tumors is characterized by dysregulation of MITF, TFE3, or TFEB and includes melanoma, clear cell sarcoma, translocation-associated (papillary) renal cell carcinomas, and alveolar soft part sarcoma.[104] C-met seems to be strongly over-expressed and constitutively activated (without mutation) in some of these tumors, presumably as a consequence of residing directly downstream of the dysregulated MITF-related transcription factor. Suppression of c-MET using siRNA or small-molecule inhibitors seems to be highly toxic and thus represents an attractive therapeutic strategy.[105]

Bcl2 is another MITF target gene that plays a central role in melanocyte survival, and is thus an attractive melanoma drug target. Although earlier attempts using antisense technology did not obtain FDA approval for treatment of metastatic melanoma, additional clinical studies are currently underway. In addition a small-molecule BH3 analog that antagonizes Bcl2 seems to be effective at increasing apoptosis, particularly in the context of cytostatic MEK inhibition.[106] This compound is under early clinical investigation for other malignancies, but will hopefully be examined for melanoma as well.

It is likely that strategies to target individual components of the machinery that controls MITF expression, or individual targets of MITF, may exhibit limited clinical activity, because of the alternative survival pathways that may arise, particularly if the direct drug target is not the mutated oncogene itself. In such cases, it is most likely that clinical success will require combinatorial drug approaches. Although conceptually simple, combinatorial approaches carry the hazard of combinatorial toxicity to normal tissues. Therefore, it will remain crucial to understand melanoma-specific survival/proliferation pathways to harness drug/target combinations that exhibit appropriate tumor selectivity.

SUMMARY

Transcriptional regulation in melanoma is a complex process that tends to hijack the normal melanocyte signaling pathways involved in melanocyte development, pigmentation, and survival. At the center of these often overlapping networks of transcriptional activation and repression is MITF, a melanocyte lineage marker that increases pigment production and exhibits diverse effects on cell survival, proliferation, and cell cycle arrest. The particular conditions that allow MITF to produce these potentially contradictory roles have not yet been fully elucidated, but analysis of the pathways involved provides opportunities to learn about new therapeutic strategies. Optimism is clearly warranted because recent evidence has shown that appropriate targeting of mutant c-Kit is therapeutically effective in melanoma patients. Thus, even melanoma is capable of efficient, predictable, clinically meaningful drug responses. However, major challenges remain to optimize the c-Kit effects into durable responses, and to broaden the therapeutic efficacy to other tumors that are driven by other oncogenic factors, many of which may not be as readily responsive to drugs. Through appropriate targeting of vital, tumor-selective regulators of melanoma survival, strategies may be devised that help turn the tide against this deadly disease.

REFERENCES

1. American Cancer Society. Cancer facts and figures, 2008. Washington, DC: American Cancer Society; 2008.
2. Levy C, Khaled M, Fisher DE. MITF: master regulator of melanocyte development and melanoma oncogene. Trends Mol Med 2006;12(9):406–14.
3. Steingrimsson E, Copeland NG, Jenkins NA. Melanocytes and the microphthalmia transcription factor network. Annu Rev Genet 2004;38:365–411.
4. The neural crest. In: Le Douarin NM, KC, editors. Developmental and cell biology series. 2nd edition. Cambridge, UK: Cambridge University Press; 1999.

5. Park Hee-Young PM, Lee Jin, Yaar Mina. Biology of melanocytes. In: Wolff K, GL, Katz SI, et al, editors. Fitzpatrick's dermatology in general medicine. 7th edition. New York: McGraw-Hill; 2008.

6. Cornell RA, Eisen JS. Delta/Notch signaling promotes formation of zebrafish neural crest by repressing Neurogenin 1 function. Development 2002;129(11):2639–48.

7. Moriyama M, Osawa M, Mak SS, et al. Notch signaling via Hes1 transcription factor maintains survival of melanoblasts and melanocyte stem cells. J Cell Biol 2006;173(3):333–9.

8. Aubin-Houzelstein G, Djian-Zaouche J, Bernex F, et al. Melanoblasts' proper location and timed differentiation depend on Notch/RBP-J signaling in postnatal hair follicles. J Invest Dermatol 2008;128(11):2686–95.

9. Bedogni B, Warneke JA, Nickoloff BJ, et al. Notch1 is an effector of Akt and hypoxia in melanoma development. J Clin Invest 2008;118(11):3660–70.

10. Hoek K, Rimm DL, Williams KR, et al. Expression profiling reveals novel pathways in the transformation of melanocytes to melanomas. Cancer Res 2004; 64(15):5270–82.

11. Balint K, Xiao M, Pinnix CC, et al. Activation of Notch1 signaling is required for beta-catenin-mediated human primary melanoma progression. J Clin Invest 2005;115(11):3166–76.

12. Liu ZJ, Xiao M, Balint K, et al. Notch1 signaling promotes primary melanoma progression by activating mitogen-activated protein kinase/phosphatidylinositol 3-kinase-Akt pathways and up-regulating N-cadherin expression. Cancer Res 2006;66(8):4182–90.

13. Klaus A, Birchmeier W. Wnt signalling and its impact on development and cancer. Nat Rev Cancer 2008;8(5):387–98.

14. Dorsky RI, Moon RT, Raible DW. Control of neural crest cell fate by the Wnt signalling pathway. Nature 1998;396(6709):370–3.

15. Dorsky RI, Raible DW, Moon RT. Direct regulation of nacre, a zebrafish MITF homolog required for pigment cell formation, by the Wnt pathway. Genes Dev 2000;14(2):158–62.

16. Takeda K, Yasumoto K, Takada R, et al. Induction of melanocyte-specific microphthalmia-associated transcription factor by Wnt-3a. J Biol Chem 2000;275(19): 14013–6.

17. Yasumoto K, Takeda K, Saito H, et al. Microphthalmia-associated transcription factor interacts with LEF-1, a mediator of Wnt signaling. EMBO J 2002;21(11): 2703–14.

18. Saito H, Yasumoto K, Takeda K, et al. Melanocyte-specific microphthalmia-associated transcription factor isoform activates its own gene promoter through physical interaction with lymphoid-enhancing factor 1. J Biol Chem 2002; 277(32):28787–94.

19. Schepsky A, Bruser K, Gunnarsson GJ, et al. The microphthalmia-associated transcription factor Mitf interacts with beta-catenin to determine target gene expression. Mol Cell Biol 2006;26(23):8914–27.

20. Rubinfeld B, Robbins P, El-Gamil M, et al. Stabilization of beta-catenin by genetic defects in melanoma cell lines. Science 1997;275(5307):1790–2.

21. Rimm DL, Caca K, Hu G, et al. Frequent nuclear/cytoplasmic localization of beta-catenin without exon 3 mutations in malignant melanoma. Am J Pathol 1999;154(2):325–9.

22. Widlund HR, Horstmann MA, Price ER, et al. β–Catenin-induced melanoma growth requires the downstream target *Microphthalmia*-associated transcription factor. J Cell Biol 2002;158(6):1079–87.

23. Kunisada T, Yoshida H, Yamazaki H, et al. Transgene expression of steel factor in the basal layer of epidermis promotes survival, proliferation, differentiation and migration of melanocyte precursors. Development 1998;125(15):2915–23.
24. Ezoe K, Holmes SA, Ho L, et al. Novel mutations and deletions of the KIT (steel factor receptor) gene in human piebaldism. Am J Hum Genet 1995;56(1):58–66.
25. Hemesath TJ, Price ER, Takemoto C, et al. MAP kinase links the transcription factor Microphthalmia to c-Kit signalling in melanocytes. Nature 1998; 391(6664):298–301.
26. Price ER, Horstmann MA, Wells AG, et al. α-Melanocyte-stimulating hormone signaling regulates expression of *microphthalmia*, a gene deficient in Waardenburg syndrome. J Biol Chem 1998;273(49):33042–7.
27. Wu M, Hemesath TJ, Takemoto CM, et al. c-Kit triggers dual phosphorylations, which couple activation and degradation of the essential melanocyte factor Mi. Genes Dev 2000;14(3):301–12.
28. Curtin JA, Busam K, Pinkel D, et al. Somatic activation of KIT in distinct subtypes of melanoma. J Clin Oncol 2006;24(26):4340–6.
29. Hodi FS, Friedlander P, Corless CL, et al. Major response to imatinib mesylate in KIT-mutated melanoma. J Clin Oncol 2008;26(12):2046–51.
30. Lutzky J, Bauer J, Bastian BC. Dose-dependent, complete response to imatinib of a metastatic mucosal melanoma with a K642E KIT mutation. Pigment Cell Melanoma Res 2008;21(4):492–3.
31. Verastegui C, Bille K, Ortonne JP, et al. Regulation of the microphthalmia-associated transcription factor gene by the Waardenburg syndrome type 4 gene, SOX10. J Biol Chem 2000;275(40):30757–60.
32. Lang D, Lu MM, Huang L, et al. Pax3 functions at a nodal point in melanocyte stem cell differentiation. Nature 2005;433(7028):884–7.
33. Huber WE, Price ER, Widlund HR, et al. A tissue-restricted cAMP transcriptional response: SOX10 modulates α-melanocyte-stimulating hormone-triggered expression of microphthalmia-associated transcription factor in melanocytes. J Biol Chem 2003;278(46):45224–30.
34. Scholl FA, Kamarashev J, Murmann OV, et al. PAX3 is expressed in human melanomas and contributes to tumor cell survival. Cancer Res 2001;61(3):823–6.
35. Reid K, Turnley AM, Maxwell GD, et al. Multiple roles for endothelin in melanocyte development: regulation of progenitor number and stimulation of differentiation. Development 1996;122(12):3911–9.
36. Pavan WJ, Tilghman SM. Piebald lethal (sl) acts early to disrupt the development of neural crest-derived melanocytes. Proc Natl Acad Sci U S A 1994;91(15): 7159–63.
37. Baynash AG, Hosoda K, Giaid A, et al. Interaction of endothelin-3 with endothelin-B receptor is essential for development of epidermal melanocytes and enteric neurons. Cell 1994;79(7):1277–85.
38. Bittner M, Meltzer P, Chen Y, et al. Molecular classification of cutaneous malignant melanoma by gene expression profiling. Nature 2000;406(6795):536–40.
39. Van Raamsdonk CD, Bezrookove V, Green G, et al. Frequent somatic mutations of GNAQ in uveal melanoma and blue naevi. Nature 2009;457(7229): 599–602.
40. Opdecamp K, Nakayama A, Nguyen MT, et al. Melanocyte development in vivo and in neural crest cell cultures: crucial dependence on the Mitf basic-helix-loop-helix-zipper transcription factor. Development 1997;124(12):2377–86.
41. Hornyak TJ, Hayes DJ, Chiu LY, et al. Transcription factors in melanocyte development: distinct roles for Pax-3 and Mitf. Mech Dev 2001;101(1–2):47–59.

42. Hertwig P. Neue Mutationen und Kopplungsgruppen bei der Hausmaus [New mutations and linkage groups in the house mouse]. Z Indukt Abstamm Vererbungsl 1942;80:220–46 [in German].
43. Stechschulte DJ, Sharma R, Dileepan KN, et al. Effect of the mi allele on mast cells, basophils, natural killer cells, and osteoclasts in C57Bl/6J mice. J Cell Physiol 1987;132(3):565–70.
44. Hodgkinson CA, Moore KJ, Nakayama A, et al. Mutations at the mouse microphthalmia locus are associated with defects in a gene encoding a novel basic-helix-loop-helix-zipper protein. Cell 1993;74(2):395–404.
45. Hemesath TJ, Steingrimsson E, McGill G, et al. microphthalmia, a critical factor in melanocyte development, defines a discrete transcription factor family. Genes Dev 1994;8(22):2770–80.
46. Steingrimsson E, Moore KJ, Lamoreux ML, et al. Molecular basis of mouse microphthalmia (mi) mutations helps explain their developmental and phenotypic consequences. Nat Genet 1994;8(3):256–63.
47. Waardenburg PJ. A new syndrome combining developmental anomalies of the eyelids, eyebrows and nose root with pigmentary defects of the iris and head hair and with congenital deafness. Am J Hum Genet 1951;3(3):195–253.
48. Read AP, Newton VE. Waardenburg syndrome. J Med Genet 1997;34(8):656–65.
49. Edery P, Attie T, Amiel J, et al. Mutation of the endothelin-3 gene in the Waardenburg-Hirschsprung disease (Shah-Waardenburg syndrome). Nat Genet 1996;12(4):442–4.
50. Puffenberger EG, Hosoda K, Washington SS, et al. A missense mutation of the endothelin-B receptor gene in multigenic Hirschsprung's disease. Cell 1994;79(7):1257–66.
51. Tassabehji M, Newton VE, Read AP. Waardenburg syndrome type 2 caused by mutations in the human microphthalmia (MITF) gene. Nat Genet 1994;8(3):251–5.
52. Hughes AE, Newton VE, Liu XZ, et al. A gene for Waardenburg syndrome type 2 maps close to the human homologue of the microphthalmia gene at chromosome 3p12-p14.1. Nat Genet 1994;7(4):509–12.
53. Amiel J, Watkin PM, Tassabehji M, et al. Mutation of the MITF gene in albinism-deafness syndrome (Tietz syndrome). Clin Dysmorphol 1998;7(1):17–20.
54. Sanchez-Martin M, Rodriguez-Garcia A, Perez-Losada J, et al. SLUG (SNAI2) deletions in patients with Waardenburg disease. Hum Mol Genet 2002;11(25):3231–6.
55. Price ER, Fisher DE. Sensorineural deafness and pigmentation genes: melanocytes and the Mitf transcriptional network. Neuron 2001;30(1):15–8.
56. Hershey CL, Fisher DE. Genomic analysis of the Microphthalmia locus and identification of the MITF-J/Mitf-J isoform. Gene 2005;347(1):73–82.
57. Chin L, Garraway LA, Fisher DE. Malignant melanoma: genetics and therapeutics in the genomic era. Genes Dev 2006;20(16):2149–82.
58. Widlund HR, Fisher DE. Microphthalamia-associated transcription factor: a critical regulator of pigment cell development and survival. Oncogene 2003;22(20):3035–41.
59. Tachibana M, Takeda K, Nobukuni Y, et al. Ectopic expression of MITF, a gene for Waardenburg syndrome type 2, converts fibroblasts to cells with melanocyte characteristics. Nat Genet 1996;14(1):50–4.
60. Aksan I, Goding CR. Targeting the microphthalmia basic helix-loop-helix-leucine zipper transcription factor to a subset of E-box elements in vitro and in vivo. Mol Cell Biol 1998;18(12):6930–8.

61. Cui R, Widlund HR, Feige E, et al. Central role of p53 in the suntan response and pathologic hyperpigmentation. Cell 2007;128(5):853–64.
62. Bentley NJ, Eisen T, Goding CR. Melanocyte-specific expression of the human tyrosinase promoter: activation by the microphthalmia gene product and role of the initiator. Mol Cell Biol 1994;14(12):7996–8006.
63. Yasumoto K, Yokoyama K, Shibata K, et al. Microphthalmia-associated transcription factor as a regulator for melanocyte-specific transcription of the human tyrosinase gene. Mol Cell Biol 1994;14(12):8058–70.
64. Veis DJ, Sorenson CM, Shutter JR, et al. Bcl-2-deficient mice demonstrate fulminant lymphoid apoptosis, polycystic kidneys, and hypopigmented hair. Cell 1993;75(2):229–40.
65. Nishimura EK, Granter SR, Fisher DE. Mechanisms of hair graying: incomplete melanocyte stem cell maintenance in the niche. Science 2005;307(5710): 720–4.
66. McGill GG, Horstmann M, Widlund HR, et al. Bcl2 regulation by the melanocyte master regulator Mitf modulates lineage survival and melanoma cell viability. Cell 2002;109(6):707–18.
67. McGill GG, Haq R, Nishimura EK, et al. c-Met expression is regulated by Mitf in the melanocyte lineage. J Biol Chem 2006;281(15):10365–73.
68. Beuret L, Flori E, Denoyelle C, et al. Up-regulation of MET expression by alpha-melanocyte-stimulating hormone and MITF allows hepatocyte growth factor to protect melanocytes and melanoma cells from apoptosis. J Biol Chem 2007; 282(19):14140–7.
69. Du J, Widlund HR, Horstmann MA, et al. Critical role of CDK2 for melanoma growth linked to its melanocyte-specific transcriptional regulation by MITF. Cancer Cell 2004;6(6):565–76.
70. Carreira S, Liu B, Goding CR. The gene encoding the T-box factor Tbx2 is a target for the microphthalmia-associated transcription factor in melanocytes. J Biol Chem 2000;275(29):21920–7.
71. Vance KW, Carreira S, Brosch G, et al. Tbx2 is overexpressed and plays an important role in maintaining proliferation and suppression of senescence in melanomas. Cancer Res 2005;65(6):2260–8.
72. Carreira S, Goodall J, Aksan I, et al. Mitf cooperates with Rb1 and activates p21Cip1 expression to regulate cell cycle progression. Nature 2005; 433(7027):764–9.
73. Loercher AE, Tank EM, Delston RB, et al. MITF links differentiation with cell cycle arrest in melanocytes by transcriptional activation of INK4A. J Cell Biol 2005; 168(1):35–40.
74. Hussussian CJ, Struewing JP, Goldstein AM, et al. Germline p16 mutations in familial melanoma. Nat Genet 1994;8(1):15–21.
75. Kamb A, Shattuck-Eidens D, Eeles R, et al. Analysis of the p16 gene (CDKN2) as a candidate for the chromosome 9p melanoma susceptibility locus. Nat Genet 1994;8(1):23–6.
76. Carreira S, Goodall J, Denat L, et al. Mitf regulation of Dia1 controls melanoma proliferation and invasiveness. Genes Dev 2006;20(24):3426–39.
77. Busca R, Berra E, Gaggioli C, et al. Hypoxia-inducible factor 1{alpha} is a new target of microphthalmia-associated transcription factor (MITF) in melanoma cells. J Cell Biol 2005;170(1):49–59.
78. Miller AJ, Du J, Rowan S, et al. Transcriptional regulation of the melanoma prognostic marker melastatin (TRPM1) by MITF in melanocytes and melanoma. Cancer Res 2004;64(2):509–16.

79. Duncan LM, Deeds J, Hunter J, et al. Down-regulation of the novel gene melastatin correlates with potential for melanoma metastasis. Cancer Res 1998;58(7): 1515–20.

80. Wellbrock C, Rana S, Paterson H, et al. Oncogenic BRAF regulates melanoma proliferation through the lineage specific factor MITF. PLoS ONE 2008;3(7): e2734.

81. Cook AL, Donatien PD, Smith AG, et al. Human melanoblasts in culture: expression of BRN2 and synergistic regulation by fibroblast growth factor-2, stem cell factor, and endothelin-3. J Invest Dermatol 2003;121(5):1150–9.

82. Bemis LT, Chen R, Amato CM, et al. MicroRNA-137 targets microphthalmia-associated transcription factor in melanoma cell lines. Cancer Res 2008;68(5): 1362–8.

83. Grabacka M, Placha W, Urbanska K, et al. PPAR gamma regulates MITF and beta-catenin expression and promotes a differentiated phenotype in mouse melanoma S91. Pigment Cell Melanoma Res 2008;21(3):388–96.

84. Jacquemin P, Lannoy VJ, O'Sullivan J, et al. The transcription factor onecut-2 controls the microphthalmia-associated transcription factor gene. Biochem Biophys Res Commun 2001;285(5):1200–5.

85. Takeda K, Takemoto C, Kobayashi I, et al. Ser298 of MITF, a mutation site in Waardenburg syndrome type 2, is a phosphorylation site with functional significance. Hum Mol Genet 2000;9(1):125–32.

86. Levy C, Nechushtan H, Razin E. A new role for the STAT3 inhibitor, PIAS3: a repressor of microphthalmia transcription factor. J Biol Chem 2002;277(3): 1962–6.

87. Miller AJ, Levy C, Davis IJ, et al. Sumoylation of MITF and its related family members TFE3 and TFEB. J Biol Chem 2005;280(1):146–55.

88. Larribere L, Hilmi C, Khaled M, et al. The cleavage of microphthalmia-associated transcription factor, MITF, by caspases plays an essential role in melanocyte and melanoma cell apoptosis. Genes Dev 2005;19(17):1980–5.

89. Sato S, Roberts K, Gambino G, et al. CBP/p300 as a co-factor for the Microphthalmia transcription factor. Oncogene 1997;14(25):3083–92.

90. de la Serna IL, Ohkawa Y, Higashi C, et al. The microphthalmia-associated transcription factor requires SWI/SNF enzymes to activate melanocyte-specific genes. J Biol Chem 2006;281(29):20233–41.

91. Garraway LA, Widlund HR, Rubin MA, et al. Integrative genomic analyses identify MITF as a lineage survival oncogene amplified in malignant melanoma. Nature 2005;436(7047):117–22.

92. Wellbrock C, Marais R. Elevated expression of MITF counteracts B-RAF-stimulated melanocyte and melanoma cell proliferation. J Cell Biol 2005;170(5):703–8.

93. King R, Weilbaecher KN, McGill G, et al. Microphthalmia transcription factor. A sensitive and specific melanocyte marker for MelanomaDiagnosis. Am J Pathol 1999;155(3):731–8.

94. Salti GI, Manougian T, Farolan M, et al. Micropthalmia transcription factor: a new prognostic marker in intermediate-thickness cutaneous malignant melanoma. Cancer Res 2000;60(18):5012–6.

95. Duncan LM, Deeds J, Cronin FE, et al. Melastatin expression and prognosis in cutaneous malignant melanoma. J Clin Oncol 2001;19(2):568–76.

96. Ugurel S, Houben R, Schrama D, et al. Microphthalmia-associated transcription factor gene amplification in metastatic melanoma is a prognostic marker for patient survival, but not a predictive marker for chemosensitivity and chemotherapy response. Clin Cancer Res 2007;13(21):6344–50.

97. Hoek KS, Schlegel NC, Brafford P, et al. Metastatic potential of melanomas defined by specific gene expression profiles with no BRAF signature. Pigment Cell Res 2006;19(4):290–302.
98. Yokoyama S, Feige E, Poling LL, et al. Pharmacologic suppression of MITF expression via HDAC inhibitors in the melanocyte lineage. Pigment Cell Melanoma Res 2008;21(4):457–63.
99. Barker N, Clevers H. Mining the Wnt pathway for cancer therapeutics. Nat Rev Drug Discov 2006;5(12):997–1014.
100. Liu S, Breit S, Danckwardt S, et al. Downregulation of Notch signaling by gamma-secretase inhibition can abrogate chemotherapy-induced apoptosis in T-ALL cell lines. Ann Hematol 2008;doi:10.1007/s00277-008-0646-x.
101. Tsai J, Lee JT, Wang W, et al. Discovery of a selective inhibitor of oncogenic B-Raf kinase with potent antimelanoma activity. Proc Natl Acad Sci U S A 2008;105(8):3041–6.
102. Zou HY, Li Q, Lee JH, et al. An orally available small-molecule inhibitor of c-Met, PF-2341066, exhibits cytoreductive antitumor efficacy through antiproliferative and antiangiogenic mechanisms. Cancer Res 2007;67(9):4408–17.
103. Davis IJ, Kim JJ, Ozsolak F, et al. Oncogenic MITF dysregulation in clear cell sarcoma: defining the MiT family of human cancers. Cancer Cell 2006;9(6): 473–84.
104. Davis IJ, Fisher DE. MiT transcription factor associated malignancies in man. Cell Cycle 2007;6(14):1724–9.
105. Tsuda M, Davis IJ, Argani P, et al. TFE3 fusions activate MET signaling by transcriptional up-regulation, defining another class of tumors as candidates for therapeutic MET inhibition. Cancer Res 2007;67(3):919–29.
106. Cragg MS, Jansen ES, Cook M, et al. Treatment of B-RAF mutant human tumor cells with a MEK inhibitor requires Bim and is enhanced by a BH3 mimetic. J Clin Invest 2008;118(11):3651–9.

Progress in Melanoma Histopathology and Diagnosis

Adriano Piris, MD[a],*, Martin C. Mihm, Jr, MD[b]

KEYWORDS

- Melanoma • Histopathology • Borderline lesions
- Prognosis • Dermal mitoses

In this article, we discuss the recent developments in the histopathological interpretation of primary malignant melanoma, including the evolving significance of prognostic factors. Although great strides have been made in the fields of immunohistochemistry and molecular biology, most of the criteria used in diagnosis and prognostication of melanoma derive from a thorough histopathological evaluation of the primary lesion.

The greatest advances in the field of melanoma morphology started approximately 40 years ago when Clark and colleagues, McGovern, and Breslow independently made major contributions in the understanding of these lesions.[1–5] Clark and McGovern, almost simultaneously, described the different subtypes of melanoma and established prognostic parameters, whereas Breslow described a method to measure these lesions under the microscope. Since then, the cornerstone of the histopathological evaluation of malignant melanoma relies on the pattern of growth, microscopic levels of invasion, and thickness of the lesion. These concepts revolutionized the understanding of this neoplasm that until then was considered a death sentence to the patient with only palliative excision as treatment option, which consisted almost always of radical mutilating surgery.

Following these milestones in melanoma diagnosis, several elements of the primary tumor were described and correlated to prognosis, finessing even more the management of patients with malignant melanoma.[6–10] The conjunction of these morphological elements that have prognostic significance represents the "prognostic factors" currently used to guide management, and some of them are key elements of the American Joint Committee on Cancer (AJCC) staging system.[11]

[a] Department of Pathology, Massachusetts General Hospital, Harvard Medical School, 55 Fruit Street, Warren 820, Boston, MA 02114, USA
[b] Department of Pathology and Dermatopathology, Massachusetts General Hospital, Harvard Medical School, 55 Fruit Street, Warren 820, Boston, MA 02114, USA
* Corresponding author.
E-mail address: apiris@partners.org (A. Piris).

Hematol Oncol Clin N Am 23 (2009) 467–480
doi:10.1016/j.hoc.2009.03.012
0889-8588/09/$ – see front matter © 2009 Elsevier Inc. All rights reserved.

hemonc.theclinics.com

PRIMARY MALIGNANT MELANOMA

From a microscopic point of view, malignant melanomas present a spectrum of morphological changes that include benign-appearing lesions, classic malignant melanoma morphology, and poorly differentiated variants. In general, melanomas presenting with a classic morphology do not constitute a diagnostic challenge. In addition, the poorly differentiated variants can be diagnosed with the use of immunohistochemical markers of melanocytic lineage. However, the lesions that mimic benign counterparts, such as spindle and spitzoid melanomas, remain a constant challenge. Despite much effort to refine diagnostic morphological criteria, a significant level of difficulty remains in categorizing some lesions as benign or malignant. Therefore, besides outright "benign" and "malignant" pigmented lesions, a third category exists, in which the lesions are designated depending on the author as borderline lesions or melanocytic tumors of uncertain malignant potential (MEL-TUMP).[12] In 2004 and 2006, advances in the field of molecular pathology have been applied to the study of these borderline lesions with the goal to obtain better diagnostic accuracy.[13,14] These new approaches are still at an early stage as diagnostic tools, and except for a few anecdotal cases, diagnosis and management of these borderline lesions are still driven by a detailed morphological analysis.

The main classification of malignant melanoma has its own section in this publication. We limit ourselves to citing the 4 main types that include superficial spreading, lentigo maligna, acral lentiginous, and nodular melanoma. In 2005, a previously unrecognized variant was described, namely the "lentiginous melanoma."[15] This entity is characterized by the presence of a confluent growth of nests and single cells consistently present in rete ridges with preserved architecture, which gives rise to an invasive component. It occurs in the elderly, and because of its peculiar pattern of growth, it can be misinterpreted as an atypical lentiginous nevus or a dysplastic nevus. The lentiginous melanomas are large, greater than 1 cm in size, and occur most commonly on the upper back and neck but also on the trunk and arms.

New classification schemes are currently being developed based on morphology, genotype of the primary lesion, and its relationship to anatomic site and pattern of sun exposure.[16] So far, most of the new findings correlate well with the classic types, and the new information serves as a complement to the current knowledge, with the added benefit of potentially adding more accuracy to current classification schemes, improving prognostic significance and broadening therapeutic options.

THE EVOLVING CONCEPT OF RADIAL AND VERTICAL GROWTH PHASE

Malignant melanomas can exhibit one or two components according to their pattern of growth and developmental stage.[17] These components are described as radial growth phase and vertical growth phase. Malignant melanoma in situ and early invasive melanoma exhibit only radial growth phase. Nodular melanomas, on the other hand, show only a vertical growth phase. This is characterized by an expansive invasive component without a noticeable radial growth phase. The remaining of the lesions will show both components. The radial growth phase represents the initial stage of melanoma development and is characterized by a prolonged intraepidermal or microinvasive growth (**Fig. 1**). Once the lesion has acquired a more aggressive invasive component, it is considered to have entered the vertical growth phase. Therefore, the vertical growth phase represents a more advanced stage in melanoma development, with emergence of cells that have the capacity to form expansile growth with a predominant invasive component, with or without mitotic activity, and with architectural distortion of the papillary dermis (**Fig. 2**). Lesions presenting only with the radial

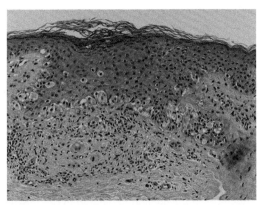

Fig. 1. Malignant melanoma in radial growth phase (microinvasive). The cytology and size of the nests in the epidermis are similar to that of the invasive component in the superficial dermis.

growth phase usually have an excellent prognosis and are virtually curable by excision.[18,19] Once the lesion acquires a vertical growth phase, it is considered to have metastatic potential and poor prognosis. As described by Clark, the distinction of these compartments relies only on cytology and architecture of the tumoral cells. A lesion is considered to be in radial growth phase when it is either in situ or with a small invasive dermal component that is cytologically and architecturally similar to the cells and nests of the intraepidermal compartment. On the other hand, when the cells in the dermis acquire a different morphology and the nests become larger than those of the intraepidermal component, the lesion is considered to have entered the vertical growth phase. Therefore, the lesions in the radial growth phase are either in situ (Clark's level I) or microinvasive (Clark's level II), whereas the lesions in the vertical growth phase are always at least Clark level III. This concept correlates well with the Breslow thickness of the tumor. However, despite these very astute observations with good prognostic correlations, there are thin melanomas that morphologically lack a dermal expansile component but that still metastasize in the absence of a

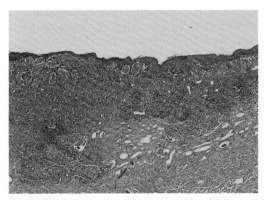

Fig. 2. Malignant melanoma in vertical growth phase. This lesion is deeply invasive with large expansile nests in the dermis. Note the predominance of the dermal component, especially on the left side of the picture.

well-developed vertical growth phase. Four main concepts help explain this phenomenon. They are the presence of the so-called "early vertical growth phase," and the presence of dermal mitosis, ulceration, and significant regression.

Early vertical growth phase is a term coined by Clark to describe the first recognizable features of a vertical growth phase in early lesions that were only Clark level II or incipient level III. In these early cases, the criteria of different cytology and size of the nests also apply when comparing the invasive and intraepidermal components to establish the presence of the vertical growth phase. Therefore, in the early vertical growth phase, there will be 1 or a few dermal nodules slightly larger than the intraepidermal ones, with a different cytology and a slightly increased number of cells per nodule. In this early stage of aggressive behavior, there is still no architectural disruption of the superficial dermal component. Mitoses may or may not be present. The presence of an early vertical growth phase is associated with 10% risk of metastasis with a follow-up of 8 years.[18] In the section dedicated to prognostic factors, we elaborate on the significance of dermal mitoses, ulceration, and regression. Despite the recent validation of these additional prognostic features as predictors of metastatic potential, Clark's description of the radial and vertical growth phase components remains the cornerstone for the morphological evaluation of primary melanomas.

SEVERELY ATYPICAL/BORDERLINE MELANOCYTIC TUMORS

Most of the lesions that fall under this category represent spindle cell melanocytic lesions with spitzoid morphology. In the most recent edition of Lever's histopathology of the skin, Elder and colleagues[20] present a table with the most useful diagnostic criteria to differentiate atypical Spitz nevi from melanoma. For benign lesions, besides benign nuclear features and the presence of prominent and confluent Kamino bodies, the salient architectural features include small size (<6 mm), symmetry, presence of maturation from top to bottom of the lesion, coexistence of epidermal hyperplasia, little or no pagetoid spread, no extension of the epidermal component beyond the dermal component, uniform ovoid nests with a perpendicular orientation to the epidermal surface, as well as little or no pigment. In addition, in benign lesions, dermal mitotic figures will be either absent or present in a small number and limited to the superficial aspect of the lesion. The malignant lesions, however, will usually show the following features: size larger than 6 mm, asymmetry, lack of maturation, minimal epidermal reaction, obvious pagetoid spread extending to the shoulders of the lesion, nests in different shape, size, and orientation, and prominent pigmentation with irregular distribution. Malignant spitzoid lesions will also have numerous mitoses, usually with atypical forms and involving the entire lesion, including the deep aspect of the tumor. It has been reported that mitotic figures within 0.25 mm of the deep tissue edge should be considered a poor prognostic indicator.[21]

Some of these lesions will present with a more or less equal number of benign and malignant features, making it impossible to call them entirely benign or malignant. These cases are designated either as borderline spitzoid melanocytic proliferations, Spitz tumor with severe atypia, or MELTUMP.[12] The likelihood of metastasis in these lesions is clinically relevant. However, the significance of positive nodes remains unclear, because even in the presence of metastatic disease, these patients can have prolonged survival.[22,23] Many authorities in the field will recommend a sentinel lymph node biopsy when such lesions show the same factors that would lead to that procedure in fully malignant cases. If the sentinel lymph node is positive, then a completion lymphadenectomy should be considered to attempt eradication or control of the tumor burden of a disease with unpredictable behavior. The issue of adjuvant therapy is more controversial, and there is divided opinion in the community with regard to considering that these patients have either metastatic melanoma or metastasizing Spitz tumors.

Another interesting entity that, even when metastatic, follows an indolent course is the "pigmented epithelioid melanocytoma." This term was coined in 2004 in the course of a study of borderline lesions with markedly hyperpigmented melanocytes and features similar to the so-called "animal-type melanoma" and the epithelioid blue nevus of Carney Complex.[24] More recently, the pigmented epithelioid melanocytomas were found to have lost expression of the protein kinase regulatory subunit type 1α coded by the *PRKAR1 A* gene, whereas melanoma and other melanocytic lesions did not show such loss.[25]

IMMUNOHISTOCHEMISTRY OF PIGMENTED LESIONS

The S100 protein is a calcium-binding protein with a role in cell surface transport and in RNA polymerase activity.[26,27] Therefore, it is present in the nucleus and cytoplasm of several cells types. The S100 positive cells include Schwann cells, melanocytes, glial cells, chondrocytes, adipocytes, myoepithelial cells, macrophages, Langerhans cells, dendritic cells, as well as their benign or malignant neoplastic counterparts. Despite its low specificity, the stain is highly sensitive and is positive in almost all melanomas.[28] To consider the stain unequivocally positive, there must be reaction of the nuclear and cytoplasmic components.

HMB45 is an antibody against the gp-100 protein, a glycoprotein considered to be part of the premelanosome complex.[29] This antibody is more specific but less sensitive than S100. Its specificity, however, is somewhat limited. Other tumors that can also mark for HMB45 include angiomyolipoma, lymphangiomyomatosis, and clear cell "sugar" tumor.

Anti–MART-1 and anti–Melan-A are two antibodies directed against the same melanocyte differentiation antigen.[30] This antigen is recognized by T cells in melanoma patients, and it represents a transmembrane protein associated with the pigmentary apparatus. These markers are more specific than S100 and HMB45, and its sensitivity is somewhat greater than that of HMB45. Anti–Mart-1 is considered to be a superior antibody to HMB45. The genes encoding MART-1/Melan-A are transcribed only by melanocytes.

Other markers used to identify tumors of melanocytic origin include microphthalmia-associated transcription factor, melanoma-associated antigen, and tyrosinase. Used as panels or cocktails, different combinations of these markers are very useful in determining the melanocytic origin of an undifferentiated neoplasm, but they are very limited in their utility in determining the benign or malignant nature of these lesions.

PROGNOSTIC FACTORS
Clark's Levels

The Clark's levels of invasion represent a description of the extent of invasion of the tumor through the different microscopic levels of the skin from the epidermis to the subcutaneous tissue. They are enumerated as follows:

Level I: Intraepidermal (melanoma in situ).
Level II: Partial involvement of the papillary dermis by single cells or small nests.

Level III: Expansile nodule filling the papillary dermis and widening it, impinging upon the reticular dermis. A few cells may infiltrate the superficial reticular dermis.

Level IV: Extension of multiple cells across a broad front into the reticular dermis.

Level V: Extension into the subcutaneous fat.

The level of Clark is no longer the primary determinant of T staging. However, in the sixth edition of the AJCC staging system, it is used to stratify patients with a Breslow thickness of 1 mm or less.[11] A primary melanoma that is 1 mm or less in thickness is considered a "T1a" lesion if the Clark's level is I or II, and "T1b," if the Clark's level is III or IV. In other words, thin lesions with Clark's level greater than III have a worse prognosis than lesions of the same thickness with a Clark's level of III or less. This stratification of patients with thin melanoma according to Clark's level, however, may not continue in the upcoming AJCC staging system, because several new reports have found that mitotic rates have a better correlation with prognosis in these early lesions. Nevertheless, the determination of the Clark's level is a useful exercise in understanding the biology of a given melanoma, as it describes the capacity of the tumoral cells to interact with the surrounding stroma and infiltrate through the different microanatomic barriers of the skin. In this regard, the Clark's level serves as a morphological yardstick to better understand several biological markers, such as adhesion molecules and matrix metalloproteinases, which are currently being studied in the context of melanoma development and progression.

Breslow Thickness

Breslow described a method of objective measurement of tumor thickness using a micrometer.[5] The measurement of tumor thickness according to his method resulted in one of the most significant microscopic parameters to predict metastasis. In the initial report, lesions that measured less than 0.76 mm did not metastasize. Currently, the AJCC considers the following thresholds for T staging:

T1: 1.0 mm or less
T2: 1.1 to 2.0 mm
T3: 2.1 to 4.0 mm
T4: more than 4.0 mm

The Breslow thickness is obtained by measuring from the top of the granular cell layer to the deepest tumor cell. If an ulcer is present, the measurement starts from the depth of the ulcer. Large junctional nests that push deeply into the papillary dermis should not be considered. Tumor cells associated with adnexal structures are also not considered in the measurement by the Breslow's method. It is, however, our experience that adventitial dermal nests located deeper than the remaining of the tumor also represent an important factor when predicting the likelihood of metastasis in individual cases. In the consultation service of one of the authors (M. C. M Jr.), a significant number of T1 tumors show positive sentinel lymph node when adnexal involvement extends beyond 1 mm (Martin C. Mihm, Jr, MD, unpublished data, 2009).

Ulceration

The presence of ulceration in the primary tumor is associated with aggressive behavior.[31] A true ulcer is microscopically defined as full-thickness interruption of the epidermis by the tumor without history of prior surgery or trauma at the site and accompanied by reactive changes, such as inflammation and fibrin deposition. Applying this strict definition, ulceration of the primary tumor represents the second criterion used by the AJCC for T staging. Based on the absence or presence of ulceration, the AJCC designates each T category as "a" or "b." The presence of ulceration within a given T category immediately lowers the survival rate of a patient compared with those without ulceration.[11]

Mitotic Rate

It has been long known that the number of dermal mitoses in the invasive component of the primary tumor is an important prognostic indicator.[6,32,33] In the model of Clark, the number of mitoses was determined per squared millimeter. In his cohort, he found survival rates of 95%, 79.4%, and 38.2%, respectively, for mitotic counts of zero, one to six, and greater than six per mm[2]. Recent studies have emphasized the importance of the mitotic count in determining melanoma prognosis. The "Pigmented Lesion Group" from the University of Pennsylvania has recently demonstrated through a series of studies, that in thin melanomas, the presence of even a single dermal mitosis is an independent prognostic factor.[34,35] Furthermore, current data from the AJCC show a highly significant correlation between mitotic rate and poor prognosis. The upcoming edition of the AJCC will include mitotic rate as part of the melanoma staging system.

The mitotic count should be performed in the invasive component of the melanoma starting in the area of major mitotic activity, designated as the "hot spot" (**Fig. 3**). Depending on the microscope used, the number of high-power fields required to obtain 1 mm[2] will vary. Therefore, it is recommended that each instrument be calibrated to obtain the exact number of fields required.

In addition to the mitotic count of the H&E slide, the proliferative activity of the tumor can also be measured using the proliferation marker Mib-1 (Ki-67). The Ki67 proliferation index, estimated as a percentage of positive nuclei within the tumor cells, has also been found to have prognostic significance.[35] The Ki-67 stain is also used in borderline lesions to better predict their biologic potential, but its value as a diagnostic marker is far less established than its prognostic significance.

Regression

Regression is defined as the focal absence of tumor in the epidermis and dermis flanked on one or both sides by intraepidermal and/or dermal tumor cells (**Fig. 4**). This area is characterized by the presence of a thin epidermis with underlying fibroplasia,

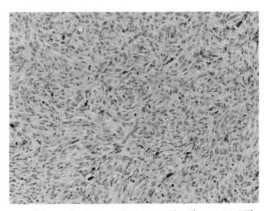

Fig. 3. A conglomerate of dermal mitoses represents the "hot spot." The mitotic figures are identified by the pycnotic (dark blue) "horse-shoe" shaped structures.

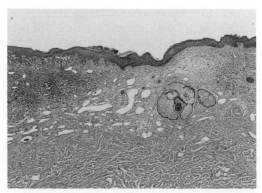

Fig. 4. Lower-power view of a partially regressed malignant melanoma. On the left, the residual intraepidermal and invasive components can be appreciated, partially obscured by inflammation. The center and the right aspects of the photograph show marked vascular ectasia and inflammation with absence of tumoral cells. The organoid structure in the midddle of the regression represents an entrapped adnexal structure.

inflammatory cells, melanophages, and prominent vasculature. These vessels are usually in a perpendicular orientation to the long axis of the epidermis. Several reports showed poor prognosis associated with the finding of regression.[6,36] However, there is controversy as to its significance, especially considering that the phenomenon of host immune response discussed later is considered to infer better prognosis.

Host Immune Response

Documentation of the presence, absence, and distribution of lymphocytes within the tumoral compartment is an important part of the current microscopic evaluation of malignant melanoma. The term "tumor infiltrating lymphocytes" (TILs) is strictly defined as infiltration of lymphocytes within the substance of the tumor, where they are in direct contact with the tumor cells. The categories of TILs are classically described as follows:

Brisk: when the TILs infiltrate diffusely throughout the substance of the tumor, or when there is infiltration across the entire base of the tumor
Nonbrisk: when there is focal or multifocal infiltration
Absent: when there are no lymphocytes within the substance of the tumor

Following this classification, Clark and colleagues[6] and Clemente and colleagues[37] found that the prognosis is better with a "brisk" infiltrate and declines progressively with the "nonbrisk" and absent categories. This finding correlates with the fact that the TILs are indeed cytotoxic T cells with the ultimate goal of eliminating the tumoral cells. However, despite the presence of a brisk lymphocytic infiltrate, individual patients still go on to develop metastasis and disease progression. Currently, there are several studies underway with the aim to further characterize these lymphocytes and understand the reasons for the failure of the immune response. The markers being studied include, among others, CD4, CD8, markers of cytotoxic activity, such as TIA-1, granzyme B, and perforin, and markers for lymphocytes with regulatory functions (T regs).

The concept of the host immune response in malignant melanoma, although not yet useful for staging purposes, offers great hope in the field of immunotherapy.

Therefore, it is imperative that it be reported as part of a complete pathology report. This allows documentation of one of the aspects of tumor biology that could potentially be very useful in treatment options currently under development. For example, Soiffer and colleagues[38] demonstrated that, by vaccinating patients with autologous melanoma cells engineered to secrete granulocyte-macrophage colony-stimulating factor, they were able to increase antitumor activity with resulting extensive tumor destruction after vaccination. A case study in 2008 by Hodi and colleagues[39] validates the importance of the regulatory mechanisms in blocking an effective immune response by TILs. In their report, a patient with metastatic melanoma in the central nervous system showed morphological evidence of response in the tumor mass after the administration of ipilimumab, which is a monoclonal antibody directed against the CD28/cytotoxic T-lymphocyte antigen-4, a component of the immune regulatory mechanism. A sample obtained following administration of ipilimumab showed extensive necrosis and an increased number of CD8 positive cells with only few FoxP3-positive T regulatory cells.

Microscopic Satellites

Microscopic satellites have been defined as tumor nests, greater than 0.05 mm in diameter, in the reticular dermis, panniculus, or vessels beneath the principal invasive tumor mass but separated from it by normal tissue on the section in which the Breslow measurement was taken.[40,41] Considered under this strict definition, the presence of microscopic satellites was found to be independently associated with worse prognosis.

The current AJCC classification incorporates microscopic satellites in the group of "intralymphatic metastases," along with clinical satellites and in-transit metastases.[11] Clinical satellites and in-transit metastases represent tumor foci that are separated from the primary lesion. The term "clinical satellite" is used for tumors located no further than 5 cm from the primary lesion. When these foci are located beyond 5 cm within the same region, they are designated as in-transit metastasis. Intralymphatic metastases represent one of the defining criteria for pathologic stage III melanoma.

Blood Vessel and Lymphatic Invasion

The relationship between the tumoral cells and the vessels, either blood vessels or lymphatics, is an important part of the pathologic evaluation of a primary melanoma. Although its importance as an independent prognostic indicator has not been fully established in multivariate analysis, the identification of this attribute is of crucial importance to understand the biology and metastatic potential of a given tumor.

Vascular invasion has been described in three different scenarios.[20,42,43] The first one represents the classical definition of viable tumor cells within the lumen of the vessel (**Fig. 5**). The second type is referred to as "uncertain vascular invasion," where the tumor cells are adjacent to the endothelium, in the vessel wall, without luminal involvement. The third category is represented by perivascular cuffing of the tumor cells. This is known as angiotropism or extravascular migratory metastasis. All three types of vascular involvement have been associated with poor prognosis.

Another aspect of melanoma biology correlating lymphatic vessels with the propensity to metastasis is the phenomenon of lymphangiogenesis.[44] In 2005, Dadras and colleagues analyzed tumor lymphangiogenesis by using lymphatic vessel endothelial receptor 1, a specific marker for lymphatic endothelium. They found that the extent of tumor lymphangiogenesis could be used as a predictor of sentinel lymph node metastasis and progression.[44]

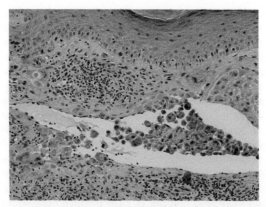

Fig. 5. Vascular invasion. Note the presence of viable malignant cells within the lumen of the vessel with partial attachment to the wall. This picture also illustrates (bottom left) the site of possible perforation of the vessel wall by the tumor.

SENTINEL LYMPH NODE BIOPSY AND COMPLETION LYMPHADENECTOMY

The sentinel lymph node is the first lymph node to receive the lymphatic drainage from a given regional lymph node basin. This is identified with the help of an injected radioactive dye in the skin surrounding the primary lesion. If the sentinel lymph node is negative, the probability that the remaining lymph nodes in the basin will harbor metastasis is very low.[45,46] This technique was developed by Morton to selectively sample the lymph node that would first be affected in case of clinically undetectable lymph node metastasis, therefore, avoiding unnecessary resection of the entire lymph node basin in case of a negative sentinel lymph node.

Once identified and dissected, the sentinel lymph node is examined by the pathologist after entirely submitting the sample in one or several blocks, followed by serial microscopic sections and obtaining sequential H&E and immunohistochemical stains. It is recommended that more than one melanocytic marker be used. Since there is no clear recommendation as to how many sections should be examined, the exact number of sections varies among institutions. It is recommended, however, that more than one series of sections be performed with each series containing one H&E slide, with a subsequent combination of two or three melanocytic markers, usually S100, Mart-1, and HMB45. A sentinel lymph node is considered positive when malignant melanoma cells are detected in the subcapsular region and/or parenchyma of the lymph node. With the combination of H&E and a cocktail of melanocytic markers, it is possible to identify minute foci of microscopic metastases, sometimes as large as one or two cells. As opposed to breast cancer, where micrometastases measuring less than 0.2 mm are considered not relevant, for malignant melanoma there is no lower threshold, and, even in the case of isolated malignant cells, the sentinel lymph node is considered positive.

Although detection of malignant cells by immunohistochemistry alone is currently accepted to designate a sentinel lymph node as positive, we strongly recommend that this be correlated when possible with the corresponding H&E slide to allow for a detailed evaluation of the morphology of the cell. The cytological criteria for malignancy, such as nuclear size, irregular chromatin distribution, and prominent nucleoli, are strictly applied to avoid overcalling histiocytes or mast cells that may cross-react with the melanocytic markers. Besides these cytological features, the architecture and location of the melanocytic nests in the lymph node are also carefully analyzed to avoid overcalling benign nevic rests. The latter show benign cytology with bland nuclear features and are located within the connective tissue of the capsule or septae, and rarely in the parenchyma of the lymph nodes.

The sensitivity for detection of these microscopic foci may be improved by using the reverse transcriptase polymerase chain reaction technique. However, the specificity may be affected, because this sophisticated technique would not be able to differentiate between malignant melanoma cells and benign nevus rests.

Detailed morphological studies of lymph nodes in patients with melanoma have revealed that there is a marked diminution in the paracortical T cell zone of sentinel nodes. In addition, there is a dramatic decrease in the number antigen-presenting cells with dendritic morphology. The otherwise normal population of "dendritic" cells is reduced, with most of the cells presenting a "so-called" veiled appearance. Indeed, these morphologic observations led to more intense study of the biology of the lymph nodes. It appears that the primary tumor secretes substances including TGFβ, which lead to a state of immunosuppression or tolerance in the lymph node.[47,48]

Once the sentinel lymph node biopsy yields a positive result, the next step is a completion lymphadenectomy. There is a dilemma, however, because only 20% of nonsentinel lymph nodes are positive. Various studies have been performed to predict nonsentinel lymph node positivity so that if possible any unnecessary node dissection with its morbidity can be avoided.[49] A study by Cochran and colleagues showed that by determining three specific criteria, namely, median thickness of the primary, percentage area of the tumor deposit in the sentinel node, and percentage area occupied by the interdigitating dendritic cells, the likelihood of positive nonsentinel lymph node could be predicted. This technique, however, is quite complex and does not lend itself to practical laboratory pathology. Another much simpler method was described by van Akkooi and colleagues,[50,51] who found that as long as the tumor burden was less than 0.1 mm, measured with a micrometer by conventional light microscopic, there were no positive nonsentinel lymph nodes. The Rotterdam group does not recommend completion lymphadenectomy in patients who have a tumor burden less than 0.1 mm.

SUMMARY

Forty years ago, the pathology report of malignant melanoma was very brief and usually implied either a death sentence and/or a serious mutilating surgical procedure. The information in this article represents the evolution of knowledge based primarily on morphology that allowed for radical changes in the diagnosis, prognosis, and therapy of this primary tumor. As longer and better follow-up of the patients is documented, the information that is forthcoming would confirm not only the value of the original descriptions more than 40 years ago but also result in continuous discovery of the nature of the tumor. Using the information at hand, we can now confidently predict favorable survival in many patients. With the onset of the genomic era, the current literature is rife with new information. However, all this new knowledge lacks coherence and validation, unless it is based on accurate morphologic observation. To our surprise the newest molecular findings are leaning toward further confirmation of the original classification of the tumor as described in the late 1960s and early 1970s.

ACKNOWLEDGMENTS

We are indebted to Dr. Carlos Nicolas Prieto Granada for contributing the images in this review.

REFERENCES

1. Clark WH Jr. A classification of malignant melanoma in man correlated with histo-genesis and biological behaviour. In: Montagna W, Hu F, editors. Advances in the biology of the skin, vol. 8. New York: Pergamon; 1967. p. 621–47.
2. Mihm MC Jr, Clark WH Jr, From L. The clinical diagnosis, classification and histo-genetic concepts of the early stages of cutaneous malignant melanomas. N Engl J Med 1971;284(19):1078–82.
3. Clark WH Jr, Mihm MC Jr. Lentigo maligna and lentigo-maligna melanoma. Am J Pathol 1969;55(1):39–67.
4. McGovern VJ. The classification of melanoma and its relationship with prognosis. Pathology 1970;2(2):85–98.
5. Breslow A. Thickness, cross-sectional area, and depth of invasion in the prog-nosis of cutanenous melanoma. Ann Surg 1970;172:902–8.
6. Clark WH Jr, Elder DE, Guerry D IV, et al. Model predicting survival in stage I melanoma base on tumor progression. J Natl Cancer Inst 1989;81:1893–904.
7. Day CL Jr, Lew RA, Mihm MC Jr, et al. A multivariate analysis of prognostic factors for melanoma patients with lesions greater than or equal to 3.65 mm in thickness. The importance of revealing alternative Cox models. Ann Surg 1982;195(1):44–9.
8. Day CL Jr, Mihm MC Jr, Lew RA, et al. Prognostic factors for patients with clinical stage I melanoma of intermediated thickness (1.51–3.39 mm). A conceptual model for tumor growth and metastasis. Ann Surg 1982;195(1):35–43.
9. Day CL Jr, Mihm MC Jr, Sober AJ, et al. Prognostic factors for melanoma patients with lesions 0.76–1.69 mm in thickness. An appraisal of "thin" level lesions. Ann Surg 1982;195(1):30–4.
10. Balch CM, Murad TM, Soong SJ, et al. A multifactorial analysis of melanoma: prognostic histopathological features comparing Clark's and Breslow's staging methods. Ann Surg 1978;188(6):732–42.
11. Balch CM, Buzaid AC, Soon SJ, et al. Final version of the American joint committee on cancer staging system for cutaneous melanoma. J Clin Oncol 2001;19:3635–48.
12. Elder DE, Xu X. The approach to the patient with a difficult melanocytic lesion. Pathology 2004;36(5):428–34.
13. Bastian BC. Molecular genetics of melanocytic neoplasia: practical applications for diagnosis. Pathology 2004;36(5):458–61, Review.
14. Bauer J, Bastian BC. Distinguishing melanocytic nevi from melanoma by DNA copy number changes: comparative genomic hybridization as a research and diagnostic tool. Dermatol Ther 2006;19(1):40–9, Review.
15. King R, Page RN, Googe PB, et al. Lentiginous melanoma: a histologic pattern of melanoma to be distinguished from lentiginous nevus. Mod Pathol 2005;18(10): 1397–401.
16. Viros A, Fridlyand J, Bauer J, et al. Improving melanoma classification by inte-grating genetic and morphologic features. PLoS Med 2008;5(6):0941–52.
17. Clark WH Jr, From L, Bernardino EA, et al. The histogenesis and biologic behavior of primary human malignant melanomas of the skin. Cancer Res 1969;29(3):705–27.
18. Clark WH Jr, Elder DE, Guerry D 4th, et al. A study of tumor progression: the precursor lesions of superficial spreading and nodular melanoma. Hum Pathol 1984;15(12):1147–65.
19. Guerry D 4th, Synnestvedt M, Elder DE, et al. Lessons from tumor progression: the invasive radial growth phase of melanoma is common, incapable of metas-tasis, and indolent. J Invest Dermatol 1993;100(3):342S–5S.

20. Elder DE, Elenitsas R, Murphy G, et al. Benign pigmented lesions and malignant melanoma. In: Elder DE, editor. Lever's histopathology of the skin. 10th edition. (PA): Lippincot Williams, and Wilkins; 2009. p. 699–789.
21. Walsh N, Crotty K, Palmer A, et al. Spitz nevus versus spitzoid malignant melanoma: an evaluation of the current distinguishing histopathologic criteria. Hum Pathol 1998;29(10):1105–12.
22. Urso C, Borgognoni L, Saieva C, et al. Sentinel lymph node biopsy in patients with "atypical Spitz tumors." A report on 12 cases. Hum Pathol 2006;37:816–23.
23. Lohmann CM, Coit DG, Brady MS, et al. Sentinel lymph node biopsy in patients with diagnostically controversial spitzoid melanocytic tumors. Am J Surg Pathol 2002;26:47–55.
24. Zembowicz A, Carney JA, Mihm MC. Pigmented epithelioid melanocytoma: a low-grade melanocytic tumor with metastatic potential indistinguishable from animal-type melanoma and epithelioid blue nevus. Am J Surg Pathol 2004;28(1):31–40. Erratum in: Am J Surg Pathol 2004 May;28(5):following table of contents.
25. Zembowicz A, Knoepp SM, Bei T, et al. Loss of expression of protein kinase a regulatory subunit 1alpha in pigmented epithelioid melanocytoma but not in melanoma or other melanocytic lesions. Am J Surg Pathol 2007;31(11):1764–75.
26. Donato R. S-100 proteins. Cell Calcium 1986;7(3):123–45.
27. Baumal R, Kahn HJ, Marks A. Role of antibody to S100 protein I diagnostic pathology. Lab Invest 1988;59(1):152–4.
28. Argenyi ZB, Cain C, Bromley C, et al. S-100 protein-negative malignant melanoma: fact or fiction? A light microscopic and immunohistochemical study. Am J Dermatopathol 1994;16:233–40.
29. Marincola FM, Hijazi YM, Fetsch P, et al. Analysis of expression of the melanoma associated antigens Mart-1 and gp-100 in metastatic melanoma cell lines and in situ lesions. J Immunother Emphasis Tumor Immunol 1996;19(3):192–205.
30. Fetsch PA, Marincola FM, Filie A, et al. A Melanoma-associated antigen recognized by T cells (MART-1). Cancer 1999;87(1):37–42.
31. Balch CM, Wilkerson JA, Murad TM, et al. The prognostic significance of ulceration of cutaneous melanoma. Cancer 1980;45(12):3012–7.
32. Azzola MF, Shaw HM, Thompson JF, et al. Tumor mitotic rate is a more powerful prognostic indicator than ulceration in patients with primary cutaneous melanoma: an analysis of 3661 patients from a single center. Cancer 2003;97:1488–98.
33. Kesmodel SB, Karakousis GC, Botbyl JD, et al. Mitotic rate as a predictor of sentinel lymph node positivity in patients with thin melanomas. Ann Surg Oncol 2005;12(6):449–58, Epub 2005 Apr 19.
34. Gimotty PA, Guerry D, Ming ME, et al. Thin primary cutaneous malignant melanoma: a prognostic tree for 10-year metastasis is more accurate than American Joint Committee on Cancer staging. J Clin Oncol 2004;22:3668–76.
35. Gimotty PA, Van Belle P, Elder DE, et al. Biologic and prognostic significance of dermal Ki67 expression, mitoses, and tumorigenicity in thin invasive cutaneous melanoma. J Clin Oncol 2005;23(31):8048–56.
36. Ronan SG, Eng AM, Briele HA, et al. Thin melanomas with regression and metastases. Arch Dermatol 1987;123(10):1326–30.
37. Clemente CG, Mihm MC Jr, Bufalino R, et al. Prognostic value of tumor infiltrating lymphocytes in the vertical growth phase of primary cutaneous melanoma. Cancer 1996;77(7):1303–10.
38. Soifer R, Hodi FS, Haluska F, et al. Vaccination with irradiated, autologous melanoma cells engineered to secrete granulocyte-macrophage colony-stimulating

factor by adenoviral–mediated gene transfer augments antitumor immunity in patients with metastatic melanoma. J Clin Oncol 2003;21(17):3343–50.

39. Hodi FS, Oble DA, Drappatz J, et al. CTLA-4 blockade with ipilimumab induces significant clinical benefit in a female with melanoma metastases to the CNS. Nat Clin Pract Oncol 2008;5(9):557–61.

40. Harrist TJ, Rigel DS, Day CL Jr, et al. "Microscopic satellites" are more highly associated with regional lymph node metastases than is primary melanoma thickness. Cancer 1984;53(10):2183–7.

41. Day CL Jr, Harrist TJ, Gorstein F, et al. Malignant melanoma. Prognostic significance of "microscopic satellites" in the reticular dermis and subcutaneous fat. Ann Surg 1981;194(1):108–12.

42. Barnhill RL, Lugassy C. Angiotropic malignant melanoma and extravascular migratory metastasis: description of 36 cases with emphasis on a new mechanism of tumour spread. Pathology 2004;36(5):485–90.

43. Barnhill R, Dy K, Lugassy C. Angiotropism in cutaneous melanoma: a prognostic factor strongly predicting risk for metastasis. J Invest Dermatol 2002;119(3):705–6.

44. Dadras SS, Lange-Asschenfeldt B, Velasco P, et al. Tumor lymphangiogenesis predicts melanoma metastasis to sentinel lymph nodes. Mod Pathol 2005;18(9):1232–42.

45. Morton DL, Cochran AJ. The case for lymphatic mapping and sentinel lymphadenectomy in the management of primary melanoma. Br J Dermatol 2004;151(2):308–19.

46. Morton DL. Sentinel lymphadenectomy for patients with clinical stage I melanoma. J Surg Oncol 1997;66(4):267–9.

47. Cochran AJ, Morton DL, Stern S, et al. Sentinel lymph nodes show profound downregulation of antigen-presenting cells of the paracortex: implications for tumor biology and treatment. Mod Pathol 2001;14(6):604–8.

48. Cochran AJ, Huang RR, Lee J, et al. Tumour-induced immune modulation of sentinel lymph nodes. Nat Rev Immunol 2006;6(9):659–70.

49. Cochran AJ, Wen DR, Huang RR, et al. Prediction of metastatic melanoma in non-sentinel nodes and clinical outcome based on the primary melanoma and the sentinel node. Mod Pathol 2004;17(7):747–55.

50. van Akkooi AC, Nowecki ZI, Voit C, et al. Sentinel node tumor burden according to the Rotterdam criteria is the most important prognostic factor for survival in melanoma patients: a multicenter study in 388 patients with positive sentinel nodes. Ann Surg 2008;248(6):949–55.

51. van Akkooi AC, de Wilt JH, Verhoef C, et al. Clinical relevance of melanoma micrometastases (<0.1 mm) in sentinel nodes: are these nodes to be considered negative? Ann Oncol 2006;17(10):1578–85.

Melanoma Early Detection

Vitaly Terushkin, BS, Allan C. Halpern, MD*

KEYWORDS

• Melanoma • Detection • Diagnosis • Dermoscopy
• Photography

Malignant melanoma continues to be a major public health concern. In 2008, it is estimated that there will be 62,480 new cases resulting in almost 8500 deaths.[1] Direct and indirect costs associated with this disease reached $3.1 billion in 2004.[2] Reducing the mortality and cost associated with melanoma can be approached in several ways. Primary prevention educational campaigns such as SunWise[3] and SunSmart[4] have been created in an attempt to reduce UV exposure; however, the anticipated benefits of these efforts may take decades to become apparent. At the other end of the disease spectrum, scientific advancements in melanoma immunology have led to novel therapeutic agents; however, metastatic disease still remains poorly responsive to systemic therapy. In contrast, early forms of melanoma are amenable to surgical cure with a 5-year survival rate of 95%.[5] It is believed that strategies aimed at recognizing early melanoma may have significant and immediate impact on decreasing mortality from this disease.[6,7] This article reviews selected components of this strategy.

EARLY DETECTION STRATEGIES

Multiple strategies have been employed to improve early detection of melanoma. These include educating patients about the importance of performing skin self-examination, increasing rates of complete skin examinations by physicians in the context of routine care, initiating mass screening campaigns, creating specialized skin cancer clinics, and developing better diagnostic tools through advances in technology.

Discovery of Melanoma by Nonphysicians

Patients play an important role in the diagnosis of melanoma. It has been reported that more than 72% of all melanomas are detected by nonphysicians; typically the patients, their families, or their friends.[8] Through increased public awareness, patients have been presenting with progressively thinner self-detected melanomas. For

Dermatology Service, Department of Medicine, Memorial Sloan-Kettering Cancer Center, 160 East 53rd Street, New York, NY 10022, USA
* Corresponding author.
E-mail address: halperna@mskcc.org (A.C. Halpern).

Hematol Oncol Clin N Am 23 (2009) 481–500
doi:10.1016/j.hoc.2009.03.001
0889-8588/09/$ – see front matter © 2009 Elsevier Inc. All rights reserved.
hemonc.theclinics.com

example, in Queensland, Australia, the proportion of thin melanomas (≤0.75 mm) detected by patients who actively examined their skin (84.6%) was greater than those found incidentally (71.2%).[9] Nonetheless, multiple studies indicate that physicians are more likely to detect thinner lesions (≤0.75 mm) compared with nonphysicians (**Table 1**).[8–12] Lack of skin awareness and poor knowledge of melanoma signs and symptoms account for delayed diagnosis and may contribute to the discrepancy between the types of lesions detected by physicians and nonphysicians.[13] These data suggest that patient education is effective and attempts to further improve patient knowledge and awareness may lead to continued improvements in the diagnosis of earlier melanomas.

A significant component of patient education is skin self-examination (SSE), which has been advocated since about 1985.[14] The potential benefits of this inexpensive and noninvasive tool have been described in several reports (**Table 2**).[15,16] SSE performers are generally diagnosed with thinner melanomas compared with nonperformers (0.77 mm vs 0.95 mm) and SSE performance is associated with diagnosis of fewer thick (>1 mm) lesions.[16] A single retrospective study suggests that SSE may have the potential to reduce mortality from melanoma by 63%.[15]

One study assessed the accuracy of SSE for detecting changes in nevi. Motivated patients who performed SSE for at least 1 year were asked to examine their backs after investigators artificially changed the diameter of an existing mole by 0, 2, or 4 mm. The sensitivity for self-detection of the 4-mm change was 75%, whereas only 58% participants correctly noticed a 2-mm change. By these standards, SSE was associated with a specificity of 62%.[17]

Although there is increasing indirect evidence for the benefits of performing SSE, a minority of at-risk individuals perform the exercise. An Italian study showed that 28.1% of patients who develop melanoma have previously performed SSE regularly.[18] In a telephone survey of 3110 residents older than 30 years in Queensland, Australia, 25.9% of participants reported SSE within the last 12 months and 33.9% within the past 3 years.[19] Another study surveyed 190 university students in the United States and found that 33.2% had ever performed SSE, with only 5.5% of individuals checking their entire body.[20] In a random-digit-dial survey of Rhode Islanders, 59% of individuals performed some form of SSE, but only 9% conducted a thorough skin examination (TSE) at least once every few months. In this study, fulfilling the TSE criteria required the examination of 8 different areas of the skin "methodically and deliberately."[21] This study underscores the varied perceptions of patients regarding SSE.

Several factors are associated with performing SSE. In a study of 200 patients, the 3 strongest predictors of SSE performance were having been diagnosed with skin cancer in the previous 3 years, attitude, and dermatology visits with skin biopsies; other predictors included knowledge, younger age, and perceived risk.[22] Predictors of performance differ by gender. Although awareness is associated with SSE in both sexes, previous benign biopsy or the presence of an abnormal mole is predictive of SSE performance in women, whereas family history of cancer, physician examination, and change in diet to reduce cancer risk are predictive of SSE performance in men.[23] Availability of a partner and a wall mirror have been found to be predictive of SSE performance in an interventional trial.[24]

Factors associated with lack of performance of SSE are manifold. In the Rhode Island study mentioned earlier, respondents noted the following: "don't think about it"; "no reason to"; "nothing there before"; "in a hurry"; "not at risk"; "hard to do/hard to see all of body"; "doctor would tell me if I needed to"; and "don't know what to look for."[21] Other potential barriers, especially in the elderly, may be related to poor vision and other health problems.

Table 1
Melanoma thickness in lesions detected by physicians and nonphysicians

Study	Mean Thickness (mm)		% Thin (≤0.75 mm) Lesions		OR or RR	Study Population
	Physician	Nonphysician	Physician	Nonphysician		
Carli et al (2003)[16]	0.68	0.90	—	—	—	816 patients consecutively diagnosed with melanoma at 11 Italian centers (1/2001 to 12/2001)
Epstein et al (1999)[10]	0.23	0.90	33.0	29.0	4.2 (RR)	102 patients diagnosed with primary melanoma at the Melanoma Center, John Hopkins Medical Institutions (6/1995 to 6/1997)
Schwartz et al (2002)[12]	0.40	1.17 (patient), 1.00 (spouse)	—	—	—	1515 consecutive patients (1/1998 to 12/1999) from the University of Michigan melanoma database
Fisher et al (2005)[11]	—	—	75.0	47.7	—	218 patients with a history of melanoma who visited the Yale Pigmented Lesion Clinic (1/1995 to 1/1996)
McPherson et al (2006)[9]	—	—	80.6	61.9	2.56 (OR)	3772 residents in Queensland, Australia, who were diagnosed with histologically confirmed melanoma between 2000 and 2003
Brady et al (2000)[8]	—	—	—	—	3.6 (OR)	471 newly diagnosed patients with melanoma (1995–1998) at Memorial Sloan-Kettering Cancer Center

Abbreviation: —, not reported.

Table 2
Melanoma thickness in skin self-examination performers versus nonperformers

Study	Mean Thickness (mm) of Melanoma		% Thin (≤0.75 mm) Lesions		Study Population
	SSE Performer	Nonperformer	SSE Performer	Nonperformer	
Carli et al (2003)[16]	0.77	0.95	–	–	816 patients consecutively diagnosed with melanoma at 11 Italian centers (1/2001 to 12/2001)
Berwick et al (1996)[15]	1.09	1.65	–	–	650 Caucasian residents of Connecticut who were newly diagnosed with melanoma (1/15/1987 to 5/15/1989)
McPherson et al (2006)[9]	–	–	71.4	60.8	3772 residents in Queensland, Australia who were diagnosed with histologically confirmed melanoma between 2000 and 2003

Abbreviation: —, not reported.

Several strategies pursued to increase performance of SSE have met with reasonable success. The randomized "Check It Out" trial demonstrated the benefit of sample photographs, an instructional video, a hand mirror, a shower card, and the American Cancer Society brochure, at increasing the performance of SSE.[25] Another study showed that an educational session targeting the patient and their partner resulted in a higher intention of performing SSE.[26] Oliveria and colleagues investigated the impact of a teaching intervention by nurses in which a randomly selected half of the patients received a book of photographs of their entire skin surface. In the teaching intervention group who did not receive a photobook, performance of SSE increased to 37% compared with 20% at baseline.[27] SSE performance was further enhanced to 61.2% for patients who were given total body photographs. These data support the need for continued effort to raise public awareness and competence for the performance of SSE, and the central role of health care providers in the process.

Finding Melanoma in Routine Care

Although patients currently identify most of their own melanomas at an early stage, physicians continue to play an important role in early detection. As noted earlier, physician-detected melanomas are, on average, detected earlier than self-detected lesions (see **Table 1**). For example, in one study, physicians detected significantly thinner melanomas compared with patients (0.23 mm vs 0.9 mm).[10] Others have reported that melanoma detected by dermatologists is associated with a significant effect on diagnosis of lesions <1 mm.[16] Fisher and colleagues[11] compared the thickness in melanomas diagnosed by dermatologists versus other physicians and found that dermatologists were more likely to diagnose lesions less than 0.75 mm in thickness.

Physicians are best positioned to detect clinically subtle melanomas and those that escape the patient's field of view. As noted earlier, physicians are also the ideal provider to educate and train patients in the performance of SSE. There is considerable evidence that there are ample opportunities for physicians to recognize early melanomas in routine care. For example, middle-aged men, who constitute a high-risk group for melanoma, are typically seen up to 4 times a year by a physician.[28]

Despite recognition that total body skin examination (TBSE) by physicians has the potential to identify early melanoma and serves as a model for patient-conducted SSE, the actual rates of TBSE during routine clinical care is low. According to the 1997 National Ambulatory Medical Care Survey (NAMCS) data, skin examinations were performed in 60 million (8.6%) of 703 million office visits, and skin cancer prevention counseling or education occurred in 12 million of those visits (1.5%).[29] In a separate NAMCS study using different search criteria, TBSEs were reportedly performed in 15.8% of all primary care visits.[30]

Additional patient survey studies provide further insight on rates of skin cancer examination. In a survey of veterans more than 40 years of age, 32% reported undergoing TBSEs by their primary care physicians (PCPs); 55% of veterans with a history of skin cancer reported skin examinations, but a larger percentage (87%) stated they would have liked their PCP to perform skin examinations regularly.[31] Using data from the 2000 and 2005 National Health Interview Survey (NHIS), LeBlanc and colleagues[32] reported that 15% of adult workers in the United States had ever had a skin examination. This value differs from the 1998 and 1992 NHIS surveys, which reported a lifetime prevalence of skin examinations in adults in the United States of 20.9% and 20.6%, respectively.[33] Based on these data, it is not surprising that although 63% of patients who later develop melanoma have seen a physician during the year before the diagnosis, only 20% report having undergone a skin examination.[34]

Results from skin cancer–specific surveys of physicians provide another perspective. In a random sample of American dermatologists, 30% (57 of 190) reported performing full-body skin cancer examinations on all adult patients; 49% reported performing examinations on high-risk patients.[35] Other studies have looked at the rates of skin cancer examinations by nondermatologists. Kirsner and colleagues[36] reported that 31% of 465 PCPs performed skin cancer examinations on all adults; a similar value, 37%, was found in another report.[37] When PCPs were asked specifically regarding their high-risk populations, 60% reported performing TBSEs.[38]

According to physician questionnaires, there are numerous barriers to performing full-body skin examinations (**Table 3**). In one survey of dermatologists, lack of time was a significant obstacle for 42% of the respondents; other barriers included embarrassment (9%) and lack of financial reimbursement (9%). In the same study, 37% of dermatologists noted that skin cancer screening was not emphasized during their

Table 3
Barriers to performing skin examinations by physicians

Study	Group	Potential Barriers	% Respondents
Federman et al (2002)[35]	Dermatologists	Lack of time	42
		Poor emphasis on skin cancer screening during training	37
		Patient embarrassment	9
		Lack of financial reimbursement	9
		Lack of evidence to support practice	4
		Inadequate lighting in examination rooms	2
Geller et al (2004)[38]	PCPs	Lack of time	70
		Patient reluctance	35
		Patient comorbidities	34
		Lack of reimbursement	19
		Lack of training	15
		Lack of confidence	7
		Lack of scientific evidence	3

medical training.[35] Similarly, lack of time was found to be the most significant barrier (70%) for PCPs to performing skin cancer examinations on their high-risk patients.[38] Others have shown that 50% of PCPs report lack of confidence as a barrier to performance of full-body skin examinations.[36] This lack of confidence may stem from inadequate coverage of the subject during medical school. Among a group of clinical competencies, 52 third year medical students at UCLA reported being least competent in performing skin cancer examinations.[39] Another barrier is that physicians do not place skin cancer examinations on the same level of importance such as pap smears and breast and digital rectal examinations and as a result, are less likely to perform them.[37]

Efforts have been made to overcome these barriers to skin examinations by physicians. In an attempt to target medical school curricula, Doshi and colleagues assessed the impact of a pilot course designed to educate medical students on the performance of skin cancer examinations. In comparing pretest to posttest scores, students showed an increase in knowledge and confidence in conducting a skin examination.[40] Several studies have focused on improving the diagnostic skills of PCPs. Following a lecture on melanoma, the sensitivity of general practitioners (GPs) to recognize malignant lesions increased from 72% to 84%.[41] Carli and colleagues evaluated the impact of a 4-hour course for 41 family physicians practicing in Florence. Following the training, the number of melanomas correctly classified increased and the number of benign lesions referred to a dermatologist decreased significantly.[42] Similarly, participation in an Internet-based continuing medical education course by PCPs resulted in an increase in specificity with a small decrease in sensitivity in the evaluation of pigmented skin lesions (PSLs).[43] Another study showed that a 2-hour basic skin cancer triage curriculum designed for PCPs resulted in a significant increase in diagnostic accuracy, triaging skills, and knowledge of skin cancer control.[44] A discussion on dermoscopy follows later, but it has been reported that a course on dermoscopy improved the accuracy of PCPs to appropriately triage suspicious lesions; significant differences were observed in referral sensitivity (from 54.1% to 79.2%) and negative predictive value (from 95.8% to 98.1%).[45]

Criteria for Skin Cancer Recognition

Whether a skin examination is performed by the physician or the patient, it is important for the examiner to be able to recognize the features concerning lesions. In the 1980s, the ABCD (Asymmetry, Border irregularity, Color variation, Diameter >5 mm) rule was developed to raise awareness of the features of skin lesion that are suggestive of melanoma.[14] This diagnostic aid has recently been modified to include E, for evolution, to capture lesions that change morphology over time but do not fulfill the ABCD criteria.[46] Brandstrom and colleagues[47] demonstrated that lay people make adequate self-referral decisions based on the ABCD criteria. Another recently publicized aid to melanoma detection has been the so-called "ugly duckling" sign which promotes recognition of morphologic outliers among pigmented lesions.[48] In a preliminary study, Scope and colleagues[49] demonstrated that clinicians and lay people can intuitively recognize lesions that stand out as distinct in color or size from a patient's many other moles and that these outliers are sensitive markers of melanoma.

Screening for Melanoma

Whereas screening is recommended for breast, prostate, cervical, and colon cancer, guidelines for periodic skin cancer examinations are inconsistent. Since 1993, the American Cancer Society has recommended skin cancer screening as part of cancer-related checkups for people aged 20 years and older. However, other groups disagree. In 2000, the Institute of Medicine issued the following statement: "the evidence of skin cancer screening is insufficient to support positive or negative conclusions about a new program of clinical screening of asymptomatic Medicare beneficiaries."[50] A similar statement followed in 2001 by the Third United States Preventive Services Task Force: "evidence is lacking that skin examination by clinicians is effective in reducing mortality or morbidity from skin cancer."[51]

Despite the lack of official guidelines, numerous screening programs have been performed in an effort to diagnose earlier forms of melanoma. Screening efforts in the United States were initiated as early as 1985 by the American Academy of Dermatology (AAD) and continue to this day. In a survey of participants with suspected melanomas in the 1992 to 1994 programs, Koh and colleagues showed that more than 90% of melanomas detected measured less than 1.5 mm in depth. Melanomas at a less advanced stage were found during screenings, in comparison to the 1990 Surveillance, Epidemiology and End Result Registry (SEERR) data. Thirty-nine percent of participants screened who were found to have melanoma indicated that they participated in the program because there was no fee.[52]

Multiple screening initiatives have also been conducted outside the United States. In a media and screening campaign in Belgium, a total of 166 melanomas were detected during a 1-month period, representing nearly one fifth of all melanomas typically diagnosed in Belgium each year.[53] In an Italian campaign, 1042 individuals were screened, resulting in the detection of 3 melanomas, 2 of which were less than 0.30 mm in thickness.[54] Similar studies have been performed in Greece[55] and Australia.[56]

Only one study to date has been able to demonstrate a possible impact of screening on mortality. Schneider and colleagues reported that an educational and screening campaign for workers at the Lawrence Livermore National Laboratory decreased melanoma-related mortality to 0. In addition, a decrease in incidence of melanomas thicker than 0.75 mm was also found.[57]

Researchers using mathematical models have demonstrated that a one-time melanoma screening of individuals greater than 50 years old is cost-effective; they have also shown that screening siblings of melanoma patients every 2 years is also cost-effective.[58] Similar results were found in an earlier analysis that supported screening of men older than 50 years every 5 years by family physicians.[59]

Although it may be ideal to conduct skin examinations on every individual who presents to a mass screening event, it has been suggested that focusing efforts on individuals with multiple risk factors may increase the number of melanomas detected, and at the same time reduce costs. Using data from the 2001 to 2005 AAD Screening program, Goldberg and colleagues[60] created the *HARMM* criteria summarizing the most statistically significant risk factors for melanoma: History of previous melanoma (OR = 3.3), Age more than 50 years (OR = 1.2), Regular dermatologist absent (OR = 1.4), Mole changing (OR = 2.0), and Male gender (OR = 1.4). Similarly, Fears and colleagues[61] created a mathematical model to predict the 5-year absolute risk of melanoma for a Caucasian man or woman between the ages of 20 and 70 years. This model uses data input that is easily obtained from a routine history and physical examination, such as tanning tendencies, freckling of the skin, and the number of small and large moles. **Table 4** summarizes these and other risk factors as well as corresponding estimated relative risks. A user-friendly online version of this tool is available at the National Cancer Institute Web site.[62] Others at increased risk for melanoma who have been considered for screening include transplant patients[63] and individuals with a history of actinic keratosis[64] and nonmelanoma skin cancer.[65,66]

Specialized Pigmented Lesion Clinic (PLC)

In recent years, specialized clinics have been created targeting patients at high risk for melanoma. PLCs employ skin cancer experts trained in advanced diagnostic techniques. With the introduction of a PLC in Scotland, 67% of patients with worrisome lesions were able to be seen within 3 months in 2001 compared with 16% in 1986.[67] Using the benign/malignant ratio as a measure of performance, Carli and colleagues[68] found a substantially lower ratio in Italian PLCs (5.8:1) compared with a large group of Australian family doctors (17:1).[69] In another study, Carli and colleagues described the sensitivity (86.7%), specificity (95.4%), positive predictive

Table 4		
Model to estimate relative risk of melanoma based on selected factors		
Gender	**Factor**	**Relative Risk Estimate**
Male	Any blistering burn	1.437
	Light complexion	1.767
	≥2 large moles	2.412
	7–16 small moles	1.935
	≥17 small moles	4.630
	More than mild freckling	1.830
	Severe solar damage	2.803
	Attributable risk	0.856
Female	Light complexion	1.802
	Light or no tan	1.926
	5–11 small moles	2.512
	≥12 small moles	5.154
	Mild freckling	2.174
	More extensive freckling	3.856
	Attributable risk	0.894

Data from Fears TR, Guerry DT, Pfeiffer RM, et al. Identifying individuals at high risk of melanoma: a practical predictor of absolute risk. J Clin Oncol 2006;24(22):3590–6.

value (13.7%), and negative predictive value (99.9%) at detecting melanoma in an Italian PLC.[70] Other investigators demonstrated a false-negative rate of 29%, 22%, and 10%, for general dermatology, plastic surgery, and pigmented lesion clinics, respectively, suggesting that PLCs outperform less specialized care.[71] The logistics of a large PLC based in the United States have been well described in the literature.[72]

Instruments to Aid in the Diagnosis of Melanoma

Recent advances in technology have provided clinicians with better in vivo imaging tools as means to detect earlier forms of melanoma. The 2 most commonly used techniques are total body photography (**Fig. 1**) and dermoscopy (**Fig. 2**, A2 and B2).

Total body photography (TBP) is useful for following patients who are at high risk for melanoma. One of the goals is to detect subtle changes over time in lesions that may otherwise go unnoticed by pure clinical examination; this is especially useful in a patient with 100s of lesions. A patient initially undergoes a series of baseline images. These photographs are then compared with the patient's examination at follow-up

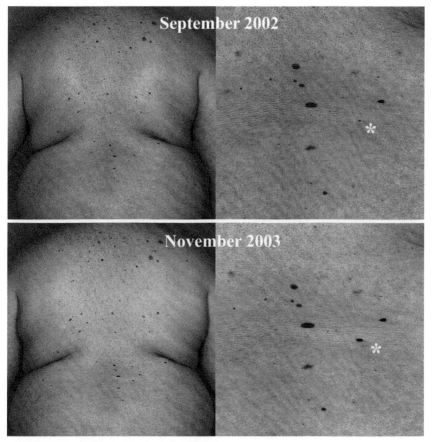

Fig. 1. Total body photography. Serial photography allows monitoring of changes in lesions that may be unnoticed during follow-up clinical examination alone. Note the change in the lesion size (*star*) from September 2002 to November 2003.

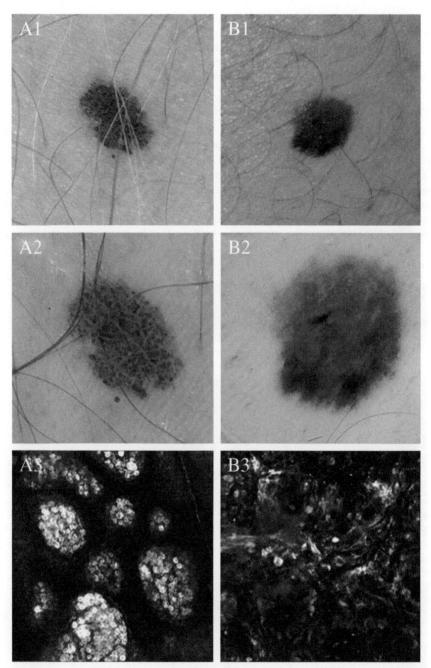

Fig. 2. Clinical, dermoscopic, and confocal images of a benign globular nevus (*A1–A3*) and melanoma (*B1–B3*).

visits. Lesions that remain the same are presumed benign, barring specific clinical or dermoscopic signs of melanoma. New and changing lesions can be further evaluated, a biopsy taken, or followed for additional change.

According to a 2002 study of academic dermatology programs, 63%[73] reported using TBP compared with 41%[74] in 1992. Nehal and colleagues[73] also reported that the establishment of a PLC correlated with the use of TBP, with 83% of programs with PLCs using TBP compared with 49% programs without PLCs.

Numerous retrospective studies have assessed the use of TBP for detecting melanoma in high-risk cohorts. Feit and colleagues reviewed the charts of 576 patients who underwent TBP. Out of 77 histologically proven melanomas, biopsies were carried out in 74% due to subtle changes from baseline and in 19% because there were new lesions. The lesions that changed from their baseline did not demonstrate the classic clinical features of melanoma.[75] In another study, 309 high-risk patients were followed for a median time of 34 months. Median melanoma thickness detected in the study was 0.39 mm compared with 0.60 mm for the general population during 1992 to 1998.[76] Wang and colleagues[77] followed a group of high-risk patients and demonstrated that 42% of detected melanomas were in situ; the mean thickness of invasive melanoma was 0.55 mm.

TBP has also been shown to have a positive impact on efficacy of SSE by patients. Oliveria and colleagues[78] demonstrated that TBP resulted in an increase in the sensitivity (from 60.2% to 96.2%) and specificity (from 72.4% to 98.4%) of patients performing self-examination of their skin. In the study by Feit and colleagues,[75] 30% of histologically proven melanomas were identified on SSEs in patients undergoing TBP.

Dermoscopy is another technique that is being increasingly adopted by physicians in the United States. In a study carried out in 2005, nearly 1 in 5 of 1200 randomly selected dermatologists in the United States reported using dermoscopy for the evaluation of PSLs.[79] According to a 2002 survey of academic dermatologists associated with residency training programs, 51% of respondents reporting using this device.[80]

In this technique, use of a magnifying lens and either polarized light or a fluid interface permits visualization of structures within the epidermis and papillary dermis invisible to the naked eye. Several diagnostic algorithms for melanoma recognition have been created in recent years; these include the Menzie's method,[81] the ABCD rule,[82] the 7-point checklist,[83] and the CASH algorithm.[84]

Multiple studies have demonstrated the positive impact that dermoscopy has made on distinguishing benign from malignant lesions. A metaanalysis of 27 studies demonstrated an improvement in diagnostic accuracy of 49%, with an increase in specificity and sensitivity of 6% and 19%, respectively.[85] In a randomized controlled trial designed to assess pigmented lesion management with the use of dermoscopy, Carli and colleagues[86] reported a reduction in the number of patients referred for biopsy (9.0% vs 15.6%). This group also demonstrated a decrease in the benign/malignant ratio from 18:1 to 4:1 following the introduction of dermoscopy into clinical practice.[87]

Dermoscopy may also be used in the follow-up of patients with suspicious lesions. Menzies and colleagues followed suspicious lesions in patients at intervals of 3 months. Melanoma was diagnosed in 11% of all changed lesions following biopsy. These melanoma cases did not demonstrate any classic features on clinical examination. The specificity for the diagnosis of melanoma in this study was reported to be 83%.[88] Others have used dermoscopy in long-term monitoring of patients at risk for melanoma, such as those with dysplastic nevus syndrome, with the goal of decreasing unnecessary excisions.[89,90] One study followed patients for a median of 25 month and although 128 (6%) lesions showed some change, only 33 were excised due to suspicious changes found on dermoscopy.[89]

To encourage widespread use of dermoscopy, proponents have demonstrated that dermoscopy adds only 72 seconds to a clinical skin examination.[91] Other supporters have shown that it is possible to easily educate nonexperts on pigmented lesions.[92,93] One study showed a significant improvement in diagnostic accuracy after nonexperts performed a web-based tutorial.[92] Similar results were found by Troyanova.[93] Short-term training of dermatology residents has also been shown to increase confidence when classifying challenging PSLs.[94]

Exciting technologies under development for improved melanoma diagnosis include teledermoscopy, reflectance confocal microscopy (RCM) (see **Fig. 2**, A3 and B3), and multispectral imaging.

Capturing and forwarding dermoscopic images by way of the Internet to a distant location for expert opinion is referred to as teledermoscopy. Numerous studies have assessed the feasibility of this tool in the diagnosis of PSLs. Piccolo and colleagues[95] demonstrated that the concordance between face-to-face diagnosis and teledermoscopy was 91%. Another study reported that the diagnostic accuracy of teledermoscopy may be superior to conventional dermoscopic diagnosis, specifically for malignant melanocytic lesions.[96] Another group evaluated teledermoscopy in skin cancer triage in a large multicenter study. In a total of 2009 teleconsultations, one group demonstrated significant intraobserver agreement for the management decision (k = 0.91) and diagnosis (k = 0.83).[97] Hsiao and colleagues reported comparable, if not better, clinical outcomes with regard to time to initial consult completion, time to biopsy, and time to surgery, for patients with skin cancer if evaluated by teledermoscopy compared with conventional referrals to dermatology clinics.[98] With regard to patient satisfaction, teledermoscopy is comparable to conventional traditional outpatient consultation.[99]

RCM is an optical imaging technique that allows in vivo visualization of structures from the epidermis through the superficial dermis, with near histologic resolution.[100] An image is created using a low-power laser beam directed onto a small point on the skin. This beam is scanned in 2 dimensions, resulting in an axial optical section below the surface similar in thickness (5 μm) and resolution (1 μm) to a histologic section of excised tissue.[100] RCM may prove especially useful for the evaluation of melanocytic lesions because melanin and melanosomes provide strong contrast in the images.[101] In contrast to histopathologic sections, RCM imaging preserves tissue architecture and allows users to repeatedly assess the same lesions over time.[102]

The use of RCM as a diagnostic tool for melanocytic lesions has been evaluated by several studies. In 2002, Busam and colleagues[103] reported that it is possible to recognize intraepidermal melanoma on RCM using the same criteria used for conventional histologic diagnosis. Features of melanoma on RCM include atypical cells, isolated nucleated cells within dermal papillae, nonedged dermal papillae, and cerebriform clusters.[104] One study assessed the sensitivity and specificity of RCM and showed that melanoma can be differentiated from other lesions with a positive predictive value of 94.2%. The interobserver agreement with regard to distinct RCM features of melanoma resulted in a k value >0.80.[105] Another study demonstrated a sensitivity of 97.5% and specificity of 99% for melanocytic lesions.[106] Langley and colleagues compared the diagnostic accuracy of in RCM to that of dermoscopy and demonstrated a higher sensitivity (97.3% vs 89.2%) but a lower specificity (83.0% vs 84.1%). The investigators concluded that these tools should be used in conjunction with one another.[107] Others recommend that RCM be used in the secondary evaluation of lesions that have been deemed suspicious by dermoscopy.[108]

Multispectral imaging is an optical technique that has been applied to the evaluation of PSLs. The technique entails analysis of images produced using multiple discreet wavelengths of light. Two commercial multispectral imaging systems are currently available: the SIAscope and Melafind. The SIAscope uses 4 different wavelengths that interact with collagen, melanin, and hemoglobin chromophores, thereby providing information on melanin distribution, skin vasculature, and collagen quantity within the skin. The resulting graphs and images are then interpreted for diagnosis. Moncrieff and colleagues[109] described features on SIAscopy that had a sensitivity of 82.7% and specificity of 80.1% for melanoma. One study evaluated the impact of SIAscopy on the triage of pigmented lesions and showed a sensitivity of 94.4% and false negative rate of 3.7% for melanoma; the investigators concluded that this tool may be useful in decreasing the number of benign lesions referred to a specialist.[110] Although SIAscopy has the potential to be an effective triaging tool, Haniffa reported that it does not provide any benefit to a dermatologist attempting to distinguish malignant from benign lesions.[111] MelaFind uses fully automated multispectral imaging to provide a rapid, nonoperator-dependent diagnosis of lesions. Elbaum and colleagues demonstrated a specificity of 68% to 85% and a sensitivity of 95% to 100% in the differentiation of malignant melanoma in situ and invasive malignant melanoma from dysplastic and other atypical nevi.[112]

Several systems, such as Dermogenius Ultra, FotoFinder, and Microderm, have been developed to use machine vision to perform automated analysis of conventional or dermoscopic images of lesions.[113] One example, SolarScan, is an automated dermoscopy image analysis system. In the diagnosis of melanoma, Menzies and colleagues[114] reported that SolarScan (sensitivity 85%, specificity 65%) performed as well as or better than experts (sensitivity 90%, specificity 59%), dermatologists (sensitivity 81%, specificity 60%), trainees (sensitivity 85%, specificity 36%), and general practitioners (sensitivity 62%, specificity 63%).

FUTURE DIRECTIONS

Much progress has been made in developing strategies for the early detection of melanoma. There have been significant advancements in diagnostic technology, increased awareness of the importance of self-examination of the skin and total body examination, and the creation of screening programs designed to detect earlier melanoma.

However, the incidence and mortality of melanoma continues to be on the increase and therefore additional efforts are necessary. Potential interventions include placing more emphasis on the educational curriculum of medical students, incorporating technology into practice, continuing to promote self-examinations of the skin by patients and total body skin examinations by physicians, and creating efficient algorithms to triage suspicious lesions effectively. The usefulness of screening should be formally tested in randomized clinical trials, but pending such data, continued attempts to screen high-risk groups seem warranted. In addition, secondary prevention efforts should be integrated with primary prevention educational campaigns.

REFERENCES

1. American Cancer Society. Cancer facts & figures 2008. Atlanta (GA): American Cancer Society; 2008.
2. Bickers DR, Lim HW, Margolis D, et al. The burden of skin diseases: 2004 a joint project of the American Academy of Dermatology Association and the Society for Investigative Dermatology. J Am Acad Dermatol 2006;55(3):490–500.

3. Kyle JW, Hammitt JK, Lim HW, et al. Economic evaluation of the US Environmental Protection Agency's SunWise program: sun protection education for young children. Pediatrics 2008;121(5):e1074–84.
4. Dobbinson SJ, Wakefield MA, Jamsen KM, et al. Weekend sun protection and sunburn in Australia trends (1987–2002) and association with SunSmart television advertising. Am J Prev Med 2008;34(2):94–101.
5. Balch CM, Buzaid AC, Soong SJ, et al. Final version of the American Joint Committee on Cancer staging system for cutaneous melanoma. J Clin Oncol 2001;19(16):3635–48.
6. Halpern AC, Lieb JA. Early melanoma diagnosis: a success story that leaves room for improvement. Curr Opin Oncol 2007;19(2):109–15.
7. Weinstock MA. Progress and prospects on melanoma: the way forward for early detection and reduced mortality. Clin Cancer Res 2006;12(7 Pt 2):2297s–300s.
8. Brady MS, Oliveria SA, Christos PJ, et al. Patterns of detection in patients with cutaneous melanoma. Cancer 2000;89(2):342–7.
9. McPherson M, Elwood M, English DR, et al. Presentation and detection of invasive melanoma in a high-risk population. J Am Acad Dermatol 2006;54(5): 783–92.
10. Epstein DS, Lange JR, Gruber SB, et al. Is physician detection associated with thinner melanomas? JAMA 1999;281(7):640–3.
11. Fisher NM, Schaffer JV, Berwick M, et al. Breslow depth of cutaneous melanoma: impact of factors related to surveillance of the skin, including prior skin biopsies and family history of melanoma. J Am Acad Dermatol 2005;53(3):393–406.
12. Schwartz JL, Wang TS, Hamilton TA, et al. Thin primary cutaneous melanomas: associated detection patterns, lesion characteristics, and patient characteristics. Cancer 2002;95(7):1562–8.
13. Oliveria SA, Christos PJ, Halpern AC, et al. Patient knowledge, awareness, and delay in seeking medical attention for malignant melanoma. J Clin Epidemiol 1999;52(11):1111–6.
14. Friedman RJ, Rigel DS, Kopf AW. Early detection of malignant melanoma: the role of physician examination and self-examination of the skin. CA Cancer J Clin 1985;35(3):130–51.
15. Berwick M, Begg CB, Fine JA, et al. Screening for cutaneous melanoma by skin self-examination. J Natl Cancer Inst 1996;88(1):17–23.
16. Carli P, De Giorgi V, Palli D, et al. Dermatologist detection and skin self-examination are associated with thinner melanomas: results from a survey of the Italian Multidisciplinary Group on Melanoma. Arch Dermatol 2003;139(5): 607–12.
17. Muhn CY, From L, Glied M. Detection of artificial changes in mole size by skin self-examination. J Am Acad Dermatol 2000;42(5 Pt 1):754–9.
18. Carli P, De Giorgi V, Palli D, et al. Self-detected cutaneous melanomas in Italian patients. Clin Exp Dermatol 2004;29(6):593–6.
19. Aitken JF, Janda M, Lowe JB, et al. Prevalence of whole-body skin self-examination in a population at high risk for skin cancer (Australia). Cancer Causes Control 2004;15(5):453–63.
20. Arnold MR, DeJong W. Skin self-examination practices in a convenience sample of U.S. university students. Prev Med 2005;40(3):268–73.
21. Weinstock MA, Martin RA, Risica PM, et al. Thorough skin examination for the early detection of melanoma. Am J Prev Med 1999;17(3):169–75.
22. Robinson JK, Fisher SG, Turrisi RJ. Predictors of skin self-examination performance. Cancer 2002;95(1):135–46.

23. Oliveria SA, Christos PJ, Halpern AC, et al. Evaluation of factors associated with skin self-examination. Cancer Epidemiol Biomarkers Prev 1999;8(11):971–8.
24. Weinstock MA, Risica PM, Martin RA, et al. Reliability of assessment and circumstances of performance of thorough skin self-examination for the early detection of melanoma in the Check-It-Out Project. Prev Med 2004;38(6):761–5.
25. Lee KB, Weinstock MA, Risica PM. Components of a successful intervention for monthly skin self-examination for early detection of melanoma: the "Check It Out" trial. J Am Acad Dermatol 2008;58(6):1006–12.
26. Robinson JK, Turrisi R, Stapleton J. Efficacy of a partner assistance intervention designed to increase skin self-examination performance. Arch Dermatol 2007; 143(1):37–41.
27. Oliveria SA, Dusza SW, Phelan DL, et al. Patient adherence to skin self-examination: effect of nurse intervention with photographs. Am J Prev Med 2004;26(2): 152–5.
28. National Center for Health Statistics. Health, United States, 2005. With chartbook and trends in the health of Americans. Hyattsville (MD): National Center for Health Statistics; 2005.
29. Feldman SR, Fleischer AB Jr. Skin examinations and skin cancer prevention counseling by US physicians: a long way to go. J Am Acad Dermatol 2000; 43(2 Pt 1):234–7.
30. Oliveria SA, Christos PJ, Marghoob AA, et al. Skin cancer screening and prevention in the primary care setting: national ambulatory medical care survey 1997. J Gen Intern Med 2001;16(5):297–301.
31. Federman DG, Kravetz JD, Tobin DG, et al. Full-body skin examinations: the patient's perspective. Arch Dermatol 2004;140(5):530–4.
32. LeBlanc WG, Vidal L, Kirsner RS, et al. Reported skin cancer screening of US adult workers. J Am Acad Dermatol 2008;59(1):55–63.
33. Saraiya M, Hall HI, Thompson T, et al. Skin cancer screening among U.S. adults from 1992, 1998, and 2000 National Health Interview Surveys. Prev Med 2004; 39(2):308–14.
34. Geller AC, Koh HK, Miller DR, et al. Use of health services before the diagnosis of melanoma: implications for early detection and screening. J Gen Intern Med 1992;7(2):154–7.
35. Federman DG, Kravetz JD, Kirsner RS. Skin cancer screening by dermatologists: prevalence and barriers. J Am Acad Dermatol 2002;46(5):710–4.
36. Kirsner RS, Muhkerjee S, Federman DG. Skin cancer screening in primary care: prevalence and barriers. J Am Acad Dermatol 1999;41(4):564–6.
37. Altman JF, Oliveria SA, Christos PJ, et al. A survey of skin cancer screening in the primary care setting: a comparison with other cancer screenings. Arch Fam Med 2000;9(10):1022–7.
38. Geller AC, O'Riordan DL, Oliveria SA, et al. Overcoming obstacles to skin cancer examinations and prevention counseling for high-risk patients: results of a national survey of primary care physicians. J Am Board Fam Pract 2004; 17(6):416–23.
39. Lee M, Hodgson CS, Wilkerson L. Predictors of self-perceived competency in cancer screening examinations. J Cancer Educ 2002;17(4):180–2.
40. Doshi DN, Firth K, Mintz M, et al. Pilot study of a skin cancer education curriculum for medical students. J Am Acad Dermatol 2007;56(1):167–9.
41. Brochez L, Verhaeghe E, Bleyen L, et al. Diagnostic ability of general practitioners and dermatologists in discriminating pigmented skin lesions. J Am Acad Dermatol 2001;44(6):979–86.

42. Carli P, De Giorgi V, Crocetti E, et al. Diagnostic and referral accuracy of family doctors in melanoma screening: effect of a short formal training. Eur J Cancer Prev 2005;14(1):51–5.

43. Harris JM, Salasche SJ, Harris RB. Can Internet-based continuing medical education improve physicians' skin cancer knowledge and skills? J Gen Intern Med 2001;16(1):50–6.

44. Mikkilineni R, Weinstock MA, Goldstein MG, et al. The impact of the basic skin cancer triage curriculum on providers' skills, confidence, and knowledge in skin cancer control. Prev Med 2002;34(2):144–52.

45. Argenziano G, Puig S, Zalaudek I, et al. Dermoscopy improves accuracy of primary care physicians to triage lesions suggestive of skin cancer. J Clin Oncol 2006;24(12):1877–82.

46. Abbasi NR, Shaw HM, Rigel DS, et al. Early diagnosis of cutaneous melanoma: revisiting the ABCD criteria. JAMA 2004;292(22):2771–6.

47. Branstrom R, Hedblad MA, Krakau I, et al. Laypersons' perceptual discrimination of pigmented skin lesions. J Am Acad Dermatol 2002;46(5):667–73.

48. Grob JJ, Bonerandi JJ. The 'ugly duckling' sign: identification of the common characteristics of nevi in an individual as a basis for melanoma screening. Arch Dermatol 1998;134(1):103–4.

49. Scope A, Dusza SW, Halpern AC, et al. The "ugly duckling" sign: agreement between observers. Arch Dermatol 2008;144(1):58–64.

50. Institute of Medicine. Extending Medicare coverage for preventive and other services. Washington, DC: National Academy Press; 2000.

51. Berg AO, Allan JD. Introducing the third US Preventive Services Task Force. Am J Prev Med 2001;20(3 Suppl):3–4.

52. Koh HK, Norton LA, Geller AC, et al. Evaluation of the American Academy of Dermatology's National Skin Cancer Early Detection and Screening Program. J Am Acad Dermatol 1996;34(6):971–8.

53. Vandaele MM, Richert B, Van der Endt JD, et al. Melanoma screening: results of the first one-day campaign in Belgium ('melanoma Monday'). J Eur Acad Dermatol Venereol 2000;14(6):470–2.

54. Carli P, De Giorgi V, Giannotti B, et al. Skin cancer day in Italy: method of referral to open access clinics and tumor prevalence in the examined population. Eur J Dermatol 2003;13(1):76–9.

55. Stratigos A, Nikolaou V, Kedicoglou S, et al. Melanoma/skin cancer screening in a Mediterranean country: results of the Euromelanoma Screening Day Campaign in Greece. J Eur Acad Dermatol Venereol 2007;21(1):56–62.

56. Aitken JF, Janda M, Elwood M, et al. Clinical outcomes from skin screening clinics within a community-based melanoma screening program. J Am Acad Dermatol 2006;54(1):105–14.

57. Schneider JS, Moore DH 2nd, Mendelsohn ML. Screening program reduced melanoma mortality at the Lawrence Livermore National Laboratory, 1984 to 1996. J Am Acad Dermatol 2008;58(5):741–9.

58. Losina E, Walensky RP, Geller A, et al. Visual screening for malignant melanoma: a cost-effectiveness analysis. Arch Dermatol 2007;143(1):21–8.

59. Girgis A, Clarke P, Burton RC, et al. Screening for melanoma by primary health care physicians: a cost-effectiveness analysis. J Med Screen 1996; 3(1):47–53.

60. Goldberg MS, Doucette JT, Lim HW, et al. Risk factors for presumptive melanoma in skin cancer screening: American Academy of Dermatology National

Melanoma/Skin Cancer Screening Program experience 2001–2005. J Am Acad Dermatol 2007;57(1):60–6.
61. Fears TR, Guerry D IV, Pfeiffer RM, et al. Identifying individuals at high risk of melanoma: a practical predictor of absolute risk. J Clin Oncol 2006;24(22): 3590–6.
62. National Cancer Institute: melanoma risk assessment tool. Available at: http://www.cancer.gov/melanomarisktool/. Accessed December 8, 2008.
63. Hollenbeak CS, Todd MM, Billingsley EM, et al. Increased incidence of melanoma in renal transplantation recipients. Cancer 2005;104(9):1962–7.
64. Ferrone CR, Ben Porat L, Panageas KS, et al. Clinicopathological features of and risk factors for multiple primary melanomas. JAMA 2005;294(13):1647–54.
65. Bower CP, Lear JT, Bygrave S, et al. Basal cell carcinoma and risk of subsequent malignancies: a cancer registry-based study in southwest England. J Am Acad Dermatol 2000;42(6):988–91.
66. Maitra SK, Gallo H, Rowland-Payne C, et al. Second primary cancers in patients with squamous cell carcinoma of the skin. Br J Cancer 2005;92(3):570–1.
67. MacKie RM, Bray CA, Leman JA. Effect of public education aimed at early diagnosis of malignant melanoma: cohort comparison study. BMJ 2003;326(7385): 367.
68. Carli P, De Giorgi V, Betti R, et al. Relationship between cause of referral and diagnostic outcome in pigmented lesion clinics: a multicentre survey of the Italian Multidisciplinary Group on Melanoma (GIPMe). Melanoma Res 2003; 13(2):207–11.
69. English DR, Burton RC, del Mar CB, et al. Evaluation of aid to diagnosis of pigmented skin lesions in general practice: controlled trial randomised by practice. BMJ 2003;327(7411):375.
70. Carli P, Nardini P, Crocetti E, et al. Frequency and characteristics of melanomas missed at a pigmented lesion clinic: a registry-based study. Melanoma Res 2004;14(5):403–7.
71. Osborne JE, Chave TA, Hutchinson PE. Comparison of diagnostic accuracy for cutaneous malignant melanoma between general dermatology, plastic surgery and pigmented lesion clinics. Br J Dermatol 2003;148(2):252–8.
72. Johnson TM, Chang A, Redman B, et al. Management of melanoma with a multidisciplinary melanoma clinic model. J Am Acad Dermatol 2000;42 (5 Pt 1):820–6.
73. Nehal KS, Oliveria SA, Marghoob AA, et al. Use of and beliefs about baseline photography in the management of patients with pigmented lesions: a survey of dermatology residency programmes in the United States. Melanoma Res 2002;12(2):161–7.
74. Shriner DL, Wagner RF Jr, Glowczwski JR. Photography for the early diagnosis of malignant melanoma in patients with atypical moles. Cutis 1992; 50(5):358–62.
75. Feit NE, Dusza SW, Marghoob AA. Melanomas detected with the aid of total cutaneous photography. Br J Dermatol 2004;150(4):706–14.
76. Banky JP, Kelly JW, English DR, et al. Incidence of new and changed nevi and melanomas detected using baseline images and dermoscopy in patients at high risk for melanoma. Arch Dermatol 2005;141(8):998–1006.
77. Wang SQ, Kopf AW, Koenig K, et al. Detection of melanomas in patients followed up with total cutaneous examinations, total cutaneous photography, and dermoscopy. J Am Acad Dermatol 2004;50(1):15–20.

78. Oliveria SA, Chau D, Christos PJ, et al. Diagnostic accuracy of patients in performing skin self-examination and the impact of photography. Arch Dermatol 2004;140(1):57–62.

79. Charles CA, Yee VS, Dusza SW, et al. Variation in the diagnosis, treatment, and management of melanoma in situ: a survey of US dermatologists. Arch Dermatol 2005;141(6):723–9.

80. Nehal KS, Oliveria SA, Marghoob AA, et al. Use of and beliefs about dermoscopy in the management of patients with pigmented lesions: a survey of dermatology residency programmes in the United States. Melanoma Res 2002;12(6):601–5.

81. Menzies SW, Ingvar C, Crotty KA, et al. Frequency and morphologic characteristics of invasive melanomas lacking specific surface microscopic features. Arch Dermatol 1996;132(10):1178–82.

82. Nachbar F, Stolz W, Merkle T, et al. The ABCD rule of dermatoscopy. High prospective value in the diagnosis of doubtful melanocytic skin lesions. J Am Acad Dermatol 1994;30(4):551–9.

83. Argenziano G, Fabbrocini G, Carli P, et al. Epiluminescence microscopy for the diagnosis of doubtful melanocytic skin lesions. Comparison of the ABCD rule of dermatoscopy and a new 7-point checklist based on pattern analysis. Arch Dermatol 1998;134(12):1563–70.

84. Henning JS, Dusza SW, Wang SQ, et al. The CASH (color, architecture, symmetry, and homogeneity) algorithm for dermoscopy. J Am Acad Dermatol 2007;56(1):45–52.

85. Kittler H, Pehamberger H, Wolff K, et al. Diagnostic accuracy of dermoscopy. Lancet Oncol 2002;3(3):159–65.

86. Carli P, de Giorgi V, Chiarugi A, et al. Addition of dermoscopy to conventional naked-eye examination in melanoma screening: a randomized study. J Am Acad Dermatol 2004;50(5):683–9.

87. Carli P, De Giorgi V, Crocetti E, et al. Improvement of malignant/benign ratio in excised melanocytic lesions in the 'dermoscopy era': a retrospective study 1997-2001. Br J Dermatol 2004;150(4):687–92.

88. Menzies SW, Gutenev A, Avramidis M, et al. Short-term digital surface microscopic monitoring of atypical or changing melanocytic lesions. Arch Dermatol 2001;137(12):1583–9.

89. Bauer J, Metzler G, Rassner G, et al. Dermatoscopy turns histopathologist's attention to the suspicious area in melanocytic lesions. Arch Dermatol 2001; 137(10):1338–40.

90. Kittler H, Guitera P, Riedl E, et al. Identification of clinically featureless incipient melanoma using sequential dermoscopy imaging. Arch Dermatol 2006;142(9):1113–9.

91. Zalaudek I, Kittler H, Marghoob AA, et al. Time required for a complete skin examination with and without dermoscopy: a prospective, randomized multicenter study. Arch Dermatol 2008;144(4):509–13.

92. Pagnanelli G, Soyer HP, Argenziano G, et al. Diagnosis of pigmented skin lesions by dermoscopy: web-based training improves diagnostic performance of non-experts. Br J Dermatol 2003;148(4):698–702.

93. Troyanova P. A beneficial effect of a short-term formal training course in epiluminescence microscopy on the diagnostic performance of dermatologists about cutaneous malignant melanoma. Skin Res Technol 2003;9(3):269–73.

94. Benvenuto-Andrade C, Dusza SW, Hay JL, et al. Level of confidence in diagnosis: clinical examination versus dermoscopy examination. Dermatol Surg 2006;32(5):738–44.

95. Piccolo D, Smolle J, Wolf IH, et al. Face-to-face diagnosis vs telediagnosis of pigmented skin tumors: a teledermoscopic study. Arch Dermatol 1999; 135(12):1467–71.

96. Braun RP, Meier M, Pelloni F, et al. Teledermatoscopy in Switzerland: a preliminary evaluation. J Am Acad Dermatol 2000;42(5 Pt 1):770–5.

97. Moreno-Ramirez D, Ferrandiz L, Nieto-Garcia A, et al. Store-and-forward teledermatology in skin cancer triage: experience and evaluation of 2009 teleconsultations. Arch Dermatol 2007;143(4):479–84.

98. Hsiao JL, Oh DH. The impact of store-and-forward teledermatology on skin cancer diagnosis and treatment. J Am Acad Dermatol 2008;59(2):260–7.

99. Collins K, Walters S, Bowns I. Patient satisfaction with teledermatology: quantitative and qualitative results from a randomized controlled trial. J Telemed Telecare 2004;10(1):29–33.

100. Rajadhyaksha M, Gonzalez S, Zavislan JM, et al. In vivo confocal scanning laser microscopy of human skin II: advances in instrumentation and comparison with histology. J Invest Dermatol 1999;113(3):293–303.

101. Rajadhyaksha M, Grossman M, Esterowitz D, et al. In vivo confocal scanning laser microscopy of human skin: melanin provides strong contrast. J Invest Dermatol 1995;104(6):946–52.

102. Aghassi D, Anderson RR, Gonzalez S. Time-sequence histologic imaging of laser-treated cherry angiomas with in vivo confocal microscopy. J Am Acad Dermatol 2000;43(1 Pt 1):37–41.

103. Busam KJ, Charles C, Lohmann CM, et al. Detection of intraepidermal malignant melanoma in vivo by confocal scanning laser microscopy. Melanoma Res 2002; 12(4):349–55.

104. Pellacani G, Cesinaro AM, Seidenari S. Reflectance-mode confocal microscopy of pigmented skin lesions – improvement in melanoma diagnostic specificity. J Am Acad Dermatol 2005;53(6):979–85.

105. Gerger A, Koller S, Weger W, et al. Sensitivity and specificity of confocal laser-scanning microscopy for in vivo diagnosis of malignant skin tumors. Cancer 2006;107(1):193–200.

106. Gerger A, Hofmann-Wellenhof R, Langsenlehner U, et al. In vivo confocal laser scanning microscopy of melanocytic skin tumours: diagnostic applicability using unselected tumour images. Br J Dermatol 2008;158(2): 329–33.

107. Langley RG, Walsh N, Sutherland AE, et al. The diagnostic accuracy of in vivo confocal scanning laser microscopy compared to dermoscopy of benign and malignant melanocytic lesions: a prospective study. Dermatology 2007;215(4): 365–72.

108. Guitera P, Pellacani G, Longo C, et al. In vivo reflectance confocal microscopy enhances secondary evaluation of melanocytic lesions. J Invest Dermatol 2009; 129(1):131–8.

109. Moncrieff M, Cotton S, Claridge E, et al. Spectrophotometric intracutaneous analysis: a new technique for imaging pigmented skin lesions. Br J Dermatol 2002;146(3):448–57.

110. Govindan K, Smith J, Knowles L, et al. Assessment of nurse-led screening of pigmented lesions using SIAscope. J Plast Reconstr Aesthet Surg 2007;60(6): 639–45.

111. Haniffa MA, Lloyd JJ, Lawrence CM. The use of a spectrophotometric intracutaneous analysis device in the real-time diagnosis of melanoma in the setting of a melanoma screening clinic. Br J Dermatol 2007;156(6):1350–2.

112. Elbaum M, Kopf AW, Rabinovitz HS, et al. Automatic differentiation of melanoma from melanocytic nevi with multispectral digital dermoscopy: a feasibility study. J Am Acad Dermatol 2001;44(2):207–18.
113. Perrinaud A, Gaide O, French LE, et al. Can automated dermoscopy image analysis instruments provide added benefit for the dermatologist? A study comparing the results of three systems. Br J Dermatol 2007;157(5):926–33.
114. Menzies SW, Bischof L, Talbot H, et al. The performance of SolarScan: an automated dermoscopy image analysis instrument for the diagnosis of primary melanoma. Arch Dermatol 2005;141(11):1388–96.

The Classification of Cutaneous Melanoma

Lyn McDivitt Duncan, MD

KEYWORDS

• Melanoma • Classification • Staging • Prognosis • *BRAF*

Melanoma is a tumor with significant impact on society, because it affects patients at a relatively young age, and when found to be metastatic, there is no reliably effective treatment. Melanoma was diagnosed in 200,000 people worldwide in 2002 and was associated with more than 40,000 deaths.[1] Nearly 2% of those who are born in the United States this year will develop melanoma during their lifetime,[2] an increase from less than 1% 2 decades ago.[3] Although most patients have localized disease at the time of diagnosis and are cured by surgical excision of the primary tumor, many patients develop metastases, and most of these patients will die of melanoma-associated causes. The classification of these tumors determines treatment plans, in particular in those patients who may be offered sentinel lymph node mapping, and adjuvant therapy.

Classification by definition involves the systematic distribution of tumors into categories that share features. Morphologic schemes rely on histologic features, and staging schemes distribute tumors into categories that share a similar prognosis. Particularly useful are classification schemes that provide a categorization that correlates with response to specific therapy. Unfortunately for patients with metastatic melanoma, although the genomic classification proposals offer some promise (eg, *BRAF*, c-KIT mutations), there is no current scheme that allows us to predict a response to therapy in more than 25% of patients in a given cohort.

Prognosis in melanoma is tightly linked to primary tumor thickness. Most patients with melanoma in developed countries are diagnosed with thin primary cutaneous tumors and are cured by local excision of the tumor with a margin of surrounding skin.[4] Nevertheless, some patients with primary melanoma less than 1 mm in maximal thickness will develop metastasis and die. The scheme originally described 40 years ago and published with few modifications in the most recent World Health Organization (WHO) classification of skin tumors allows for segregation of melanoma into subtypes based on clinical and histologic features that correlate somewhat with disease course and also with recent genomic data.[5–7] The American Joint Committee on Cancer (AJCC) staging classification scheme is a tumor-node-metastasis (TNM)

Department of Pathology, Harvard Medical School, MGH Dermatopathology Unit WRN827, Massachusetts General Hospital, 55 Fruit Street, Boston, MA 02114, USA
E-mail address: duncan@helix.mgh.harvard.edu

Hematol Oncol Clin N Am 23 (2009) 501–513
doi:10.1016/j.hoc.2009.03.013
0889-8588/09/$ – see front matter © 2009 Elsevier Inc. All rights reserved.

based clinical and histologic scheme that segregates patients into prognostic categories that are not correlated with any specific therapeutic response.[8] To date, the therapeutic response data have little to contribute to these schemes, given that the best responses are anecdotal and even the most successful clinical trials report complete responses in fewer than 25% of patients. Integration of the genomic and clinical pathologic schemes may provide a future classification scheme that segregates tumors by predicted outcome and potential response to specific therapy. This article discusses the current schemes and the interesting finding that the recently proposed genomic classifications serve to validate the original morphologic scheme described more than 40 years ago.[5]

EXISTING CLASSIFICATION SCHEMES FOR MELANOMA

The existing classification schemes for melanoma include the histologic scheme adopted by the WHO[9] and the AJCC staging scheme,[8] both based on clinical and histologic parameters and both used routinely in the diagnosis and treatment of patients diagnosed with cutaneous melanoma.[10] There have also been a handful of proposed genomic classifications, some of which have promise.[10] One of these genomic surveys yielded results that validated the original classification of melanoma into subtypes and also suggested the capacity of some histologic findings to predict genomic abnormalities.[8]

Histologic Classification of Cutaneous Melanoma

Forty years ago, detailed observations and descriptions of the clinical and histopathological features of primary cutaneous melanoma led to the initial proposal for classification of these tumors.[6,11] Today, many decades later, we still use these tools. There have been some tweaks to the classification scheme, but the basic findings as described so thoroughly in the late 1960s and early 1970s form the foundation for the currently recognized subtypes of cutaneous melanoma.[6,7,11–14] These authors described the clinical appearance of cutaneous melanoma, the anatomic site, the presence or absence of sun damage, and the patients' gender and age. These attributes were then considered alongside the histologic appearance of the tumors. The histologic features evaluated included intraepidermal pattern of growth, dermal growth pattern, cytologic appearance of the tumor cells, epidermal changes including atrophy and ulceration, the presence of solar elastosis, the anatomic level of invasion into the dermis, the maximal tumor thickness as measured perpendicular to the epidermal surface from the top of the granular cell layer, vascular invasion, mitotic activity, and the pattern and density of lymphocytic host response. Using these clinical and pathologic variables, these observers described similar classification categories for cutaneous melanoma. They recognized 3 major subtypes: malignant melanoma invasive with adjacent intraepidermal component of superficial spreading type (superficial spreading melanoma [SSM]), malignant melanoma invasive with adjacent intraepidermal component of Hutchinson's melanotic freckle type (lentigo maligna melanoma, LMM), and invasive melanoma without adjacent intraepidermal component (nodular malignant melanoma [NMM]). The adjacent intraepidermal component was defined as extending at least three rete ridges within the epidermis beyond the edge of the dermal component. Subsequently, this adjacent intraepidermal component has been further described as the radial growth component, and the dermal invasive and expansile tumor, as vertical growth phase. The following is a summary of the observations from these original reports (**Table 1**).

Superficial spreading melanoma

Clinically these tumors show a haphazard combination of color, including tan, brown, gray, black, violaceous, pink, and rarely blue or white. The lesion outline is usually sharply marginated with one or more irregular peninsula-like protrusions. The surface may have a palpable papule or a nodule that extends several millimeters above the skin surface.

Histologically SSM is characterized by the presence of an intraepidermal component that displays a pagetoid and nested growth pattern at all levels of the epidermis (**Fig. 1**A). The predominant intraepidermal tumor cell cytology is that of an epithelioid cell with abundant cytoplasm that is eosinophilic, amphophilic, or has a dusty distribution of fine cytoplasmic melanin granules. The nuclei may be large and have 1 or more

Table 1
Clinical and histologic subtypes of cutaneous melanoma

	Superficial Spreading	Lentigo Maligna	Nodular
Clinical findings			
Color	Tan, brown, gray, black, violaceous, pink Rarely blue or white	Tan, brown, black, flecks of pigment	Brown, black, blue-black
Outline	Sharply marginated Peninsula-like protrusions	Irregular outline	Plaque or nodule without surrounding flat pigmented lesion
Shape	Palpable papule or nodule	Flat, with rare papule	Smoothly surfaced nodule, ulcerated polyp, or elevated plaque
Anatomic site	Trunk, extremities	Face and neck	Trunk, extremities
Sun exposure	Intermittent	Chronic sun exposure	Intermittent sun
Histologic findings			
Intraepidermal melanocytic proliferation	Pagetoid and nested epithelioid cells with amphophilic or finely pigmented cytoplasm, prominent nucleoli common	Increased density of individual melanocytes along the dermal epidermal junction, large densely chromatic nuclei, multinucleated cells, extension down hair follicles	Minimal and only directly overlying the dermal tumor, no intraepidermal nested melanocytic proliferation more than three rete lateral to the dermal tumor
Epidermis	Hyperplasia	Atrophy	Atrophy or hyperplasia
Intradermal melanocytic proliferation	Nests of variable sizes, expansile tumor nodule, cytology similar to epidermal component	Nested or infiltrative, epithelioid or spindled cells, may be similar to SSM and NMM	Small nests and aggregates of tumor cells that form an expansile nodule

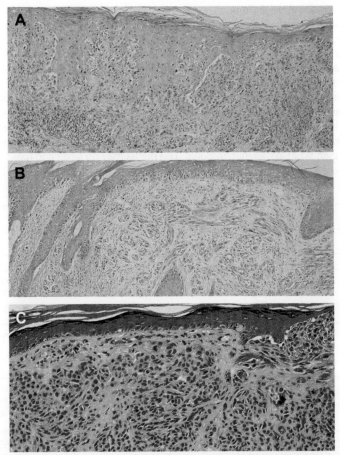

Fig. 1. Histologic features of cutaneous melanoma subtypes. (*A*) Superficial spreading melanoma. Intraepidermal tumor cells display individual cell scatter and nests of cells at all epidermal levels with associated epidermal hyperplasia. (*B*) Lentigo maligna melanoma. Intraepidermal tumor cells are localized to the base of the epidermis and extend down hair follicle epithelium with associated epidermal atrophy. (*C*) Nodular melanoma. There is minimal intraepidermal tumor with an underlying nested proliferation of melanoma cells.

prominent nucleoli. These intraepidermal tumor cells are relatively uniform in that they appear cytologically similar to one another. In the dermal invasive component, the melanoma cells have cytologic features that are similar to those of the intraepidermal tumor cells. The dermal component may also be characterized by numerous nests of variable sizes and occasionally an expansile nodule of tumor. In cases with abundant dermal tumor, the cytologic heterogeneity becomes more apparent. At times, the variation in cell morphology from one tumor nest to the next is striking.

Lentigo maligna melanoma
Clinically this is often a relatively large, mostly flat tumor that displays a variegated coloration that includes tan, brown, and black and may have flecks of black or brown on a tan background. This tumor displays more shades of brown and less of the violaceous and pink colors than those seen in SSM. The outline of the tumor is irregular,

and although the tumor is mostly flat, a focus of invasion may be detected as a slightly raised papule that may be best detected by side lighting.[15]

Histologically the intraepidermal component of LMM is characterized by a predominantly individual proliferation of cells that are localized to the basal layers of the epidermis (**Fig. 1**B). This growth pattern is described as lentiginous in both benign and malignant melanocytic tumors. The tumor cells have large densely chromatic nuclei and are occasionally multinucleated. They may be so numerous that the basal keratinocytes appear to be replaced by a continuous line of melanoma cells. The tumor cells extend down the hair follicle epithelium, maintaining the close approximation to the basal layer. Intraepidermal nests and pagetoid spread may be observed; however, these features are subtle when present, in contrast to SSM, which is characterized by a nested and pagetoid intraepidermal component. The dermal invasive component of LMM may display spindled cells and tumor cell pigmentation, and the dermal component may also show features similar to those observed in SSM and NMM.

Nodular malignant melanoma

These tumors usually have a relatively uniform brown, black, or blue-black color and may arise as a smooth-surface cutaneous nodule, an elevated plaque with irregular outlines, or as a polypoidal often ulcerated exophytic tumor. In contrast to superficial spreading and lentigo maligna types of melanoma, there is no surrounding flat, pigmented lesion associated with the tumor.

NMM is characterized by a predominance of dermal invasive tumor. An intraepidermal component may be present but directly overlies the invasive melanoma. Occasionally, the epidermal component is so minimal as to suggest the possibility that the tumor represents a dermal metastasis (**Fig. 1**C). The tumor is composed of small nests and aggregates of tumor cells that together form the overall tumor nodule.

Pathologists from the United States, Australia, Scotland, Canada, England, and France used clinical and histologic observations to devise a classification of melanoma that has persisted with minor amendments for over 40 years. Additionally, a prognostic score sheet for the diagnosis of melanoma published in 1968 bears close resemblance to the synoptic reports used by those who diagnose melanoma today.[16] There have been few revisions to these original descriptions, mostly to further define the categories and to add categories for more rarely occurring, yet histologically distinctive, tumors.

In 1982, a group of pathologists met in Sydney, Australia, to update the melanoma classification scheme formulated 10 years before. In this update, the group recommended the following six designations: melanoma with an adjacent component of one of four types, either superficial spreading, lentigo maligna, acral lentiginous, or mucosal lentiginous, or melanoma with no adjacent component, and finally melanoma of unclassifiable histogenetic type.[17] Additionally, these observers recommended that all melanoma pathology reports contain notes as to tumor thickness, ulceration, microanatomical level (Clark), mitotic rate, vascular invasion, regression, and margins.[17] These parameters are virtually identical to those included in the current synoptic reports used globally for melanoma more than 20 years later.

The segregation of melanoma into subtypes allows for the identification of clinically and histologically distinctive forms of melanoma. However, this classification does not segregate tumors into classes that differ significantly in clinical course and overall prognosis. In multivariate analysis, the prognosis for patients with cutaneous melanoma remains more tightly linked to primary tumor thickness than to these subtypes.[14,18] The AJCC system, first published in 1978, incorporated microstaging, specifically tumor thickness and Clark level, into a staging scheme that segregates tumors into categories with disparate, disease-free, and overall survival. The Melanoma Staging Committee of the AJCC has updated this staging scheme several times to include contemporary data relating to melanoma prognosis. The AJCC Melanoma Staging Committee relied on specific guidelines in developing the existing schema. This TNM classification needed to be practical, reproducible, applicable to all medical disciplines, and reflect the biology of melanoma as observed throughout the world. The criteria were required to be evidence-based prognostic factors identified in Cox multivariate regression analyses. The criteria were also selected as those that were relevant to current practice, regularly incorporated into clinical trials, and relatively easy for tumor registrars to identify in medical records.[8]

The criteria that form the basis of the AJCC staging schema include primary tumor thickness, ulceration, level of invasion, regional metastasis, and distant metastasis (**Table 2**). The T classification is based on the tumor thickness at breakpoints less than or equal to 1 mm, 1 to 2 mm, 2 to 4 mm, and greater than 4 mm. For tumors smaller than 1 mm, anatomic level greater than III upstages the tumor from T1a to T1b, and for all T stages, the presence of ulceration upstages the patient from Ta to Tb. The N classification is based on the number of lymph nodes containing metastatic tumor. Microscopic metastases detected histologically in sentinel lymph nodes are staged as Na, whereas clinically detectable lymph node metastases or microscopic evidence of extracapsular extension is staged as Nb. Patients without lymph node metastases but with in-transit metastases or satellite metastases are staged as N2c. If in-transit metastasis or satellite metastases are detected along with lymph node metastases, they are staged at N3. The M classification is based on the location of distant metastases and serum lactate dehydrogenase (LDH). In patients with a normal serum LDH, the presence of distant cutaneous, subcutaneous, or nodal metastases leads to stage M1a, lung metastases to M1b, and all other visceral metastases to M1c. Patients with elevated LDH and distant metastases of any site are staged as M1c. The combination of these TNM definitions leads to a staging schema that segregates patients based on overall survival (see **Table 2**). This scheme was the

Table 2
AJCC 2001 staging criteria and estimated 5-year survival of patients with cutaneous melanoma

Stage	TNM Stage	Pathological Features	5y survival (%)
0	Tis N0 M0	—	100
IA	T1a,b N0 M0	<1 mm	93
IB	T2a N0 M0	1–2 mm no ulcer	89
IIA	T2b N0 M0	1–2 mm + ulcer	—
	T3a N0 M0	2–3 mm no ulcer	78
IIB	T3b N0 M0	3–4 mm + ulcer	65
	T4a	>4 mm no ulcer	—
IIC	T4b N0 M0	>4 mm + ulcer	45
IIIA	T1-4a N1a, 2a, M0	Any thickness, microscopic nodal mets	67
IIIB	T4b N1a, 2a, M0	>4 mm + ulcer or	53
	T1-4 N1b, 2b, M0	macroscopic nodal mets <4	
IIIC	any T N3 M0	4+ lymph nodes or matted lymph nodes	26

result of a major collaborative study based on data regarding nearly 18,000 melanoma patients from cancer centers worldwide.[8]

The next iteration of the AJCC staging classification includes mitotic activity of the dermal tumor, now known to be a powerful predictor of outcome in patients with thin primary tumors.[19,20] There has also been attention to the prognostic utility of sentinel lymph node status in patients with tumors less than 1 mm in thickness.[21] Additionally, tumor-infiltrating lymphocytes (TILs) have been shown to have significant prognostic bearing for patients with primary cutaneous tumors greater than 2 mm in thickness.[22] Although TILs were historically not included in staging schema because of concerns regarding interobserver reproducibility, recent work indicates that this parameter may be taught and reported reliably.[23]

As a complement to the existing staging schemes, there have been several reports of decision trees and other prognostic models that use a combination of selected factors to better segregate patients into prognostically distinct groups.[24–27] For example, in patients with tumors less than 1 mm thick, the combination of mitotic rate, ulceration, male sex, and the presence of vertical growth phase predicts an increased risk of sentinel lymph node metastasis.[28] In this setting, a patient might be offered sentinel lymph node mapping despite having a tumor less than 1 mm thick.

None of these prognostic models or decision trees uses the subtype of melanoma as a factor. Most patients with cutaneous melanoma have either SSM or NMM, and these criteria have in large part been evaluated from cohorts rich in these types of tumors. Nevertheless, in clinical practice, the staging schemes and algorithms are applied to all patients, including those with acral lentiginous melanoma (ALM) and LMM, without consideration for the histologic subtype of tumor.

The current schemes are reliably effective at predicting disease-free survival and overall survival for patients diagnosed with melanoma. In recent years, much attention has been given to patients with thin melanomas who develop metastatic disease; mitotic rate and sentinel lymph node factors have contributed to a more robust staging scheme for these early stage patients.

Although these schemes serve their purpose, they are lacking in two ways: (1) they do not segregate patients based on response to specific therapy, (2) they do not incorporate any melanoma-specific biomarker or genomic information. The main reason for these differences from classification schemes in other malignancies, for example, breast cancer and lymphoma, is that (1) the factors that predict response to specific therapies remain unknown and (2) there is no biomarker or genomic signature that predicts outcome robustly and that fulfills the usability criteria for clinical practice (affordable, timely, proven in multivariate analysis, etc.).

What has happened in the melanoma classification arena between 1969 and 2009? The categories of acral lentiginous and mucosal lentiginous melanoma have been added to the schema. Additionally, many exceedingly rare forms of melanoma have been described, although most fit into an existing subtype, for example, desmoplastic melanomas are usually lentigo maligna type and nevoid melanomas are nodular type.[29–32] Exceptions include the pigmented epithelioid melanocytoma and Spitzoid melanoma;[33–42] the treatment plan for these rare tumors is based on reports of similar tumors rather than the AJCC or other schemes. Other contributions to the understanding and prognostication of melanoma include the publication of numerous algorithms, decision trees, and mathematical models based on large databases and pooled resources. In 2002, the AJCC classification scheme was revised to modify the thickness breakpoints, add ulceration, and revise the inclusion and definitions of microscopic satellites, satellite metastasis, and the extent of lymph node metastasis. Although the originally described melanoma subtypes, SSM, LMM, NMM, and so forth, are noted in the pathology report, the staging schema and therapeutic decisions are based primarily on specific factors: primary tumor thickness, mitotic rate, ulceration, and extent of metastatic disease. Melanoma patient treatment is influenced by both subtype and AJCC stage. The AJCC stage dictates those patients who will be offered sentinel lymph node sampling, adjuvant therapy, and eligibility for clinical trials. Tumor subtype may dictate clinical trial eligibility due to the recent correlation of genomic abnormalities with specific tumor subtypes, for example, the prevalence of c-Kit mutations in acral and mucosal melanomas has led to the use of imatinib mesylate in clinical trials for these patients.[43–45] In 2002, *BRAF* mutations were reported to result in constitutive kinase activity in approximately 60% of melanomas. Although clinical trials since then have enrolled melanoma patients to evaluate the effectiveness of RAF kinase inhibitors alone and in combination, the results of these trials have been disappointing to date. Nevertheless, specific *BRAF* inhibitors may yield more promising results. The mitogen-activated protein kinase (MAPK) signaling cascade is one of the many pathways being widely studied as a source of drug targets in patients with melanoma.[46,47] Tumor subtype has renewed impact, given the findings that *BRAF* mutation correlates with the histologic features that segregate melanomas into SSM, NMM, and LMM.[6]

PROPOSALS FOR MOLECULAR SCHEMES

After several decades of laboratory-based research, we now have a better understanding of some of the key pathways and potential therapeutic targets in melanoma tumor progression. Although translation of these findings from the research laboratory to clinical practice is in progress, none of these findings has led to a significant change in patient outcome or the development of a robustly effective therapy for any subset of patients with metastatic melanoma. In the future, molecular techniques will likely play an important role in the classification of melanoma. Because current techniques such as comparative genomic hybridization (CGH) and expression analysis are time consuming and expensive, they are not yet clinically useful and are for the most part confined to research protocols. Further refinements of these screening techniques and correlation with gene expression data may lead to the development of more clinically mainstream tests, such as those that incorporate in situ hybridization technology.[10] Although several authors have proposed new classification schemes for melanoma based on molecular and genomic results, analysis of large cohorts of clinically annotated melanoma specimens will be needed to determine the clinical utility of these schemes.[5,48–54]

It has been proposed that armed with a better understanding of the molecular events and pathways we could design a genomic classification of melanoma. Several interconnected pathways are known to be involved in melanoma tumor progression.[49,54] These include the MAPK extracellular signal-regulated kinase (ERK) signaling cascade, the phosphatidylinositol-3-kinase (PI3/AKT) pathway, and the retinoblastoma pathway that regulates the cell cycle via cyclin-dependent kinases (CDKs). Microphthalmia-associated transcription factor (MITF) transcription and translation are influenced by a variety of stimuli including c-KIT via the MAPK/ERK pathway and mammalian target of rapamycin and nuclear factor kappa B (NF-kB) via the PI3/AKT pathway. MITF has been described as a master melanocyte regulator of development, function, and survival by modulating various differentiation and cell-cycle progression genes.[55] The details of the known signaling pathways in melanoma are described in other articles in this issue. The MAPK/ERK signaling cascade will be described here briefly followed by a description of the correlation of *BRAF* mutations with histologic features of melanoma. Receptor tyrosine kinases (such as c-KIT) initiate the MAPK signaling at the cell membrane. Signals are transduced via RAS-GTPase, which, when activated, can bind effector proteins including *BRAF* and PI3 kinase. Activating mutations of *BRAF* kinase (common in melanocytic nevi and melanomas) drives the MAPK pathway via the phosphorylation of MAPK. Finally, the ERK is activated, leading to proliferation or survival signals via cytoplasmic protein targets, cytoskeletal targets, and nuclear transcription factors, including cMYC, cFOS and HIF-1a. In dissecting the MAPK pathway, RAS and RAF have been the focus of most studies. N-RAS and *BRAF* mutations are for the most part mutually exclusive in that tumors usually have one or the other but not both.[56] Mutations of N-RAS are observed in approximately 15% of melanomas and do not correlate with sun damage or anatomic site of the tumor. On the other hand, somatic mutations of *BRAF* have been identified in 66% of melanomas and are associated intermittent sun exposure and anatomic site. Interestingly, 82% of benign nevi also have activating mutations of *BRAF*, suggesting that activation of the MAPK signaling cascade is not sufficient for the development of melanoma.

In an analysis of 101 melanoma cell lines, using unsupervised learning methods, hierarchical clustering grouped the samples into 6 main groups based on amplifications and deletions that localized mostly to chromosomes 4q, 7q, 10, 11q, and 22q.[53] Some clusters were associated with enrichment for *BRAF* mutation, compared with *NRAS* mutation. In another study using microarray and hierarchical clustering, 31 melanomas were segregated into two subtypes based on the analysis of 22 genes;[50] other investigators used quantitative reverse transcriptase polymerase chain reaction and analyzed 30 melanoma samples for 20 genes and also found a major and minor clustering that was differentiated in part by genes of the MAPK/ERK pathway (*BRAF*, JUN, FOS).[48]

Evaluation of cutaneous melanomas using CGH to determine DNA copy number changes suggested a distinction between the subtypes of melanoma and degree of sun damage.[51,57,58] *BRAF* mutations are more common in melanomas occurring on skin subject to intermittent sun exposure (eg, SSM and NMM) and are rare in melanomas occurring on sun-protected skin (ALM) and chronically sun damaged skin (LMM). In contrast, mutation or amplification of KIT was observed in tumors at sun-protected sites (ALM) and in chronically sun-damaged sites (LMM). Acral melanomas were associated with more aberrations involving chromosomes 5p, 11q, 12q, and 15, and LMM showed more frequent loss of chromosomes 17p and 13q when compared with SSM.

MORPHOLOGIC AND GENOMIC CLASSIFICATIONS COME TOGETHER

An analysis of *BRAF* and *NRAS* mutations in coordination with histologic features revealed an aligning of certain histologic findings with *BRAF* mutation but not with *NRAS*. The primary tumors that displayed *BRAF* mutation had a higher frequency of intraepidermal single cell scatter, intraepidermal nesting, increased epidermal thickness, cytologic features that included epithelioid cells and cytoplasmic pigmentation, and a sharp circumscription of the tumor. These features are common to SSMs. This contrasts with the features of lentigo maligna and acral/mucosal lentiginous melanomas, which display less intraepidermal scatter and nesting and are characterized by a proliferation of solitary tumor cells along the base of the epidermis without sharp lateral circumscription of the tumor. These tumor cells have cytologic features of large hyperchromatic nuclei with sparse cytoplasm and minimal pigmentation, in contrast to the variably pigmented epithelioid cells characteristic of SSM.[5]

Additional studies that examine the genomic characteristics of tumors with histologic correlates may allow for the development of a morphologic classification scheme linked to genomic profiles. Subgroups of melanoma that are genetically more homogeneous than those that are known today may be defined. Such schemata may lead to better stratification of tumors with regard to outcome, including predicted patterns of metastasis and response to specific therapy.

In their original description of three distinct forms of melanoma, superficial spreading, nodular, and lentigo maligna, Clark and colleagues[6] emphasize the importance of evaluating the superficial and intraepidermal aspects of the tumors. They note that the deeply invading tumor cells may appear similar regardless of whether they are from a superficial spreading, nodular, or lentigo maligna type of melanoma. This raises an interesting point where the morphologic and genomic correlates are concerned. It is important to bear in mind two characteristics of melanoma: (1) melanoma is a heterogeneous tumor; within a primary tumor, subsets of tumor cells with different gene expression profiles may exist, and (2) melanoma may differentiate or dedifferentiate as a tumor progresses. Because of these two characteristics, we may learn that a genomically based classification scheme may not be static for a given patient's tumors. At diagnosis, a genomic profile that represents the majority of the dermal tumor cells may not be the profile of the most "malignant" tumor cells. A small subset of cells with a divergent profile may represent the tumor cells that will depart the skin, leading to metastases. After homing to the metastatic site, the metastatic focus may evolve again to form genomically distinct subsets of tumor. This hypothesis is supported by the intratumoral heterogeneity that is observed in both primary tumors and metastases.[59]

Melanoma remains one of the most drug-resistant tumors perhaps in part due to the inherent intratumoral heterogeneity. Rare patients who display long-term response to therapy may have tumors that have lost genomic diversity. A knowledge of the intratumoral heterogeneity of biomarkers related to the canonical pathways that drive melanoma tumor progression will likely contribute to future classification of this complex tumor. The most robust predictive classifications will likely incorporate histologic features, intratumoral molecular phenotype (evaluated by in situ hybridization and/or immunohistochemical analysis), and genomic profiles. Rather than relying on a few biomarkers to predict prognosis or response to therapy, the evaluation of biomarkers in concert with morphologic and genomic factors, validated in prospective clinical trials, will likely serve as the most useful clinical tools in the future care of patients with melanoma.

SUMMARY

Forty years ago a classification scheme and prognostic factors for cutaneous melanoma were described, based on detailed clinical features and histologic analysis, by an international group of authors. In addition to the subtypes—superficial spreading, nodular, lentigo maligna—prognostic factors including tumor thickness, ulceration, and mitotic activity were identified. There have been some tweaks to the classification scheme, but these basic findings form the foundation for the currently recognized subtypes of cutaneous melanoma and prognostic factors used in the AJCC staging scheme. Most notably, we still rely on a measurement with a simple ruler as the basis for staging of primary cutaneous melanoma, while the recognition of primary tumor mitotic activity and ulceration also remain significant factors. To date, no molecular marker or target has proved reliably useful in the staging or treatment of melanoma. Mutational analysis has revealed a correlation of activating mutations with these morphologic descriptors.[6] Future classification schemes may have more power in predicting response to therapy by incorporating specific genomic, intratumoral expression profiles and morphologic findings.

REFERENCES

1. Parkin DM, Bray F, Ferlay J, et al. Global cancer statistics, 2002. CA Cancer J Clin 2005;55(2):74–108.
2. Jemal A, Siegel R, Ward E, et al. Cancer statistics, 2007. CA Cancer J Clin 2007; 57(1):43–66.
3. Jemal A, Devesa SS, Hartge P, et al. Recent trends in cutaneous melanoma incidence among whites in the United States. J Natl Cancer Inst 2001;93(9):678–83.
4. Gimotty PA, Elder DE, Fraker DL, et al. Identification of high-risk patients among those diagnosed with thin cutaneous melanomas. J Clin Oncol 2007;25(9): 1129–34.
5. Viros A, Fridlyand J, Bauer J, et al. Improving melanoma classification by integrating genetic and morphologic features. PLoS Med 2008;5(6):e120.
6. Clark WH Jr, From L, Bernardino EA, et al. The histogenesis and biologic behavior of primary human malignant melanomas of the skin. Cancer Res 1969;29(3): 705–27.
7. McGovern VJ, Mihm MC Jr, Bailly C, et al. The classification of malignant melanoma and its histologic reporting. Cancer 1973;32(6):1446–57.
8. Balch CM, Soong SJ, Atkins MB, et al. An evidence-based staging system for cutaneous melanoma. CA Cancer J Clin 2004;54(3):131–49.
9. LeBoit PE, Burg G, Weedon D, Sarasin A, editors. Pathology and genetics of skin tumours; (IARC) IAfRoC, edition. World Health Organization Classification of Tumours. Lyon: IARC Press; 2006. p. 52–89.
10. Bastian BC, LeBoit PE, Pinkel D. Genomic approaches to skin cancer diagnosis. Arch Dermatol 2001;137(11):1507–11.
11. McGovern VJ. The classification of melanoma and its relationship with prognosis. Pathology 1970;2(2):85–98.
12. Mihm MC Jr, Clark WH Jr, From L. The clinical diagnosis, classification and histogenetic concepts of the early stages of cutaneous malignant melanomas. N Engl J Med 1971;284(19):1078–82.
13. Trapl J, Palecek L, Ebel J, et al. Tentative new classification of melanoma of the skin. Acta Derm Venereol 1966;46(5):443–6.
14. Breslow A. Thickness, cross-sectional area and depth of invasion in the prognosis of cutaneous melanoma. Ann Surg 1970;172:902–8.
15. Wolff K, Johnson R, Suurmond D, editors. Fitzpatrick's color atlas and synopsis of clinical dermatology. 5th edition. New York: McGraw-Hill; 2005.
16. Cochran AJ. Method of assessing prognosis in patients with malignant melanoma. Lancet 1968;2(7577):1062–4.
17. McGovern VJ, Cochran AJ, Van der Esch EP, et al. The classification of malignant melanoma, its histological reporting and registration: a revision of the 1972 Sydney classification. Pathology 1986;18(1):12–21.
18. Balch CM, Murad TM, Soong S-J, et al. A Multifactorial analysis of melanoma: prognostic histopathological features comparing Clark's and Breslow's staging methods. Ann Surg 1978;188:732–42.
19. Azzola MF, Shaw HM, Thompson JF, et al. Tumor mitotic rate is a more powerful prognostic indicator than ulceration in patients with primary cutaneous

melanoma: an analysis of 3661 patients from a single center. Cancer 2003;97(6): 1488–98.

20. Gimotty PA, Van Belle P, Elder DE, et al. Biologic and prognostic significance of dermal Ki67 expression, mitoses, and tumorigenicity in thin invasive cutaneous melanoma. J Clin Oncol 2005;23(31):8048–56.

21. Karakousis GC, Gimotty PA, Czerniecki BJ, et al. Regional nodal metastatic disease is the strongest predictor of survival in patients with thin vertical growth phase melanomas: a case for SLN Staging biopsy in these patients. Ann Surg Oncol 2007;14(5):1596–603.

22. Kruper LL, Spitz FR, Czerniecki BJ, et al. Predicting sentinel node status in AJCC stage I/II primary cutaneous melanoma. Cancer 2006;107(10):2436–45.

23. Busam KJ, Antonescu CR, Marghoob AA, et al. Histologic classification of tumor-infiltrating lymphocytes in primary cutaneous malignant melanoma. A study of interobserver agreement. Am J Clin Pathol 2001;115(6):856–60.

24. Gimotty PA, Guerry D, Ming ME, et al. Thin primary cutaneous malignant melanoma: a prognostic tree for 10-year metastasis is more accurate than American Joint Committee on Cancer staging [see comment] [erratum appears in J Clin Oncol 2005 Jan 20;23(3):656]. J Clin Oncol 2004;22(18):3668–76.

25. Clark WH Jr, Elder DE, Guerry D IV, et al. Model predicting survival in stage I melanoma based on tumor progression. J Natl Cancer Inst 1989;81:1893–904.

26. Schuchter L, Schultz DJ, Synnestvedt M, et al. A prognostic model for predicting 10-year survival in patients with primary melanoma. Ann Intern Med 1996;125: 369–75.

27. Tsai CA, Chen DT, Chen JJ, et al. An integrated tree-based classification approach to prognostic grouping with application to localized melanoma patients. J Biopharm Stat 2007;17(3):445–60.

28. Karakousis GC, Gimotty PA, Botbyl JD, et al. Predictors of regional nodal disease in patients with thin melanomas. Ann Surg Oncol 2006;13(4):533–41.

29. Wong TY, Suster S, Duncan LM, et al. Nevoid melanoma: a clinicopathological study of seven cases of malignant melanoma mimicking spindle and epithelioid cell nevus and verrucous dermal nevus. Hum Pathol 1995;26:171–9.

30. Labrecque PG, Hu CH, Winkelmann RK. On the nature of desmoplastic melanoma. Cancer 1976;38(3):1205–13.

31. Busam KJ. Cutaneous desmoplastic melanoma. Adv Anat Pathol 2005;12(2): 92–102.

32. Zembowicz A, McCusker M, Chiarelli C, et al. Morphological analysis of nevoid melanoma: a study of 20 cases with a review of the literature. Am J Dermatopathol 2001;23(3):167–75.

33. Zembowicz A, Knoepp SM, Bei T, et al. Loss of expression of protein kinase a regulatory subunit 1 alpha in pigmented epithelioid melanocytoma but not in melanoma or other melanocytic lesions. Am J Surg Pathol 2007;31(11): 1764–75.

34. Scolyer RA, Thompson JF, Warnke K, et al. Pigmented epithelioid melanocytoma. Am J Surg Pathol 2004;28(8):1114–5, author reply 1115–6.

35. Zembowicz A, Carney JA, Mihm MC. Pigmented epithelioid melanocytoma: a low-grade melanocytic tumor with metastatic potential indistinguishable from animal-type melanoma and epithelioid blue nevus. Am J Surg Pathol 2004; 28(1):31–40 [see comment] [erratum appears in Am J Surg Pathol 2004 May;28(5):following table of contents].

36. King MS, Porchia SJ, Hiatt KM. Differentiating spitzoid melanomas from Spitz nevi through CD99 expression. J Cutan Pathol 2007;34(7):576–80.

37. Mooi WJ, Krausz T. Spitz nevus versus spitzoid melanoma: diagnostic difficulties, conceptual controversies [see comment]. Adv Anat Pathol 2006;13(4):147–56.
38. Lee DA, Cohen JA, Twaddell WS, et al. Are all melanomas the same? Spitzoid melanoma is a distinct subtype of melanoma. Cancer 2006;106(4):907–13.
39. Barnhill RL. The Spitzoid lesion: rethinking Spitz tumors, atypical variants, 'Spitzoid melanoma' and risk assessment. Mod Pathol 2006;19(Suppl 2):S21–33.
40. van Dijk MC, Bernsen MR, Ruiter DJ. Analysis of mutations in B-RAF, N-RAS, and H-RAS genes in the differential diagnosis of Spitz nevus and spitzoid melanoma. Am J Surg Pathol 2005;29(9):1145–51.
41. Gill M, Cohen J, Renwick N, et al. Genetic similarities between Spitz nevus and Spitzoid melanoma in children. Cancer 2004;101(11):2636–40.
42. Crotty KA, Scolyer RA, Li L, et al. Spitz naevus versus Spitzoid melanoma: when and how can they be distinguished? [see comment]. Pathology 2002;34(1):6–12.
43. Beadling C, Jacobson-Dunlop E, Hodi FS, et al. KIT gene mutations and copy number in melanoma subtypes. Clin Cancer Res 2008;14(21):6821–8.
44. Hodi FS, Friedlander P, Corless CL, et al. Major response to imatinib mesylate in KIT-mutated melanoma. J Clin Oncol 2008;26(12):2046–51.
45. Ashida A, Takata M, Murata H, et al. Pathological activation of KIT in metastatic tumors of acral and mucosal melanomas. Int J Cancer 2009;124(4):862–8.
46. Davies H, Bignell GR, Cox C, et al. Mutations of the BRAF gene in human cancer [see comment]. Nature 2002;417(6892):949–54.
47. Smalley KS, Flaherty KT. Integrating BRAF/MEK inhibitors into combination therapy for melanoma. Br J Cancer 2009;100(3):431–5.
48. Lewis TB, Robison JE, Bastien R, et al. Molecular classification of melanoma using real-time quantitative reverse transcriptase-polymerase chain reaction. Cancer 2005;104(8):1678–86.
49. Fecher LA, Cummings SD, Keefe MJ, et al. Toward a molecular classification of melanoma. J Clin Oncol 2007;25(12):1606–20.
50. Bittner M, Meltzer P, Chen Y, et al. Molecular classification of cutaneous malignant melanoma by gene expression profiling. Nature 2000;406(6795):536–40.
51. Bastian BC, Olshen AB, LeBoit PE, et al. Classifying melanocytic tumors based on DNA copy number changes. Am J Pathol 2003;163(5):1765–70.
52. Liu W, Dowling JP, Murray WK, et al. Rate of growth in melanomas: characteristics and associations of rapidly growing melanomas [see comment]. Arch Dermatol 2006;142(12):1551–8.
53. Lin WM, Baker AC, Beroukhim R, et al. Modeling genomic diversity and tumor dependency in malignant melanoma. Cancer Res 2008;68(3):664–73.
54. Chin L, Garraway LA, Fisher DE. Malignant melanoma: genetics and therapeutics in the genomic era. Genes Dev 2006;20(16):2149–82.
55. Levy C, Khaled M, Fisher DE. MITF: master regulator of melanocyte development and melanoma oncogene. Trends Mol Med 2006;12(9):406–14.
56. Curtin JA, Fridlyand J, Kageshita T, et al. Distinct sets of genetic alterations in melanoma. [see comment]. N Engl J Med 2005;353(20):2135–47.
57. Curtin JA, Busam K, Pinkel D, et al. Somatic activation of KIT in distinct subtypes of melanoma [see comment]. J Clin Oncol 2006;24(26):4340–6.
58. Maldonado JL, Fridlyand J, Patel H, et al. Determinants of BRAF mutations in primary melanomas. J Natl Cancer Inst 2003;95(24):1878–90.
59. Zubovits J, Buzney E, Yu L, et al. HMB-45, S-100, NK1/C3, and MART-1 in metastatic melanoma. Hum Pathol 2004;35(2):217–23.

Educational and Screening Campaigns to Reduce Deaths from Melanoma

Alan C. Geller, MPH, RN

KEYWORDS

- Screening • Mortality • Early detection • Education
- Comprehensive

Incidence and mortality rates of melanoma throughout most of the developed world have risen in the past 25 years.[1] To date, however, there has been no central plan or coordinated strategy to reduce melanoma deaths.[2] This is in contrast to the nation's most common and preventable cancers, such as colorectal cancer, breast cancer, and prostate cancers, for which government-sponsored comprehensive strategic plans leading to full-scale advocacy campaigns have led to higher screening rates (**Fig. 1**) and mortality reduction.[2]

For melanoma control, patchwork recommendations have called on Americans to examine their skin regularly and seek physician care for unusual lesions;[3–5] however, the esteemed United States Preventive Services Task Force (USPSTF) states that there is insufficient evidence for population-based screening.[6] Without such evidence, screening, the potentially best means for reducing the disease, continues to be severely underused, because only 14% to 21% of Americans report ever having received a skin cancer examination.[7,8]

Episodic or haphazard planning will only maintain the status quo and do little to reverse the more than 8400 US deaths per year, many of which fall disproportionately on middle-aged and older men and persons of lower socioeconomic status (SES).[9,10] However, no population subgroups should be immune from a new public health strategy, since there has been no change in the mortality rate for US women since 1975.[1]

We propose that reduction of melanoma mortality can be bolstered by a two-fold parallel track strategy guided by experts in dermatology and oncology, cancer education and health systems research, epidemiologists and behavioral scientists, among others. First, public and professional educational campaigns should be guided by an understanding of three underlying but overlapping roots: *epidemiologic and*

Division of Public Health Practice, Harvard School of Public Health, Landmark Center, 401 Park Drive, Third Floor East, Boston, MA 02215, USA
E-mail address: ageller@hsph.harvard.edu

Hematol Oncol Clin N Am 23 (2009) 515–527
doi:10.1016/j.hoc.2009.03.008
0889-8588/09/$ – see front matter © 2009 Published by Elsevier Inc.

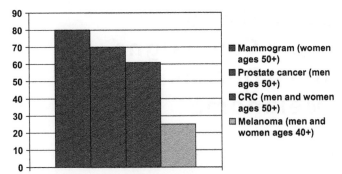

Fig. 1. Proportion of Americans reporting a cancer screen (evidence and advocacy → policy → higher rates).

preventable mortality (an understanding of who is most likely to be diagnosed with thick or late-stage melanoma), *biologic* (investigation of tumor types that are relatively common but potentially most lethal), and *sociologic* (an analysis of the changes needed in social structures to improve access to those most in need of early detection programs). We first review these major concepts and then briefly discuss the elements of a high-risk educational campaign. Second, in the absence of current proof or evidence that screening works to reduce melanoma mortality, randomized trials across a broader population should be launched to test various screening strategies. New trials could test the use of different examiners (nurses vs physicians), types of examinations (clinical examinations alone vs clinical examinations coupled with the use of new technologies, such as dermoscopy and teledermatology), or the most optimal venues (health maintenance organizations (HMOs), primary care clinics, communities, and research centers). Currently, research teams in Germany are launching a nationwide screening campaign led by family physicians (Rudiger Greinert, personal communication, 2008), investigators in Queensland are analyzing data collected from a community-based, randomized trial in 18 communities,[11-13] and US scientists are exploring whether various health systems and health providers are primed to undertake a large-scale, national trial. We elaborate on the broad tenets of a randomized screening trial and describe the "building block" benefits of a pilot screening trial.

MAGNITUDE OF MELANOMA

Both in the United States and throughout most of the world, the incidence of melanoma has been increasing steadily for at least the past 4 decades.[1,14-19] In the United States, the overall mortality rate has recently stabilized, although mortality rates have increased 28% since 1975.[1] Melanoma mortality disproportionately burdens men aged 55+ years—in fact, they remain the only demographic subgroup that has experienced increases for the past 30 to 40 years. Among all of the nations affected by the epidemic of melanoma mortality, none has reported a population-wide decrease in mortality, and to date, no nation has reported a decrease in the incidence of thick melanomas. In the absence of new treatments for melanoma and the unremitting high incidence rates for middle-aged and older men (who are also less likely to examine their skin),[20] targeted early detection and screening programs must be a vital component of a melanoma control strategy.

Epidemiology—Identifying Population Subgroups at Greatest Risk of Melanoma Mortality

There are ever-growing disparities in melanoma incidence, mortality, and survival by age and gender, social class, race and ethnicity, and geography.

Disparities by age and gender

In the United States, incidence rates (1975–2005) have risen in all age groups and in men and women; however, men aged 60 years have experienced more than a 4-fold increase (19.1–86.1 per 100,000), and rates have risen more than 5-fold in men aged 70 years (23.2–109.1 per 100,000) (**Table 1**).[1,10]

During the same period, melanoma mortality decreased by 23% in women aged 20 through 54 years and by 11% in men of the same age. In contrast, mortality rates rose 15% in women aged 55 through 64 years and 64% in men of the same age (**Fig. 2**). In all, nearly 50% of US melanoma deaths are in white men aged 50 years and older,[1,10] and persons aged 55 years and older comprise nearly 75% of all deaths.

Internationally, mortality rates are highest (in order) in New Zealand, Australia, Norway, Denmark, and South Africa, among others, with more than 6/100,000 deaths per year in New Zealand and Australia.[21–23] In all of these countries, mortality rates in men are higher than those in women. Rates are rising worldwide most sharply in older men, with women of the same age experiencing smaller increases. Mortality rates are decreasing or stabilizing for younger women, and rates among younger men vary by country. For example, mortality has plateaued in Sweden since the mid-1980s, and in particular, a statistically significant downward trend was observed for women.[24]

Men are less likely than women to examine their skin for melanoma or to proactively request physician examinations.[25] However, among men with a strong interest in detection, tumor thickness is markedly decreased. In a recent multi-institutional study of men diagnosed with thin (n = 170) and thick (n = 57) melanoma, thinner tumors were significantly correlated with men who had: heard of melanoma, paid attention to their health, regularly taken interest in reading or watching stories about health topics, believed it was important to have a doctor examine their skin for signs of melanoma, and carefully paid attention to information about skin cancer detection.[26]

Social class

Disparities in access to screening and those by social class, race and ethnicity, and geography are also profound. We also briefly review the rising disparity in survival between developed and less developed regions of the world.

Table 1
Age- and gender-specific incidence rates per 100,000 persons, United States, 1975–2005 (Connecticut and SEER)

Age (y)	Incidence		Incidence	
	Men 1975–79	Men 2001–05	Women 1975–79	Women 2001–05
30	5.9	8.6	7.7	15.1
40	12.3	19.8	12.0	23.6
50	15.8	39.1	18.8	28.9
60	19.1	86.1	12.0	39.0
70	23.2	109.1	13.0	45.8
80	21.4	145.3	17.3	50.4

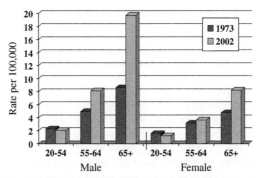

Fig. 2. Melanoma mortality among whites, 1973 and 2002, by age and gender.

Although all studies agree that melanoma is more commonly diagnosed in fair-skinned individuals with higher education and income, individuals with lower SES experience higher case-fatality rates, later-stage disease, and decreased survival. SES has been measured at the individual level (occupation) or in the aggregate via well-established measures, such as median household income, education, socioeconomic deprivation, or poverty percentage.[9] Lower SES is also associated with less knowledge and awareness of melanoma, and patients with lower SES or without health insurance are less likely to undergo either self-examination or physician screening.[25] Similar to differences by gender, greater awareness of warning signs of melanoma and access to primary care/dermatologists by SES may account for disparities in the report of late-stage diagnoses between persons of moderate-high SES and lower SES.[27–29]

Most recently, Reyes-Ortiz linked the tumor registry records from the US Surveillance Epidemiology and End Results (SEER) program and Medicare claims from the Centers for Medicare and Medicaid Services. After adjustment for sociodemographic variables, stage at diagnosis, comorbidities, and tumor thickness, residing in low-income areas was found to be an independent poor prognostic factor in melanoma survival.[9,27] A US population-based study found that men and women with invasive melanoma residing in poor areas had lower survival rates than those living in wealthier areas.[30] A population-based study in Massachusetts found that advanced stage and higher case fatality of melanoma were associated with lower census tract or zip code.[31] Reyes-Ortiz and colleagues[9,27] speculated that low SES influenced melanoma survival in 3 separate ways: biologic features of the tumor, stage or thickness at diagnosis, and host factors. For example, at the biologic level, nodular tumors, which are normally aggressive, have been found to be more frequent in persons who have the least education.[32]

Race and ethnicity

Although diagnoses are rare in persons of color, the latest examination of the US SEER registry found that the overall 5-year survival was noticeably less for minorities (72%–81%) than that for whites (89.6%).[1] The anatomic location and the severity of disease in low SES populations, particularly the high rates of acral melanoma in African Americans[33–35] and recently found among Hispanics in California,[36] may make these lesions harder to discover at an earlier, curable stage.

Melanoma is very uncommon in African Americans (1.0 per 100,000), comprising less than 1/20th of the rates of Caucasians.[1] Although rates of invasive melanoma for Hispanic men are far less than those for non-Hispanic men in California (2.8 per

100,000 compared with 17.2 per 100,000), estimated annual percent change rates increased 1.8 per year for Hispanic men between 1988 and 2001. Thicker lesions (greater than 1. 5 mm) were more common in Hispanic men (35%) than in non-Hispanic men (24%). Hispanic men and women experienced sharper increases in thick tumors than for thin (<0.75 mm) or moderate (0.75–1.49 mm) tumors.[36]

Biologic-Histologic Features Associated with Late-Stage Disease

Throughout the United States, Europe, and Australia, superficial spreading melanoma (SSM) comprises approximately two-thirds of all invasive melanoma but less than 10% of all melanoma greater than 2 mm.[37] Conversely, nodular melanoma (NM) comprises less than 10% of all melanoma but at least 50% of all melanoma greater than 2 mm.[37] The ability to identify population subgroups and early clinical signs of NM and to then translate these into meaningful warning signs for the public and professionals is a vital control strategy.

Results from a recent population-based study in Queensland demonstrated significant associations between NM of the extreme thickness categories (T1 and T4) and revealed that respondents aged 60 to 75 years were nearly three times more likely to have a T4 NM than a T1 NM compared with respondents aged 40 to 59 years. Compared with respondents who had a clinical skin examination (CSE) in the last 3 years, respondents who did not have a CSE were nearly four times more likely to have a T4 NM than a T1 NM. In comparison with respondents whose NM was detected by a doctor, those with self-detected melanoma were nearly five times more likely to be T4 than T1.[32]

Compared with thicker NM, patients with thinner NM were nearly twice as likely to report a change in color (46.2% versus 25.8%), 5 times more likely to observe an irregular shape, and far more likely to report brown pigmentation (47.4% versus 27.2%). Compared with thinner NM and all SSMs, thicker NMs were less common on the back of the trunk but more common on the scalp and neck.[32]

Three observations emerged from this analysis of the Queensland population-based cancer registry. There have been few reports of the presentation of thinner NM—herein, 57% of NMs were diagnosed to be less than or equal to 2.0 mm. This report coupled with a similar finding from the US SEER registry bodes well for identifying a significant subset of NM that can be detected relatively early. Second, warning signs traditionally thought to be features only of SSM, such as change in color and brown pigment, were also found among patients diagnosed with thinner NM. Third, older age, male gender, and the absence of a physician skin examination in the 3 years before diagnosis were also associated with thicker NM.[32]

Using well-established sources for professional and public education has been the hallmark for education on early detection. Less than 7% and 5% of all SSMs diagnosed in the United States and Queensland, respectively, are greater than 2 mm.[37,38] However, in both US and Queensland population-based cancer registries, NM is about one-sixth as common as SSM but 6 times more likely to result in thick melanoma.[37,38] The fact that a significant minority of Queensland patients diagnosed with thin NM reported a change in a lesion highlights the need for broad-scale but sharpened initiatives to increase public and professional attention to immediate attention to changing moles.

Sociologic and Structural Barriers

Many salient factors point to the need for restructuring health systems and medical education to enable high-risk Americans to have greater access to expert dermatologic care. Fewer than half of US medical students ever practice a single skin cancer examination during their 4 years of education, and rates during residency fare no better.[39] Scant attention to the skin cancer examination among their preceptors is borne out by low rates of skin surveillance for at-risk Americans.[7,8,40] For the public, self-reported rates of physician skin cancer examinations have improved little and hover at 20% to 25% in consecutive series of large-scale federal surveys conducted during the past 12 years.[7,8]

The overriding question within this section is how to create new models or paradigms that encourage greater access to skilled examinations. Limited access to care is likely to be associated with poor outcomes, including late-stage melanoma and decreased survival. Moreover, inequalities between low-SES patients and those of moderate/higher SES include underinsurance, lack of access to dermatologists and/or primary care physicians, and barriers, such as travel.[9]

In an ecological analysis, Roetzheim and colleagues strongly suggested that physician workforce issues could impact health outcomes in melanoma. They found that with each additional dermatologist per a population of 10,000, there was a 39% increased odds of earlier diagnosis.[41] How specialty and physician workforce issues are associated with earlier diagnosis is rife with complexity and requires further investigation. First, it is likely that a community presence of more dermatologists might facilitate and expedite referrals from primary care physicians. Other possible added benefits of more dermatologists in a community include prompt removal of atypical moles and one-to-one expert education regarding self-screening and family screening.

Researchers in Nova Scotia used a billing system within their province to examine access to and continuity with family practitioners and their association with melanoma thickness. Patients with multiple visits to the same physician (rather than to many different providers) had a lower risk for having a thicker than 0.75 mm melanoma at the time of diagnosis.[42] Access to care is also illustrated by recent studies using Medicare data finding that diagnosis by a dermatologist (as opposed to nondermatologist physicians) predicts melanoma survival at 2 years.[43] In a study of 42 counties in North Carolina (including many rural counties)[44] Stitzenberg and colleagues found that greater distance from home to a dermatologist predicted melanoma Breslow thickness. They suggested that proximity to dermatologic care was an indicator of local health resources and observed that patients who lived in counties with at least one dermatologist traveled less for care than communities with fewer dermatologists.[44] In the United States, mortality rates of melanoma appeared to be higher in states with the lowest ratio of dermatologists to the public.[45]

Suggested steps for improving access to skilled examinations

Educational efforts to overcome disparities must expand public outreach and education, educate health care providers and the public, and recruit new screeners in light of the shortage of medical dermatologists in high-risk areas. New screeners could include not only nurses and nurse practitioners and physician assistants but also medical students and residents who have not been formally trained.

Increasing the availability of free screenings for individuals previously unscreened should be the lynchpin of national campaigns led by the American Academy of Dermatology and rapidly proliferating US melanoma foundations, which have heretofore emphasized sun protection to the exclusion of early detection. Professional education programs with physicians and physicians-in-training must alert them not only to well-established risks such as adverse sun exposure for their patients but also to the disproportionate burden of late-stage disease related to social class and gender.

Patient navigation systems that have drawn increased attention for other "early detectable" cancers[46] should be used to assist patients with significant risk factors for melanoma. Such patients could be identified and provided personal teaching in skin self-examination (SSE), encouraged to promptly follow through after diagnosis of presumptive melanomas, and to avoid delay in postreferral surgical care. In more impoverished areas, novel patient navigation systems may enhance high-risk patients' opportunities to access skilled and expert evaluations.

Improved screening and outreach for underserved individuals will be best accomplished through a concerted combination of the following: (1) policy changes to provide melanoma screening as a benefit of health care, (2) chart reminders to encourage physicians to provide first-time screening to at-risk patients, and (3) advocacy for legislation to support melanoma screening.[2] However, well before such initiatives become a mainstay of US primary care, proof via large-scale randomized trials must show the efficacy of the clinician total-body screen for melanoma. In the next section, we review the current screening efforts and propose various strategies for the United States.

Mass Screening Campaigns and Trials

Fatal melanoma is generally visible on the surface of the skin at a curable phase in its evolution, presenting a theoretical opportunity in almost all cases to prevent death through early detection.[47,48] The high-risk group for death from melanoma are adults older than 45 or 50 years of age, and among that group, population-based mortality rates continue to increase.[1,10] There is an urgent and important need to promptly reverse this trend.

The USPSTF finds that there is insufficient evidence to recommend for or against screening for melanoma based on the absence of randomized trials, indicating an impact of screening on mortality.[6] Few physicians report being skilled in the skin cancer examination, and most medical students are not specifically taught skin cancer examination during training.[39] Given this lack of expertise, the lack of formal recommendations for screening, and the growing time pressures of clinical practice, it is not surprising that current rates of melanoma screening are very low. It can be anticipated that they will remain very low barring the development of a standardized melanoma screening procedure and randomized trial data supporting the efficacy of melanoma screening. To address this large gap between rates of disease and less than optimal screening rates, the US House and Senate Appropriations Committee endorsed the Strategic Plan for Melanoma and asked the National Cancer Institute to consider a national screening study for early melanoma detection.

There is much precedent for the development of new screening trials. Researchers in Australia (where such a study is more feasible because of higher rates of melanoma) planned and began to implement a randomized trial of population screening.[11–13] Although the plan called for eventually randomizing 44 Queensland communities, 18 were initially randomized to intervention (n = 9) and control (n = 9) towns. The trial's 3 components included (1) a community education component, which aimed to provide accurate information about melanoma and screening to residents, (2) an education and support component for medical practitioners, which aimed to increase awareness of the program and to improve doctors' skills in screening for and diagnosing melanoma, and (3) the provision of free skin screening services.[11–13] Uptake of the whole-body skin cancer examination was measured by surveys of residents in intervention and control towns. Baseline rates were similar in intervention and control towns (11.2% and 11.3%); however, rates for full-body examinations increased within 2 years to 34.8% in intervention towns compared with 13.9% in control communities.[11–13] Screenings were performed generally by general practitioners and special screening services. More than 16,000 whole-body examinations had been conducted in 18 communities, with the following confirmed diagnoses: 33 melanomas, 259 basal cell carcinomas, and 97 squamous cell carcinomas with the probability of detecting any type of skin cancer of 2.4%.[11–13] The overall specificity of the skin examination for melanoma was 86.1%. Unfortunately, because of the lack of governmental funding, the study was not expanded to the 44 communities and was disbanded. Data are forthcoming on the effect of screening on tumor thickness among screened individuals.

A recent report of the experience of the Lawrence Livermore National Laboratories describes an early detection program associated with the reduction of melanoma deaths to zero among all employees.[49] A case-control study associated monthly SSE with substantially reduced melanoma mortality.[50] In people with multiple primary melanomas, who receive close clinician surveillance as well as education and training in SSE after their first primary melanoma, second primaries were noted to be thinner.[51] Dermatologist skin examinations are also associated with thinner melanoma lesions,[52] and physician-detected melanomas in general are thinner, likely, with a better prognosis.[53] Using computer modeling, melanoma early detection procedures have been projected to be cost-effective in appropriate demographic groups.[54,55]

In response to the compelling need to demonstrate the efficacy of screening for reducing melanoma mortality, and in anticipation of possible funding for such a trial in response to recommendations in the 2008 US Congressional appropriations bill, a group of investigators, the Melanoma Screening Group (MSG), has been working toward creating a Melanoma Early Detection (MED) Trial. During the past year, the MSG has conducted an extensive review of the cancer screening literature, consulted with members of its advisory panel, held regular conference calls to determine a plan of action, elaborated on key study design features, and established important contacts with a major potential screening site, the HMO Cancer Research Network.

Several key points and broad principles were derived from these efforts with particular attention given to the scope of a large trial and the need for a pilot trial to test the feasibility, recruitment strategies, throughput, and sensitivity and specificity for a larger trial.

1. Current lack of primary care physician expertise in skin cancer detection and the limited availability of dermatologists preclude the use of physician examiners as the only mode of population-based routine melanoma screening.
2. Significant preliminary data support the potential utility of specially trained nurses as melanoma screeners.[56] One can draw lessons from screening for colorectal cancer in which nurse practitioners have been reported to show equal proficiency as gastroenterologists for the sigmoidoscopy.[57]
3. Established but not thoroughly tested technologies, including dermoscopy and teleconsultation, are available for use by and support of nurse screeners.
4. Unlike most other cancers, including breast cancer, the earliest stages of melanoma are readily visible and amenable to detection by self-examination, and hence training in self-detection should be a component of melanoma screening.
5. The costs and morbidity associated with the screening procedure will need to be assessed in addition to the mortality end points. The extent to which the screening procedure results in additional skin surgery and other morbidity and resource use will be determined to the extent possible from routinely collected data in the health systems in which the participants were recruited.

For economy and practicality in conducting the MED trial, recruitment could occur in HMOs and/or Veterans Affairs Medical Centers/affiliated Community-Based Outpatient Centers. This has the added advantage that all participants will have access to health care in the health system from which they were recruited for any melanoma that is discovered.

Based on current melanoma incidence and mortality, a randomized trial of melanoma screening with a 20% impact on mortality will require a screened study population of 350,000 Americans (and 700,000 controls) aged 45 years and older, with a 4-year intervention period and 8 years passive follow-up at an estimated cost of $30 to 40 million. Traditionally, large-scale trials have used mortality as proper end point. However, with compelling data confirming the usefulness of tumor thickness and stage of disease as a proxy for mortality, exploring the concept of melanoma severity should be addressed as part of any cost projections.

The purpose of this proposed trial is to test the effect of early detection intervention on melanoma mortality by exploiting the notion of a proof of principle that captures the synergy between SSE, clinician skin examination, and advances in technology. Teaching of the SSE can be woven into the clinician examination and augmented by video instruction and personalized reminders.

Pilot trial

Various study designs have been considered, including (1) standard care control versus (2) a nurse-led clinical examination and SSE teaching versus (3) a robust arm that would include nurse clinical examination, SSE teaching, dermoscopy, and teledermatology. In a 4- to 5-year pilot trial, multiple experiments on the frequency with which screenees receive examinations can be tested. Modules for standardized training of nurses in the conduct of dermoscopically assisted screening examinations and for the assessment of the proficiency of trained examiners in terms of diagnostic accuracy and patient acceptance will be constructed. In addition to providing a standardized and optimized screening examination for the ensuing clinical trial, the modules developed with this aim will be applicable for the training, testing, certification, and credentialing of the many physician extenders currently being used for skin cancer detection in the absence of any national standards.

Choosing an appropriate end point for a pilot trial that can serve as a useful surrogate for early detection of melanoma is challenging, because it is expected that there would be few melanomas in an appropriate sample of 2000 of 3000 subjects, most likely the size of a pilot trial. Some degree of at least moderate atypia would be the likely candidate for a reasonable outcome, and this should allow researchers to test the sensitivity and specificity for such an examination.

The early detection procedure and training for it will be drafted by a core group and will be evaluated and revised in collaboration with a larger advisory committee of clinicians (including primary care physicians, dermatologists, nurses, and others), scientists with relevant expertise, and educators assembled for that purpose. The final early detection intervention should be applicable to training at multiple sites. This procedure must combine the key components of early detection for melanoma, including history, visual examination, and dermoscopic examination with selected use of imaging and teledermoscopy and combined with thorough SSE counseling and training. Since board-certified dermatologists are generally viewed as the "gold standard" for melanoma diagnosis, it must be demonstrated that a group of nurses can perform with high sensitivity and reasonable specificity in a screening context so they can reliably provide the initial screen. This performance can be measured by testing the trained nurses using an established digital archive of high-resolution, total body, and individual skin lesion images as well as with live patients.

There will be many other issues in conducting a large trial, and some of these can be answered in a pilot trial that allows researchers to examine questions of feasibility. These could include:

1. the number of recruitment calls and mailings needed to get one person coming for a screening
2. differences among participants who complete one round of screening versus those who participate in multiple screenings
3. the number of staff needed to screen and provide counseling
4. the ease with which positive screenees can be seen by dermatologists and biopsies can be obtained if necessary
5. the ability to track patients through first follow-up as well as reminder systems for second- and third-year screenings
6. the ability to obtain screening results via pathology laboratories and to track case and death reports via cancer registries and the National Death Index
7. the establishment of a tracer organization that locates people who leave their current HMOs
8. the standardization of procedures for obtaining and processing all study information
9. the unit cost for follow-up treatments.

International Trends for Melanoma Survival and Mortality

Although developing screening and educational programs is of paramount importance for highly industrialized nations with high incidence rates, there are a number of countries with far worse mortality and survival rates. For these countries, a far greater understanding of their health care systems is needed before planning can proceed. Herein, we present data on the strong disparities between nations.

Although 5-year survival rates in many countries, such as the United States, Scotland, Australia, and Sweden, surpass 90%, worldwide melanoma control must be a priority, because a number of countries have not benefited from early detection and educational programs.[58,59] Very low 5-year survival rates have been found among men in Northern Ireland (53.5), Cracow (55.8), the Czech Republic (60.3), and Slovenia (60.6) equaling survival rates in the United States and Australia from more than 40 years ago. Survival rates for women generally fared no better in these 4 countries (58).

Four Eastern European countries (Croatia, Slovenia, Macedonia, and the Slovak Republic) are the 10 nations in the world with the highest melanoma mortality rates in men; 5 nations (Latvia, Estonia, Lithuania, Slovak Republic, and Macedonia) are among the 10 nations with the highest mortality rates in women.[58] For women, mortality/incidence ratios (MIR) are 0.460 for less developed regions and 0.179 for more developed regions. In fact, for three countries with more than 200 cases per year among women (Ethiopia, Zaire, and Indonesia), the MIR exceeds 60%. In contrast, the US MIR is less than 15%.[1]

Notably, 5-year survival rates are also low in Croatia, and a 20-year epidemiologic study of one of the more populous districts in Croatia found strong disparities in late-detected melanoma. For example, NM made up 35% of all diagnoses, more than three-fold found in countries with higher melanoma survival. Most of the lesions were thicker than 1.50 mm. The authors called for more effective community information and a commitment to mass education.[59]

REFERENCES

1. Surveillance, Epidemiology, and End Results (SEER) Program. Limited-Use Data (1973–2005), National Cancer Institute, DCCPS, Surveillance Research Program, Cancer Statistics Branch, released April 2008, based on the November 2007 submission. Available at: www.seer.cancer.gov.
2. Geller AC, Miller DR, Swetter SM, et al. A call for the development and implementation of a targeted national melanoma screening program [see comment] [editorial]. Arch Dermatol 2006;142:504–7.
3. Skin Cancer Foundation. Available at: http://www.skincancer.org/. Accessed December 28, 2008.
4. American Cancer Society. Available at: http://www.cancer.org/docroot/home/index.asp. Accessed December 28, 2008.
5. American Academy of Dermatology. Available at: http://www.aad.org/default.htm. Accessed December 28, 2008.
6. US Preventive Services Task Force. Screening for skin cancer: US Preventive Services Task Force recommendation statement. Ann Intern Med 2009;150:188–93.
7. Saraiya M, Hall HI, Thompson T, et al. Skin cancer screening among U.S. adults from 1992, 1998, and 2000 National Health Interview Surveys. Prev Med 2004;39:308–14.
8. Santmyire BR, Feldman SR, Fleischer AB Jr. Lifestyle high-risk behaviors and demographics may predict the level of participation in sun-protection behaviors and skin cancer primary prevention in the United States: results of the 1998 National Health Interview Survey. Cancer 2001;92:1315–24.
9. Reyes-Ortiz CA, Goodwin JS, Freeman JL, et al. Socioeconomic status and survival in older patients with melanoma. J Am Geriatr Soc 2006;54:1758–64.
10. Geller AC, Miller DR, Annas GD, et al. Melanoma incidence and mortality among US whites, 1969–1999. JAMA 2002;288:1719–20.
11. Aitken JF, Elwood JM, Lowe JB, et al. A randomised trial of population screening for melanoma. J Med Screen 2002;9:33–7.
12. Aitken JF, Janda M, Elwood M, et al. Clinical outcomes from skin cancer screening clinics within a community-based melanoma screening program. J Am Acad Dermatol 2006;54:105–14.
13. Aitken JF, Youl PH, Janda M, et al. Increase in skin cancer screening during a community-based randomized intervention trial. Int J Cancer 2006;118:1010–6.
14. Crocetti E, Capocaccia R, Casella C, et al. Population-based incidence and mortality cancer trends (1986–1997) from the network of Italian cancer registries. Eur J Cancer Prev 2004;13:287–95.
15. Marrett LD, Nguyen HL, Armstrong BK. Trends in the incidence of cutaneous malignant melanoma in New South Wales, 1983–1996. Int J Cancer 2001;92:457–62.
16. Lindholm C, Andersson R, Dufmats M, et al. Swedish Melanoma Study Group. Invasive cutaneous malignant melanoma in Sweden, 1990–1999. A prospective, population-based study of survival and prognostic factors. Cancer 2004;101:2067–78.
17. MacKie RM, Bray CA, Hole DJ, et al. Scottish Melanoma Group. Incidence of and survival from malignant melanoma in Scotland: an epidemiological study. Lancet 2002;360:587–91.
18. de Vries E, Bray FI, Eggermont AM, et al. European Network of Cancer Registries. Monitoring stage-specific trends in melanoma incidence across Europe reveals

the need for more complete information on diagnostic characteristics. Eur J Cancer Prev 2004;13:387–95.

19. de Vries E, Bray FI, Coebergh JW, et al. Changing epidemiology of malignant cutaneous melanoma in Europe 1953–1997: rising trends in incidence and mortality but recent stabilizations in western Europe and decreases in Scandinavia. Int J Cancer 2003;107:119–26.

20. Koh HK, Miller DR, Geller AC, et al. Who discovers melanoma? Patterns from a population-based survey. J Am Acad Dermatol 1992;26:914–9.

21. Ferlay JBF, Pisani P, Parkin DM. GLOBOCAN 2002. Cancer incidence, mortality and prevalence worldwide. Lyon (France): IARC Press; 2004.

22. Diepgen TL, Mahler V. The epidemiology of skin cancer. Br J Dermatol 2002; 146(Suppl 61):1–6.

23. Severi G, Giles GG, Robertson C, et al. Mortality from cutaneous melanoma: evidence for contrasting trends between populations. Br J Cancer 2000;82: 1887–91.

24. Cohn-Cedermark G, Mansson-Brahme E, Rutqvist LE, et al. Trends in mortality from malignant melanoma in Sweden, 1970–1996. Cancer 2000;89:348–55.

25. Miller DR, Geller AC, Wyatt SW, et al. Melanoma awareness and self-examination practices: results of a United States survey. J Am Acad Dermatol 1996;34:962–70.

26. Swetter Sm JT, Miller DR, Layton CJ, et al. Melanoma in Middle-Aged and Older Men: a multi-institutional survey study of factors related to tumor thickness. Arch Dermatol, in press.

27. Koh HK, Geller AC, Miller DR, et al. Who is being screened for melanoma/skin cancer? Characteristics of persons screened in Massachusetts. J Am Acad Dermatol 1991;24:271–7.

28. Ortiz CA, Goodwin JS, Freeman JL. The effect of socioeconomic factors on incidence, stage at diagnosis and survival of cutaneous melanoma. Med Sci Monit 2005;11:RA163–72.

29. Geller AC, Koh HK, Miller DR, et al. Use of health services before the diagnosis of melanoma: implications for early detection and screening. J Gen Intern Med 1992;7:154–7.

30. Singh GK, Miller BA, Hankey BF, et al. Area socioeconomic variations in U.S. cancer incidence, mortality, stage, treatment, and survival, 1975–1999. NCI Cancer Surveillance Monograph Series, Number 4. Bethesda (MD): National Cancer Institute; 2003. NIH Publication No. 03-5417.

31. Geller AC, Miller DR, Lew RA, et al. Cutaneous melanoma mortality among the socioeconomically disadvantaged in Massachusetts. Am J Public Health 1996; 86:538–43.

32. Geller AC, Elwood M, Swetter SM, et al. Factors related to the presentation of thin and thick nodular melanoma from a population-based cancer registry in Queensland Australia. Cancer 2009;115:1318–27.

33. Cress RD, Holly EA. Incidence of cutaneous melanoma among non-Hispanic whites, Hispanics, Asians, and blacks: an analysis of California cancer registry data, 1988–93. Cancer Causes Control 1997;8:246–52.

34. Byrd KM, Wilson DC, Hoyler SS, et al. Advanced presentation of melanoma in African Americans. J Am Acad Dermatol 2004;50:21–4 [discussion: 142–3].

35. Hemmings DE, Johnson DS, Tominaga GT, et al. Cutaneous melanoma in a multi-ethnic population: is this a different disease? Arch Surg 2004;139:968–72 [discussion: 972–3].

36. Cockburn MG, Zadnick J, Deapen D. Developing epidemic of melanoma in the Hispanic population of California. Cancer 2006;106:1162–8.

37. Demierre MF, Chung C, Miller DR, et al. Early detection of thick melanomas in the United States: beware of the nodular subtype. Arch Dermatol 2005;141:745–50.
38. Queensland Cancer Registry. Available at: http://www.cancerqld.org.au/research/qcr/qld_cancerReg.asp.
39. Moore MM, Geller AC, Zhang Z, et al. Skin cancer examination teaching in US medical education. Arch Dermatol 2006;142:439–44.
40. Coups EJ, Manne SL, Heckman CJ. Multiple skin cancer risk behaviors in the US population. Am J Prev Med 2008;34:87–93.
41. Roetzheim RG, Pal N, van Durme DJ, et al. Increasing supplies of dermatologists and family physicians are associated with earlier stage of melanoma detection. J Am Acad Dermatol 2000;43:211–8.
42. Di Quinzio ML, Dewar RA, Burge FI, et al. Family physician visits and early recognition of melanoma. Can J Public Health 2005;96:136–9.
43. Pennie ML, Soon SL, Risser JB, et al. Melanoma outcomes for Medicare patients: association of stage and survival with detection by a dermatologist vs a nonder-matologist. Arch Dermatol 2007;143:488–94.
44. Stitzenberg KB, Thomas NE, Dalton K, et al. Distance to diagnosing provider as a measure of access for patients with melanoma. Arch Dermatol 2007;143:991–8.
45. Geller AC, Swetter SM, Brooks K, et al. Screening, early detection, and trends for melanoma: current status (2000–2006) and future directions. J Am Acad Dermatol 2007;57:555–72 [quiz 573–6].
46. Freeman HP. Patient navigation: a community centered approach to reducing cancer mortality. J Cancer Educ 2006;21:S11–4.
47. Weinstock MA. Progress and prospects on melanoma: the way forward for early detection and reduced mortality. Clin Cancer Res 2006;12(7 Pt 2):2297s–300s.
48. Koh HK. Cutaneous melanoma. N Engl J Med 1991;325:171–82.
49. Schneider JS, Moore DH III, Mendelsohn ML. Screening program reduced melanoma mortality at the Lawrence Livermore National Laboratory, 1984 to 1996. J Am Acad Dermatol 2008;58:741–9.
50. Berwick M, Begg CB, Fine JA, et al. Screening for cutaneous melanoma by skin self-examination [see comment]. J Natl Cancer Inst 1996;88:17–23.
51. DiFronzo LA, Wanek LA, Morton DL. Earlier diagnosis of second primary melanoma confirms the benefits of patient education and routine postoperative follow-up. Cancer 2001;91:1520–4.
52. Fisher NM, Schaffer JV, Berwick M, et al. Breslow depth of cutaneous melanoma: impact of factors related to surveillance of the skin, including prior skin biopsies and family history of melanoma. J Am Acad Dermatol 2005;53:393–406.
53. Epstein DS, Lange JR, Gruber SB, et al. Is physician detection associated with thinner melanomas? JAMA 1999;281:640–3.
54. Losina E, Walensky R, Geller AC, et al. Visual screening for malignant melanoma. A cost-effectiveness analysis. Arch Dermatol 2007;143:21–8.
55. Girgis A, Campbell EM, Redman S, et al. Screening for melanoma: a community survey of prevalence and predictors. Med J Aust 1991;154:338–43.
56. Govindan K, Smith J, Knowles L, et al. Assessment of nurse-led screening of pigmented lesions using SIAscope. J Plast Reconstr Aesthet Surg 2007;60:639–45.
57. Kelly SB, Murphy J, Smith A, et al. Nurse specialist led flexible sigmoidoscopy in an outpatient setting. Colorectal Dis 2008;10:390–3.
58. Globocan. Available at: http://www-dep.iarc.fr/globocan/downloads.html.
59. Zamolo G, Gruber F, Jonjic A, et al. A 20-year epidemiological study of cutaneous melanoma in the Rijeka district of Croatia. Clin Exp Dermatol 2000;25:77–81.

BRAF Signaling and Targeted Therapies in Melanoma

Nathalie Dhomen, BSc, PhD, Richard Marais, BSc, PhD*

KEYWORDS

- BRAF • Melanoma • MAPK signaling • Targeted therapies
- Small molecule inhibitors

The past decade has seen significant advances in our understanding of the cell signaling pathways that drive melanoma in humans. These studies have demonstrated that the RAS/RAF/MEK/ERK pathway is hyperactivated in the majority of human melanomas and that this pathway plays a critical role in regulating melanoma cell proliferation, invasion, and survival. This pathway has therefore emerged as a major player in the induction and maintenance of melanoma and has been validated as a therapeutic target in this disease. The availability of new drugs to the components of this pathway means that targeted therapies are fast becoming a real option in the clinical management of melanoma. Clinical trials using the first-generation inhibitors of this pathway have been completed and trials using the second-generation inhibitors are currently underway. Here we discuss what we have learned about targeting this pathway in melanoma.

THE RAS/RAF/MEK/ERK SIGNALING PATHWAY

The RAS and RAF genes were identified over 25 years ago; since then, the pathway has been studied in enormous detail. RAS is a small G-protein that binds to the inner surface of the plasma membrane, and RAF, MEK, and ERK are protein kinases that form a three-tiered kinase cascade. In the canonical pathway (**Fig. 1**), RAS initiates RAF activation and then RAF phosphorylates and activates MEK, which in turn phosphorylates and activates ERK. ERK regulates gene expression, metabolism, and cytoskeletal functions to control cell functions from proliferation to differentiation and senescence to death. As drawn, the representation in **Fig. 1** is a naïve view of the pathway, because in reality it has a considerably more complex architecture. There are three RAS genes (HRAS, KRAS, NRAS), three RAF genes (ARAF, BRAF, CRAF),

This work was supported by Cancer Research UK (C107/A10433) and the Institute of Cancer Research.

Section of Cell and Molecular Biology, Institute of Cancer Research, 237 Fulham Road, London SW3 6JB, UK

* Corresponding author.

E-mail address: richard.marais@icr.ac.uk (R. Marais).

Hematol Oncol Clin N Am 23 (2009) 529–545
doi:10.1016/j.hoc.2009.04.001
0889-8588/09/$ – see front matter © 2009 Elsevier Inc. All rights reserved.

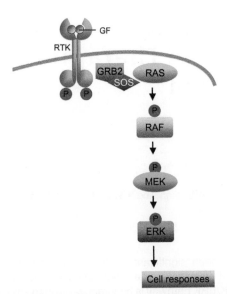

Fig. 1. Overview of the RAS/RAF/MEK/ERK signaling pathway. Upon binding of growth factors (GF) to receptor tyrosine kinases (RTK), RAS becomes activated at the plasma membrane via GRB2 and SOS. Activated RAS recruits RAF to the plasma membrane where it in turn becomes activated. RAF phosphorylates and activates MEK, which in turn phosphorylates and activates ERK. Activated ERK mediates various cellular responses, such as proliferation, survival, and differentiation.

two MEKs (MEK1, MEK2) and two ERKs (ERK1, ERK2). In addition, a variety of scaffold proteins enhance or restrict interactions between the components to provide exquisite regulation of the signaling through the pathway.[1] Importantly, the cellular consequences of ERK signaling depend on the intensity and duration of the ERK signal, on which other pathways are active in the cell, and on intrinsic and extrinsic cell factors. Together, this network enables this pathway to participate in such apparently contradictory cellular outcomes.

A major breakthrough in melanoma biology came in 2002, when large-scale resequencing of ERK pathway components revealed a high frequency of mutations in BRAF in human melanoma.[2] NRAS mutations were already known to occur in melanoma, but subsequent large-scale resequencing campaigns revealed BRAF to be mutated in approximately 44% of melanomas (**Table 1**), NRAS to be mutated in 21% of cases, KRAS in 2% of cases, and HRAS in 1% of cases. No mutations have been seen in ARAF, CRAF, MEK, or ERK, but the receptor tyrosine kinase c-KIT and the heterotrimeric G-protein α-subunit GNAQ, both of which also signal through ERK, are mutated in a high proportion of mucosal and acral, and uveal melanomas, respectively.[3,4] As a consequence of these mutations, ERK (which is normally only activated downstream of receptor tyrosine kinases, cytokine receptors and heterotrimeric G-protein coupled receptors), is constitutively activated in melanoma cells.

Over 65 mutations affecting over 30 codons have been identified in BRAF in malignant melanoma (see **Table 1**) and most cluster in two regions of the kinase domain—the glycine-rich loop and the activation segment—and involve residues that stabilize the inactive form of the kinase.[5] Thus, most of the mutations are thought to destabilize the inactive conformation, allowing the active conformation to prevail. The majority of these mutations activate BRAF from 1.5 to 700 fold, although a small number actually are inactivating.[5] However, even these inactive mutants can activate ERK because they can bind to and activate CRAF, which then activates MEK.[5,6]

The most common mutation in BRAF in melanoma is a glutamic acid for valine substitution at position 600 (V600E). This mutation, which activates BRAF 500-fold, accounts for over 90% of those that occur in melanoma. BRAF[V600E] stimulates constitutive ERK signaling in cultured melanocytes, driving cell transformation and allowing the cells to proliferate in a growth factor-independent manner in vitro and as tumors in nude mice.[7] Furthermore, recent transgenic mouse models have been developed that allow regulated expression of BRAF[V600E] off the endogenous mouse gene in mature melanocytes.[8,9] Expression of BRAF[V600E] induces melanoma and, when combined with loss of the PTEN phosphatase, the mice develop metastatic disease with 100% penetrance and short latency. In human melanoma cells, RNA interference and small molecule inhibitors of BRAF and MEK have been used to show that BRAF[V600E] drives constitutive ERK and NFκB activity and stimulates proliferation and survival.[10–14] In mice, targeting BRAF or MEK suppresses human melanoma xenograft tumor growth, decreases vasculogenesis by suppressing VEGF production, and reduces seeding of melanoma cells to the lungs in a model of metastatic tumor growth.[15–17]

Together, these data demonstrate that BRAF mutations can be founder events in melanomagenesis and establish that BRAF[V600E] is required for melanoma maintenance and progression, and, as mutational activation of BRAF is the most common genetic lesion in melanoma, these data validate BRAF as an important therapeutic target in melanoma. Consequently, a number of BRAF drug discovery programs have been initiated.

FIRST-GENERATION INHIBITORS

The first-generation inhibitors of the MAP kinase pathway were not designed to target oncogenic BRAF, because they were developed before the BRAF mutations had been discovered. The initial interest in this pathway was predicated on the fact that RAS is mutated in up to 20% of human cancers, thus identifying RAS as a therapeutic target in cancer.[18] However, attempts to perturb RAS interactions with the exchange factor son-of-sevenless (SOS), its upstream activator, or to target the interaction between SOS and the adaptor protein GRB2, have not generated any viable drug candidates.[19] More promising were the farnesyltransferase inhibitors (FTIs) that were designed to block an essential posttranslational modification of RAS, thereby disrupting RAS localization to the plasma membrane and perturbing its signaling function.[20] Preclinical studies demonstrated that FTIs compromise neoplastic transformation and tumor growth in mice, and Phase I trials revealed these compounds to be relatively well tolerated.[21,22] However, the Phase II trial results were disappointing and it has now become clear that these drugs are rather unspecific and that their antineoplastic activity is due to off-target effects on other farnesylated proteins.[20] Furthermore, in the presence of FTIs, KRAS becomes geranyl-geranylated, a modification that substitutes for farnesylation and allows KRAS to escape the action of these drugs.[23]

Because RAS has proven to be such an intractable target, alternative approaches to targeting this pathway were sought and the focus turned to its downstream effetors. In particular, the RAF/MEK/ERK and phosphatidylinositol 3-kinase (PI3K) pathways were selected, in part because they were the first pathways to be identified downstream of RAS, but also because they were shown to regulate proliferation in cancer cells. However, before BRAF was shown to be mutated in cancer, CRAF was thought to be the important isoform that transmits proliferation signals downstream of RAS,

Table 1
Summary of reported incidence of BRAF mutations in malignant melanoma samples

Amino Acid	Coding Variants	Freq (%)	Sample Source (Incidence)
K439	Q	0.05	primary (1)
R444	W	0.05	surgery–fixed (1)
G464	R	0.05	primary (1)
G466	A,E,R,V	0.42	primary (6), metastasis (1), surgery–fixed (1)
S467	L	0.05	surgery–fixed (1)
G469	E,R,S,V	0.62	surgery–fixed(6), surgery–NOS (1), metastasis (3), primary (1), cell line (1)
K475	M	0.05	secondary (1)
N581	I	0.05	fixed–NOS (1)
I582	M	0.05	primary (1)
L584	F	0.05	surgery–NOS (1)
E586	K	0.10	cell line(1), surgery–fixed (1)
D587	E,N	0.10	surgery–fixed (2)
L588	P,R	0.10	surgery–fixed(2)
I592	M,V	0.16	primary (2), surgery–fixed (1)
D594	E,G,N,V	0.26	primary (3), surgery–NOS (2)
F595	L, S	0.10	surgery–fixed (1), primary (1)
G596	S	0.05	surgery–fixed (1)
L597	Q,R,S,V	0.52	metastasis(4), short-term culture (2), primary (1), cell line (1), surgery–NOS (1), surgery–fixed(1)
A598	V	0.05	surgery–fixed (1)
T599	I	0.05	primary (1)
T599 insertion	Two amino acid insertion (TT)	0.16	primary (1), mestastasis (1), surgery–NOS (1)
T599 insertion	Amino acid insertion (V)	0.05	surgery–fresh/frozen (1)
V600	D,E,G,K,M,R	95.16	surgery–fixed (438), cell line (221), metastasis (338), primary (328), secondary (11), blood–bone marrow (58), fixed–NOS (5), NS (122), recurrent (1), short-term culture (14), surgery–NOS (209), surgery–fresh/frozen (83), fixed–NOS (1)
V600 ins/del	Two amino acids replaced by a glutamic acid	0.05	primary (1)
V600 ins/del	Six amino acids replaced by an aspartic acid	0.05	primary (1)
K601	E,I,N	0.52	primary (3), metastasis (2), surgery–fixed (2), surgery–NOS (2), surgery–fresh/frozen (1)

(continued on next page)

Table 1
(continued)

Amino Acid	Coding Variants	Freq (%)	Sample Source (Incidence)
W604	G,S	0.10	primary (1), surgery–NOS (1)
S605	F,G,N,R	0.26	surgery–fixed (2), surgery–NOS (1), primary (2)
G606	E	0.05	primary (1)
S607	P	0.05	surgery–fixed (1)
H608	R	0.05	primary (1)
Q609	R	0.05	surgery–fixed (1)
E611	D	0.05	surgery–fixed (1)
S614	P	0.10	primary (1), surgery–fixed (1)
G615	R	0.05	primary (1)
S616	P	0.05	primary (1)
I617	T	0.05	surgery–fixed(1)
L618	S	0.10	primary (2)
W619	R	0.05	surgery–fixed (1)

Of 4274 melanoma samples analyzed, 1884 (44%) had BRAF mutations.
Column 1 lists the mutations described in BRAF in melanoma.
Column 2 shows the residues to which they are mutated (coding variant).
Column 3 provides the frequency with which each residue is mutated with respect to reported BRAF mutations. These data are compiled from 194 publications with over 1900 BRAF mutation–positive tumor samples and cell lines. Due to editorial limitations, we are unable to cite all the references used to compile this table and we apologize to the authors of those papers not cited. For a detailed description of the BRAF mutations in cancer, please see the COSMIC Web site (www.sanger.ac.uk/genetics/CGP/cosmic/).
Column 4 lists the sample source in which the mutations were identified. Incidence refers to the total number of times the mutations at the indicated position have been identified in the reported samples.

and BRAF was thought to regulate differentiation.[24] Although it is now known that both isoforms transmit proliferation signals, this early misconception focused the early cancer drug discovery programs on CRAF.

The first viable compound to emerge from these efforts was sorafenib (BAY 43-9006), which was developed in a classical medicinal chemistry optimisation program using CRAF as the target.[25,26] Sorafenib inhibits CRAF with an IC_{50} of 12 nM and in cell-based assays it inhibits RAF-mediated pathway activation in colon, pancreatic, and breast tumor cell lines expressing mutant KRAS. It also inhibits tumor cell proliferation and transformation in vitro, and once daily oral dosing of sorafenib demonstrated broad-spectrum antitumor activity in colon, breast, and non–small-cell lung cancer xenograft models.[27] Sorafenib was subsequently found to inhibit purified BRAF^{V600E} with an IC_{50} of 40 nM, although its activity in cells is less impressive at about 5 μM.[10] Nevertheless, it suppresses the growth of melanoma xenografts in nude mice.[10]

Based on these results, melanoma patients were actively recruited to an existing multicenter phase II randomized discontinuation trial (RDT) with sorafenib.[28] Subjects who had advanced disease received a 12-week run-in of sorafenib and were then assessed. Those subjects whose tumors had grown more than 25% were judged to be nonresponders and were removed from the study. Subjects whose tumors shrank more than 25% were judged to be responding and continued on open-label sorafenib.

However, to determine whether the remaining subjects were responding, they were randomized to sorafenib or placebo for a further 12 weeks. If their tumors started to grow, the code was broken and if that subject had been randomized to placebo, it was clear that the drug was active against their tumor and they were switched back to sorafenib.

Thirty-seven melanoma subjects were enrolled. Seven (19%) achieved stable disease (SD) (n = 1 open-label; n = 6 randomized), 23 (62%) had progressive disease (PD) and 7 (19%) could not be evaluated. No complete responses (CR) were observed. The overall median progression-free survival (PFS) was 11 weeks. DNA was extracted from the tumors of 17 of 22 subjects and six were shown to harbor mutations in BRAF[V600E]. Of these, four had PD, one SD, and one could not be evaluated. Of the 11 subjects whose tumors did not have BRAF mutations (none had RAS mutations), nine had PD, one SD, and one could not be evaluated. Thus, although this study demonstrated that sorafenib is well tolerated, it also showed that single-agent sorafenib is ineffective in melanoma and that BRAF mutations do not predict for response.

Despite these unpromising results, sorafenib was combined with conventional chemotherapy in melanoma patients. In one trial of 105 subjects, sorafenib was combined with paclitaxel and carboplatin. Disease control was achieved in 85% (CR + PR + SD) of subjects and a median PFS of 8.8 months was observed.[29] A second study yielded one CR and nine PR amongst 24 subjects and, most important, these responses appeared durable.[30] However, there was no correlation between clinical response and BRAF mutation status in either study. Nevertheless, due to the encouraging responses, randomized phase III trials were performed to assess this combination. One study involved 270 subjects who had failed dacarbazine (DTIC) or temozolomide (TMZ)-based treatments, but there was no improvement in PFS or overall response rate comparing sorafenib-plus-paclitaxel-and-carboplatin with paclitaxel-and-carboplatin alone (17.9 versus 17.4 weeks[31]). In a second, larger trial, 800 subjects who had not received previous chemotherapy were randomized to carboplatin-and-paclitaxel with placebo or with sorafenib (http://clinicaltrials.gov/ct/show/NCT00110019). This trial is now closed and the primary endpoint is overall survival. The results are expected in April 2010.

Sorafenib has also been combined with DTIC or TMZ. Sorafenib and DTIC are well tolerated, but, once again, BRAF mutation status did not predict response[32] and in a single-arm phase II study, subjects who had advanced metastatic disease achieved a median PFS of 14.6 weeks,[33] compared with a published PFS of 6 weeks for DTIC alone.[34] Similarly, in a randomized, double-blind, placebo-controlled multicenter study with 101 chemotherapy-naïve subjects who had stage III (unresectable) or stage IV melanoma, the median PFS in the sorafenib-plus-DTIC arm was 21.1 weeks versus 11.7 weeks in the placebo-plus-DTIC arm (hazard ratio [HR], 0.665; $P = .068$). There were statistically significant improvements in PFS at 6 and 9 months, and in time-to-progression (TTP; median, 21.1 versus 11.7 weeks; HR, 0.619) in favor of the sorafenib-containing arm. However, no difference was observed in overall survival (median, 51.3 versus 45.6 weeks comparing placebo-plus-DTIC with sorafenib-plus-DTIC; HR, 1.022).[35] Finally, in a randomized phase II study of TMZ and sorafenib in advanced melanoma, subjects received either extended dose (75 mg/m^2 every day for 6 out of 8 weeks) or standard dose (150 mg/m^2 every day for 5 out of 28 days) TMZ together with sorafenib. Additional separate cohorts were available for subjects who had brain metastases or prior treatment with TMZ. Initial results suggest the combination of drugs is superior to either drug alone and that this combination is active in subjects who have brain metastases. However, as with all the other studies, BRAF mutational status did not appear to predict for response rate or PFS.[36]

In all of the trials described above, a common theme is the lack of correlation between BRAF mutation status and responses to sorafenib. This result could be interpreted to imply that BRAF is not a good therapeutic target in melanoma. However, a more likely explanation is that sorafenib is insufficiently potent to target BRAF^{V600E} in melanoma patients. We have already mentioned that sorafenib is not particularly active against BRAF^{V600E} in cells[10] and there are no published data to demonstrate consistent inhibition of oncogenic BRAF by sorafenib in subject samples. However, sorafenib can clearly enter cells, because it inhibits vascular endothelial growth factor (VEGF) receptor signaling in cells with an IC_{50} of 100 nM[27] and it shows excellent clinical activity against renal cell carcinoma and hepatocellular carcinoma, two highly angiogenic cancers that do not typically harbor mutations in BRAF. Sorafenib is a broad-specificity drug that inhibits many kinases, including the VEGF and platelet-derived growth factor (PDGF) receptors, Flt-3 and c-KIT receptor tyrosine kinases, nonreceptor tyrosine kinases such as LCK, and serine/threonine specific kinases such as p38 MAPK.[27] Together, these data argue that the clinical target of sorafenib is likely to be the VEGF and possibly the (PDGF) receptors and therefore sorafenib is an antiangiogenic and not a BRAF drug.

MEK INHIBITORS IN MELANOMA

The other major approach to targeting the RAF/MEK/ERK pathway has been to develop MEK inhibitors. MEK1 and MEK2 are highly homologous (80% identity) and phosphorylate ERK with similar kinetics.[37] They are activated by a limited number of upstream kinases and their only known substrate is ERK,[38] so they occupy a strategic position in the pathway. This makes them desirable targets because their inhibition should produce highly specific responses. A number of selective inhibitors to these kinases have been developed, originally for use in cancers in which RAS is mutated. However, it has subsequently emerged that melanoma cells in which BRAF is mutant are more sensitive to MEK inhibition than cells in which RAS is mutated.[39] As RAS and RAF both signal through MEK, this suggests that the activation of additional signaling pathways by RAS makes melanoma cells less dependent on MEK, or, conversely, BRAF mutant cells are more "addicted" to MEK signaling, implying that BRAF mutant tumors will respond more readily to MEK inhibition than will RAS mutant tumors. Consequently, most studies with MEK inhibitors now focus on BRAF mutant cancers.

The difluorobenzamide CI-1040 (PD184352) was the first MEK inhibitor shown to be capable of eliciting oral anticancer activity in preclinical cancer models[40] and the first to be tested in patients.[41] CI-1040, the related compound PD0325901, and the benzimidazole AZD6244, possess similar potency (IC_{50} CI-1040: 17 nM; PD0325901: 1 nM; AZD6244: 14 nM[40,42,43]) and one feature of these compounds is their extraordinary selectivity toward MEK, due in part to their intriguing mechanism that involves binding in a binary complex with ATP.[44] They all inhibit in vitro proliferation, soft-agar colony formation, and matrigel invasion of BRAF^{V600E} mutant human melanoma cells.[39,45] They are also effective against BRAF^{V600E} melanoma xenografts in mice.

Phase I trials with CI-1040 indicated a good safety profile at drug levels resulting in 70% inhibition of MAPK activation in tumor biopsies.[46] Mild (grade 1 or 2) adverse events, including diarrhea and skin rash, were experienced by approximately 60% of subjects. The first trial, with 77 subjects, including 6 melanoma subjects, produced some encouraging signs of clinical activity, with a PR in a pancreatic cancer subject and SD lasting a median of 5 months in an additional 19 subjects who had breast, colon, and non–small-cell lung cancer. However, phase II trials against advanced colorectal, breast, non–small-cell lung, and pancreatic cancer were disappointing[47] and, coupled with its poor bioavailability and poor metabolism that necessitated frequent administration of high doses of drug,[46] the clinical development of this drug has been abandoned.

In vivo, PD0325901 exhibits longer-lasting biologic effects at significantly reduced doses compared with CI-1040 and exhibits both metabolic stability and high bioavailability.[48] Phase I trials with this compound have shown early signs of clinical activity, with two PR in melanoma subjects and eight subjects having SD that lasted 3–7 months.[48–50] However, the toxicities associated with PD0325901 are more severe than with CI-1040, and the visual disturbances (which occurred with lower frequency and shorter duration with CI-1040) caused particular concern.[51] These toxicity concerns resulted in this drug also being abandoned.[52]

AZD6244 is considerably more selective for BRAF mutant cancer cell lines, which is reflected in its in vivo activity, whereby BRAF mutant xenografts are more sensitive than NRAS or KRAS mutant xenografts.[53] Blurred vision was also reported during phase I evaluation of AZD6244, but was resolved on dose-lowering. The maximum tolerated dose was established at 100 mg twice daily.[54,55] During expanded phase I testing, the subject cohort was enriched to include 50% melanoma subjects. After two cycles, the overall incidence of SD was 49% (19/37,[48,55] with nine of the 19 subjects, including six melanoma subjects, achieving SD for 5–14 months). Although encouraging, initial results from a randomized phase II study comparing AZD6244 monotherapy with the alkylating agent TMZ for first-line treatment of melanoma showed no apparent difference in efficacy between the two agents using PFS as the primary endpoint.[56]

Thus, while PD0325901 and AZD6244 represent a step forward in the development of effective MAPK pathway inhibitors, the promise of MEK inhibition has not yet been realized. The ocular toxicity seen with these agents is a particular concern, because its severity correlates with drug potency against MEK, suggesting that it is mechanism-based and, if so, may have implications for all agents that target this pathway, such as the BRAF inhibitors described below. Clearly, future development and trial design with inhibitors of this pathway will need to take account of these toxicities, and patients with predisposing factors for retinopathy in particular will need to be carefully monitored.

NEXT-GENERATION RAF INHIBITORS

With the discovery of BRAF mutations in melanoma, there has been intense interest in developing selective and potent BRAF inhibitors. Some compounds are in preclinical development or have entered clinical trials. Promising preclinical studies suggest these compounds will be significantly more effective than sorafenib in melanoma. The compound RAF-265 was developed as a fast follower to sorafenib and was shown to selectively inhibit all RAF isoforms, including $BRAF^{V600E}$. However, as with sorafenib, RAF-265 also inhibits VEGFR-2, c-KIT, and PDGFRβ with IC_{50} values less than 100 nM. In cell-based assays, this drug appears to target $BRAF^{V600E}$ and VEGFR-2 most potently and in xenograft models, RAF-265 induces tumor regression and displays an antiangiogenic effect.[57] These data suggest that RAF-265 has antitumorigenic and antiangiogenic activities; it is currently in phase I clinical trial in melanoma subjects (http://clinicaltrials.gov).

We have also developed inhibitors of BRAF based on a disubstituted pyrazine scaffold and achieved IC_{50} values against $BRAF^{V600E}$ in the 300–500 nM range.[58,59] These compounds show 5- to 86-fold selectivity for $BRAF^{V600E}$ compared with wild-type BRAF and, more recently, we have designed and synthesized mutant BRAF inhibitors containing pyridoimidazolone as a new hinge-binding scaffold. Compounds have been obtained that have low nanomolar potency for mutant BRAF, (IC$_{50}$ values down to 12 nM) and low micromolar cellular potency against a mutant BRAF melanoma cell line.[60] Importantly, our most promising inhibitors have low metabolism, a favorable PK profile, are orally bioavailable, and induce tumor regressions in nude mice, and they are currently in preclinical testing.

Another highly potent BRAF inhibitor (IC$_{50}$ 0.26 nM) is the triarylimidazole SB-590885.[61] This compound is highly selective. It distinguishes BRAF^{V600E} from CRAF and shows over 3000-fold selectivity for BRAF^{V600E} against 46 other kinases. In vitro, SB-590885 displays selective inhibition of ERK, proliferation and transformation in malignant cells expressing oncogenic BRAF, and in an in vitro spheroid cell system it induced cell death. In vivo, SB-590885 caused decreased growth of human melanoma xenografts in immunocompromised mice.[61] This compound is important because it demonstrates the feasibility of producing highly selective BRAF inhibitors and demonstrated an excellent correlation between cell response and the presence of oncogenic BRAF in those cells, but its clinical development is yet unclear.

Finally, PLX4720 is another highly selective and potent BRAF^{V600E} inhibitor that has an IC$_{50}$ of 13 nM. It only inhibits one other kinase from a panel of 65 that represent all the families of the human kinome and it is up to100-fold more selective for mutated BRAF than for wild type BRAF in cell lines.[62] PLX4720 showed strong and selective antiproliferative activity in BRAF mutant cells, with IC$_{50}$ values in the low nanomolar range.[63] It also induced cell death in BRAF mutant cells and was found to cause regression in mouse tumor xenograft models carrying the BRAF^{V600E} mutation.[62,63] These encouraging preclinical data have resulted in the initiation of phase I clinical trials with PLX4720 and its structural analog PLX4032 (www.clinicaltrials.gov).

WHICH COMPONENTS SHOULD WE TARGET?

As our understanding of cell signaling increases, it is becoming apparent that signaling pathways exist within highly complex networks, rather than being the simple linear pathways depicted in **Fig. 1**. Consequently they possess many built-in checkpoints and compensatory pathways, and also a number of feedforward and feedback mechanisms that affect the overall responses of cells to oncogenic protein signaling. Thus, although many new therapeutic targets have been identified, we need to fully understand the biology of the signaling networks that surround a specific pathway if we are to achieve clinical responses to targeted therapies. This is nicely exemplified with the RAS/RAF/MEK/ERK pathway in melanoma.

Although oncogenic BRAF binds to and directly activates CRAF,[6] CRAF is not required for ERK activation in BRAF mutant melanoma cells.[10] However, depletion of CRAF using RNA interference does suppress proliferation of these cells,[64] suggesting that CRAF has ERK-independent functions. It is unclear whether these functions require CRAF kinase activity, or how effective a therapeutic target CRAF will prove to be in BRAF mutant melanoma, but it has recently been shown that elevated CRAF expression mediates resistance to BRAF inhibitors in BRAF^{V600E} melanoma cells.[65] Furthermore, in RAS mutant melanoma cells, CRAF is essential because oncogenic RAS signals through CRAF and does not use BRAF.[66] Taken together, these data demonstrate a role for CRAF both in BRAF and RAS mutant melanomas and suggest that highly specific BRAF inhibitors will be ineffective in RAS mutant melanomas or BRAF mutant melanomas whose resistance is mediated by CRAF upregulation, suggesting that pan-RAF inhibitors will be needed for these patients.

Another important consideration is the mode of drug binding. The crystal structures of the BRAF kinase domain reveal that BRAF adopts a fold that is characteristic of all protein kinase domains (**Fig. 2**). There is a small N-terminal domain that is composed largely of β-sheet, but contains a single α-helix (the so-called "αC-helix") and a large C-terminal domain, composed mostly of α-helix. These domains are separated by the catalytic cleft. Notably, when sorafenib binds to BRAF, there is an unusual interaction between the glycine-rich loop and the activation segment (see **Fig. 2**A).[5] This interaction disrupts a region called the "DFG motif," placing it into the so-called "out" position, and generating a structure that is incompatible with catalytic activity. Thus, sorafenib binds to the inactive conformation. In contrast, SB-590885 binds to the active conformation.[61] The glycine-rich loop and activation segment do not interact, allowing the activation segment to refold and the DFG motif to adopt the "in" position (see **Fig. 2**B). Curiously, PLX4720 can bind to both conformations, although it strongly prefers the active conformation.[62]

These findings are important because experience with drugs that target tyrosine kinases has shown that, although patients initially respond, most relapse on treatment due to the acquisition of secondary mutations within the target kinase that prevent drug binding. Thus, in chronic myelogenous leukemia, mutations in the ABL kinase domain of BCR-ABL fusions block imatinib binding.[67] Similarly, mutations in the kinase domain of the receptor tyrosine kinases c-KIT block imatinib binding in gastrointestinal stromal tumors,[68] and in lung cancer, mutations in the EGF receptor block binding of erlotinib and gefitinib.[69] It therefore seems likely that resistance will be seen in BRAF in melanoma, but there is a good chance that mutations affecting drugs of one binding class will not affect drugs of the other binding class. This should then allow alternative treatments to be offered to patients who develop clinical resistance. Alternatively, patients who develop resistance to BRAF drugs could be offered MEK drugs and vice versa. It may even be possible to suppress or delay the emergence of resistance if drugs with different binding modes, or that target BRAF and MEK, are co-administered.

RATIONAL DRUG COMBINATIONS

It is clear that melanoma is driven by multiple genetic lesions that disrupt signaling through several pathways and, because these pathways are embedded within

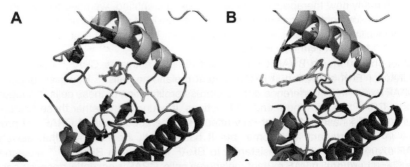

Fig. 2. BRAF drugs have different binding modes. The crystal structure of the catalytic cleft of BRAF bound to sorafenib (*A*) or SB-590885 (*B*) is shown. BRAF adopts a classical kinase fold. The small lobe is shown in magenta, with the glycine-rich loop highlighted in green and αC-helix shown in fawn. The large lobe is shown in blue, with the activation segment shown in red and the DFG motif in yellow. The drugs are shown in marine. Note the different positions occupied by the activation segment and DFG motifs in the two structures.

complex networks that influence each other's activity, it is likely that effective treatments will require simultaneous targeting of several pathways. It may even be necessary to target a single pathway at multiple points to achieve effective treatment. The rational design of the most effective combinations require in-depth understanding of the biology underlying the disease and drugs may even need to be tailored to the specific lesions with an individual's tumor (BRAF drugs in BRAF mutant melanoma; CRAF drugs in RAS mutant melanoma). Even then, patients metabolize drugs at different rates, and individual cells within a tumor may respond differently. Thus, treatments will need to be personalized to individual patients, presenting a major challenge for the future.

One of the most compelling combinations suggested by present knowledge is to combine BRAF/MEK inhibitors with inhibitors of the PI3K pathway. As mentioned, this pathway is activated downstream of RAS, but it is also activated by loss of the phosphatase PTEN in a high proportion of BRAF mutant melanomas.[70] One study has shown that, while inhibition of BRAF/ERK or PI3K signaling alone blocked melanoma cell growth in cell monolayers in tissue culture plastic, cell growth in a 3D spheroid culture system was effectively inhibited only when both pathways were targeted simultaneously.[71] Similarly, a recent study suggests that BRAF[V600E] and AKT3 (a component of the PI3K pathway) cooperate in the early stages of tumor development, arguing that, in the absence of elevated PI3K signaling, BRAF[V600E] can only drive nevus formation.[72] Furthermore, targeting both BRAF[V600E] and AKT3 in laboratory-generated and animal skin through use of nanoliposomal–small interfering RNA confirms a synergistic inhibitory effect.[73] PI3K signaling is elevated in many forms of cancer and so a great deal of effort has been made to develop effective drugs that target this pathway.[74] It now seems logical to combine inhibitors of this pathway with RAF or MEK inhibitors in melanoma.

The AMP-activated protein kinase (AMPK) has also recently been identified as a potentially important therapeutic target in BRAF mutant melanoma cells. AMPK is the major sensor of metabolic stress in eukaryotic cells.[75] When activated, it blocks cell growth by favoring catabolic (energy producing) over anabolic (energy consuming) processes. Intriguingly, even though melanoma cells are under metabolic stress, BRAF[V600E] suppresses AMPK activation through ERK and another downstream kinase called RSK, both of which can phosphorylate AMPK in the presence of BRAF[V600E],[76] suggesting that BRAF[V600E] promotes proliferation even under unfavorable metabolic conditions. This suggests that antidiabetic drugs such as metformin, which activate AMPK through indirect mechanisms, may provide antitumor activity in melanoma.[77] However, since AMPK is effectively on the same pathway as BRAF[V600E], it is unclear whether AMPK activators should be used in combination with, or instead of, BRAF/MEK inhibitors.

Another area that needs to be considered with respect to BRAF-targeting drugs is the immune system, particularly cytokine signaling. It has been shown that BRAF or MEK inhibition in BRAF mutant melanoma cells induces cell death through apoptosis.[10,11] However, cells that are simultaneously treated with tumor necrosis factor (TNF)-α do not succumb to this apoptotic signal, but survive and re-enter the cell cycle.[78] This phenomenon is dependent on nuclear factor-κB (NF-κB), a transcription factor that is implicated in various cell responses, including survival, angiogenesis, and metastasis. The TNF-α response appears to be highly specific because TNF-α does not rescue cells treated with DNA-damaging agents or drugs such as thapsigargin. Furthermore, the TNF-α antagonist etanercept (Enbrel) blocks the prosurvival signal and other cytokines are unable to substitute for TNF-α. Thus, TNF-α appears to provide a rescue pathway that antagonizes cell-killing mediated by BRAF/MEK drugs. Cells of the immune system, particularly macrophages and mast cells, infiltrate melanomas and secrete a cadre of cytokines, including TNF-α, IL-1, and IL-6,[79–81] so these findings have important clinical implications as they suggest that the immune responses will block the effectiveness of BRAF/MEK drugs in patients.

The data above suggest that a combination of BRAF/MEK drugs with agents that target TNF-α/NF-κB may be an effective therapy in melanoma. They may also point to a wider role of inflammation and potential therapeutic opportunities in this disease. For example, the phenomenon of oncogene-induced senescence (OIS) is thought to provide protection against the acquisition of oncogenic mutations in genes such as BRAF and NRAS[82–86] and benign nevi harboring oncogenic BRAF mutations are thought to be examples of OIS in vivo.[78,82] Recently, it was shown that senescent melanocytes secrete the cytokine IL-6,[87] a pleiotropic cytokine that functions as an autocrine or paracrine tumorigenic and promitogenic factor. However, in senescent cells it appears to be necessary to implement and then maintain cell-cycle arrest in an autocrine, cell-autonomous manner, possibly through its ability to induce expression of the cell-cycle inhibitor p15^{INK4b}. Notably, depletion of IL-6 abolishes senescence in melanocytic cells. IL-8 is also upregulated in response to oncogenic stress in melanocytes, and in growth-arrested human colon adenoma cells it is associated with expression of p16^{INK4a}. These studies suggest that an inflammatory transcriptome may play a role in preventing melanoma progression, but further studies are required to determine whether this offers any therapeutic opportunities.

It has also been suggested that a protein called IGFBP7 may be important.[88] IGFBP7 is a secreted protein found in normal human sera, amniotic fluid, CSF, and urine.[89] In melanocytes, BRAF^{V600E} induces IGFBP7 expression and this induces senescence and apoptosis, the latter due to IGFBP7-mediated upregulation of BNIP3L, a pro-apoptotic BCL2 family protein. Recombinant IGFBP7 (rIGFBP7) induces apoptosis in BRAF^{V600E}-positive human melanoma cell lines, and systemically administered rIGFBP7 suppresses the growth of BRAF^{V600E}-positive xenografts in mice.

Taken together, these various studies offer tantalizing insight into rational combinations that could be effective in melanoma cells, particularly if combined with BRAF/MEK inhibitors. Clearly, further studies are required to validate these combinations, and also to identify new targets and combinations that could be effective.

SUMMARY

We are entering an exciting time in melanoma research. The last decade has seen an explosion in our understanding of the genetic basis of this disease and several tractable therapeutic targets have now been identified. Clearly, BRAF^{V600E} is important because it is the most commonly mutated oncogene in melanoma, but other targets are already having more immediate effects. The identification of c-KIT mutations in a large proportion of mucosal and acral melanomas[3] led to rapid trials with imatinib, the early results of which are very encouraging.[90,91] This bodes well for the potential of the BRAF and MEK drugs that have already entered, or are soon to enter, the clinic and the results from these studies are eagerly awaited. In the interim, ongoing studies improve our understanding of how best to combine BRAF/MEK drugs with other agents to achieve the best therapeutic outcome. Absolutely critical in these trials is patient preselection so that appropriate drug cocktails can be matched to the genetic lesions that drive the individual's tumor. We have made significant advances in our ability to achieve these ends and now appear to be on the verge of knowing how best to do this where it really matters—in melanoma patients.

REFERENCES

1. Kolch W. Coordinating ERK/MAPK signalling through scaffolds and inhibitors. Nat Rev Mol Cell Biol 2005;6:827–37.
2. Davies H, Bignell GR, Cox C, et al. Mutations of the BRAF gene in human cancer. Nature 2002;417:949–54.
3. Curtin JA, Busam K, Pinkel D, et al. Somatic activation of KIT in distinct subtypes of melanoma. J Clin Oncol 2006;24:4340–6.
4. Van Raamsdonk CD, Bezrookove V, Green G, et al. Frequent somatic mutations of GNAQ in uveal melanoma and blue naevi. Nature 2009;457:599–602.
5. Wan PT, Garnett MJ, Roe SM, et al. Mechanism of activation of the RAF-ERK signaling pathway by oncogenic mutations of B-RAF. Cell 2004;116:855–67.
6. Garnett MJ, Rana S, Paterson H, et al. Wild-type and mutant B-RAF activate C-RAF through distinct mechanisms involving heterodimerization. Mol Cell 2005;20:963–9.
7. Wellbrock C, Ogilvie L, Hedley D, et al. V599EB-RAF is an oncogene in melanocytes. Cancer Res 2004;64:2338–42.
8. Dhomen ND, Reis-Filho JS, Da Rocha Dias S, et al. Oncogenic Braf induces melanocyte senescence and melanoma in mice. Cancer Cell 2009;15:294–303.
9. Dankort D, Curley DP, Cartlidge RA, et al. BRafV600E cooperates with Pten silencing to elicit metastatic melanoma. Nat Genet 2009;41:544–52.
10. Karasarides M, Chiloeches A, Hayward R, et al. B-RAF is a therapeutic target in melanoma. Oncogene 2004;23:6292–8.
11. Hingorani SR, Jacobetz MA, Robertson GP, et al. Suppression of BRAF(V599E) in human melanoma abrogates transformation. Cancer Res 2003;63:5198–202.
12. Ikenoue T, Hikiba Y, Kanai F, et al. Functional analysis of mutations within the kinase activation segment of B-Raf in human colorectal tumors. Cancer Res 2003;63:8132–7.
13. Ikenoue T, Hikiba Y, Kanai F, et al. Different effects of point mutations within the B-Raf glycine-rich loop in colorectal tumors on mitogen-activated protein/extracellular signal-regulated kinase kinase/extracellular signal-regulated kinase and nuclear factor kappaB pathway and cellular transformation. Cancer Res 2004;64:3428–35.
14. Houben R, Becker JC, Kappel A, et al. Constitutive activation of the Ras-Raf signaling pathway in metastatic melanoma is associated with poor prognosis. J Carcinog 2004;3:6.
15. Sharma A, Trivedi NR, Zimmerman MA, et al. Mutant V599EB-Raf regulates growth and vascular development of malignant melanoma tumors. Cancer Res 2005;65:2412–21.
16. Sharma A, Tran MA, Liang S, et al. Targeting mitogen-activated protein kinase/extracellular signal-regulated kinase kinase in the mutant (V600E) B-Raf signaling cascade effectively inhibits melanoma lung metastases. Cancer Res 2006;66:8200–9.
17. Hoeflich KP, Gray DC, Eby MT, et al. Oncogenic BRAF is required for tumor growth and maintenance in melanoma models. Cancer Res 2006;66:999–1006.
18. Bos JL. Ras oncogenes in human cancer: a review. Cancer Res 1989;49:4682–9.
19. Tanaka T, Rabbitts TH. Interfering with protein-protein interactions: potential for cancer therapy. Cell Cycle 2008;7:1569–74.
20. Sousa SF, Fernandes PA, Ramos MJ. Farnesyltransferase inhibitors: a detailed chemical view on an elusive biological problem. Curr Med Chem 2008;15:1478–92.

21. Hahn SM, Bernhard E, McKenna WG. Farnesyltransferase inhibitors. Semin Oncol 2001;28:86–93.
22. Baum C, Kirschmeier P. Preclinical and clinical evaluation of farnesyltransferase inhibitors. Curr Oncol Rep 2003;5:99–107.
23. Lerner EC, Zhang TT, Knowles DB, et al. Inhibition of the prenylation of K-Ras, but not H- or N-Ras, is highly resistant to CAAX peptidomimetics and requires both a farnesyltransferase and a geranylgeranyltransferase I inhibitor in human tumor cell lines. Oncogene 1997;15:1283–8.
24. Hagemann C, Rapp UR. Isotype-specific functions of Raf kinases. Exp Cell Res 1999;253:34–46.
25. Lyons JF, Wilhelm S, Hibner B, et al. Discovery of a novel Raf kinase inhibitor. Endocr Relat Cancer 2001;8:219–25.
26. Wilhelm S, Chien DS. BAY 43-9006: preclinical data. Curr Pharm Des 2002;8: 2255–7.
27. Wilhelm SM, Carter C, Tang L, et al. BAY 43-9006 exhibits broad spectrum oral antitumor activity and targets the RAF/MEK/ERK pathway and receptor tyrosine kinases involved in tumor progression and angiogenesis. Cancer Res 2004;64: 7099–109.
28. Eisen T, Ahmad T, Flaherty KT, et al. Sorafenib in advanced melanoma: a Phase II randomised discontinuation trial analysis. Br J Cancer 2006;95:581–6.
29. Flaherty KT, Brose M, Schuchter LM, et al. Sorafenib combined with carboplatin and paclitaxel for metastatic melanoma: progression-free survival and response versus B-RAF status. Ann Oncol 2006;17 [abstract 0.1110].
30. Flaherty KT, Schiller J, Schuchter LM, et al. A phase I trial of the oral, multikinase inhibitor sorafenib in combination with carboplatin and paclitaxel. Clin Cancer Res 2008;14:4836–42.
31. Agarwala SS, Keilholz U, Hogg D, et al. Randomized phase III study of paclitaxel plus carboplatin with or without sorafenib as second-line treatment in patients with advanced melanoma. J Clin Oncol 2007;25 [abstract 8510].
32. Eisen T, Ahmad T, Gore ME, et al. Phase I trial of BAY 43-9006 (sorafenib) combined with dacarbazine (DTIC) in metastatic melanoma patients. J Clin Oncol 2005;23 [abstract 7508].
33. Eisen T, Marais R, Affolter A, et al. An open-label phase II study of sorafenib and dacarbazine as first-line therapy in patients with advanced melanoma. J Clin Oncol 2007;25 [abstract 8529].
34. Bedikian AY, Millward M, Pehamberger H, et al. Bcl-2 antisense (oblimersen sodium) plus dacarbazine in patients with advanced melanoma: the Oblimersen Melanoma Study Group. J Clin Oncol 2006;24:4738–45.
35. McDermott DF, Sosman JA, Gonzalez R, et al. Double-blind randomized phase II study of the combination of sorafenib and dacarbazine in patients with advanced melanoma: a report from the 11715 Study Group. J Clin Oncol 2008;26:2178–85.
36. Amaravadi R, Schuchter LM, McDermott DF, et al. Updated results of a randomized phase II study comparing two schedules of temozolomide in combination with sorafenib in patients with advanced melanoma. J Clin Oncol 2007;25 [abstract 8527].
37. Haystead TA, Dent P, Wu J, et al. Ordered phosphorylation of p42mapk by MAP kinase kinase. FEBS Lett 1992;306:17–22.
38. Seger R, Ahn NG, Posada J, et al. Purification and characterization of mitogen-activated protein kinase activator(s) from epidermal growth factor-stimulated A431 cells. J Biol Chem 1992;267:14373–81.

39. Solit DB, Garraway LA, Pratilas CA, et al. BRAF mutation predicts sensitivity to MEK inhibition. Nature 2006;439:358–62.
40. Sebolt-Leopold JS, Dudley DT, Herrera R, et al. Blockade of the MAP kinase pathway suppresses growth of colon tumors in vivo. Nat Med 1999;5:810–6.
41. Sebolt-Leopold JS. Advances in the development of cancer therapeutics directed against the RAS-mitogen-activated protein kinase pathway. Clin Cancer Res 2008;14:3651–6.
42. Sebolt-Leopold JS, Herrera R. Targeting the mitogen-activated protein kinase cascade to treat cancer. Nat Rev Cancer 2004;4:937–47.
43. Yeh TC, Marsh V, Bernat BA, et al. Biological characterization of ARRY-142886 (AZD6244), a potent, highly selective mitogen-activated protein kinase kinase 1/2 inhibitor. Clin Cancer Res 2007;13:1576–83.
44. Davies SP, Reddy H, Caivano M, et al. Specificity and mechanism of action of some commonly used protein kinase inhibitors. Biochem J 2000;351:95–105.
45. Haass NK, Sproesser K, Nguyen TK, et al. The mitogen-activated protein/extra-cellular signal-regulated kinase kinase inhibitor AZD6244 (ARRY-142886) induces growth arrest in melanoma cells and tumor regression when combined with docetaxel. Clin Cancer Res 2008;14:230–9.
46. Lorusso PM, Adjei AA, Varterasian M, et al. Phase I and pharmacodynamic study of the oral MEK inhibitor CI-1040 in patients with advanced malignancies. J Clin Oncol 2005;23:5281–93.
47. Rinehart J, Adjei AA, Lorusso PM, et al. Multicenter phase II study of the oral MEK inhibitor, CI-1040, in patients with advanced non-small-cell lung, breast, colon, and pancreatic cancer. J Clin Oncol 2004;22:4456–62.
48. Wang D, Boerner SA, Winkler JD, et al. Clinical experience of MEK inhibitors in cancer therapy. Biochim Biophys Acta 2007;1773:1248–55.
49. Menon SS, Whitfield LR, Sadis SS, et al. Pharmacokinetics (PK) and pharmaco-dynamics (PD) of PD 0325901, a second generation MEK inhibitor after multiple oral doses of PD 0325901 to advanced cancer patients. J Clin Oncol 2005;23 [abstract 3066].
50. Lorusso PM, Krishnamurthi S, Rinehart J, et al. A phase 1-2 clinical study of a second generation oral MEK inhibitor, PD 0325901 in patients with advanced cancer. J Clin Oncol 2005;23 [abstract 3011].
51. Lorusso PM, Krishnamurthi S, Rinehart J, et al. Clinical aspects of a phase I study of PD-0325901, a selective oral MEK inhibitor, in patients with advanced cancer. Mol Cancer Ther 2007;6 [abstract B113].
52. Ramnath N, Adjei AA. Inhibitors of Raf kinase and MEK signaling. Update Cancer Ther 2007;2:111–8.
53. Davies BR, Logie A, McKay JS, et al. AZD6244 (ARRY-142886), a potent inhibitor of mitogen-activated protein kinase/extracellular signal-regulated kinase kinase 1/2 kinases: mechanism of action in vivo, pharmacokinetic/pharmacodynamic relationship, and potential for combination in preclinical models. Mol Cancer Ther 2007;6:2209–19.
54. Chow LQM, Eckhardt SG, Reid J, et al. A first in human dose-ranging study to assess the pharmacokinetics, pharmacodynamics, and toxicities of the MEK inhibitor ARRY-142886 (AZD6244) in patients with advanced solid malignancies. AACR-NCI-EORTC International Conference on Molecular Targets and Cancer Therapeutics. Philadelphia, November 14–18, 2005.
55. Adjei AA, Cohen RB, Franklin WA, et al. Phase I pharmacokinetic and pharmacodynamic study of the MEK inhibitor AZD6244 (ARRY-142886).

AACR-NCI-EORTC International Conference on Molecular Targets and Cancer Therapeutics. Prague, Czech Republic, November 7–10, 2006.

56. Drummer R, Robert C, Chapman P, et al. AZD6244 (ARRY-142886) vs temozolomide (TMZ) in patients (pts) with advanced melanoma: an open-label, randomized, multicenter, phase II study. J Clin Oncol 2008;26 [abstract 9033].

57. Stuart D, Aardalen K, Venetsanakos E, et al. RAF265 is a potent Raf kinase inhibitor with selective anti-proliferative activity in vitro and in vivo. 99th AACR Annual Meeting. San Diego, California, April 12–16, 2008.

58. Niculescu-Duvaz I, Roman E, Whittaker SR, et al. Novel inhibitors of B-RAF based on a disubstituted pyrazine scaffold. Generation of a nanomolar lead. J Med Chem 2006;49:407–16.

59. Niculescu-Duvaz I, Roman E, Whittaker SR, et al. Novel inhibitors of the v-raf murine sarcoma viral oncogene homologue B1 (BRAF) based on a 2,6-disubstituted pyrazine scaffold. J Med Chem 2008;51:3261–74.

60. Niculescu-Duvaz D, Gaulon C, Dijkstra HP, et al. Pyridoimidazolones as novel potent inhibitors of v-Raf murine sarcoma viral oncogene homologue B1 (BRAF). J Med Chem 2009;52:2255–64.

61. King AJ, Patrick DR, Batorsky RS, et al. Demonstration of a genetic therapeutic index for tumors expressing oncogenic BRAF by the kinase inhibitor SB-590885. Cancer Res 2006;66:11100–5.

62. Tsai J, Lee JT, Wang W, et al. Discovery of a selective inhibitor of oncogenic B-Raf kinase with potent antimelanoma activity. Proc Natl Acad Sci U S A 2008;105: 3041–6.

63. Sala E, Mologni L, Truffa S, et al. BRAF silencing by short hairpin RNA or chemical blockade by PLX4032 leads to different responses in melanoma and thyroid carcinoma cells. Mol Cancer Res 2008;6:751–9.

64. Gray-Schopfer VC, da Rocha Dias S, Marais R. The role of B-RAF in melanoma. Cancer Metastasis Rev 2005;24:165–83.

65. Montagut C, Sharma SV, Shioda T, et al. Elevated CRAF as a potential mechanism of acquired resistance to BRAF inhibition in melanoma. Cancer Res 2008;68: 4853–61.

66. Dumaz N, Hayward R, Martin J, et al. In melanoma, RAS mutations are accompanied by switching signaling from BRAF to CRAF and disrupted cyclic AMP Signaling. Cancer Res 2006;66:9483–91.

67. Bianchini M, De Brasi C, Gargallo P, et al. Specific assessment of BCR-ABL transcript overexpression and imatinib resistance in chronic myeloid leukemia patients. Eur J Haematol 2009;82:292–300.

68. Nishida T, Kanda T, Nishitani A, et al. Secondary mutations in the kinase domain of the KIT gene are predominant in imatinib-resistant gastrointestinal stromal tumor. Cancer Sci 2008;99:799–804.

69. Bean J, Riely GJ, Balak M, et al. Acquired resistance to epidermal growth factor receptor kinase inhibitors associated with a novel T854A mutation in a patient with EGFR-mutant lung adenocarcinoma. Clin Cancer Res 2008;14:7519–25.

70. Goel VK, Lazar AJ, Warneke CL, et al. Examination of mutations in BRAF, NRAS, and PTEN in primary cutaneous melanoma. J Invest Dermatol 2006;126:154–60.

71. Smalley KS, Haass NK, Brafford PA, et al. Multiple signaling pathways must be targeted to overcome drug resistance in cell lines derived from melanoma metastases. Mol Cancer Ther 2006;5:1136–44.

72. Cheung M, Sharma A, Madhunapantula SV, et al. Akt3 and mutant V600E B-Raf cooperate to promote early melanoma development. Cancer Res 2008;68:3429–39.

73. Tran MA, Gowda R, Sharma A, et al. Targeting V600EB-Raf and Akt3 using nano-liposomal-small interfering RNA inhibits cutaneous melanocytic lesion development. Cancer Res 2008;68:7638–49.
74. Ihle NT, Powis G. Take your PIK: phosphatidylinositol 3-kinase inhibitors race through the clinic and toward cancer therapy. Mol Cancer Ther 2009;8:1–9.
75. Hardie DG. Roles of the AMP-activated/SNF1 protein kinase family in the response to cellular stress. Biochem Soc Symp 1999;64:13–27.
76. Zheng B, Jeong JH, Asara JM, et al. Oncogenic B-RAF negatively regulates the tumor suppressor LKB1 to promote melanoma cell proliferation. Mol Cell 2009; 33:237–47.
77. Martin MJ, Carling D, Marais R. Taking the stress out of melanoma. Cancer Cell 2009;15:163–4.
78. Gray-Schopfer VC, Cheong SC, Chong H, et al. Cellular senescence in naevi and immortalisation in melanoma: a role for p16? Br J Cancer 2006;95:496–505.
79. Brocker EB, Zwadlo G, Holzmann B, et al. Inflammatory cell infiltrates in human melanoma at different stages of tumor progression. Int J Cancer 1988;41:562–7.
80. Duncan LM, Richards LA, Mihm MC Jr. Increased mast cell density in invasive melanoma. J Cutan Pathol 1998;25:11–5.
81. Torisu H, Ono M, Kiryu H, et al. Macrophage infiltration correlates with tumor stage and angiogenesis in human malignant melanoma: possible involvement of TNFalpha and IL-1alpha. Int J Cancer 2000;85:182–8.
82. Michaloglou C, Vredeveld LC, Soengas MS, et al. BRAFE600-associated senescence-like cell cycle arrest of human naevi. Nature 2005;436:720–4.
83. Chen Z, Trotman LC, Shaffer D, et al. Crucial role of p53-dependent cellular senescence in suppression of Pten-deficient tumorigenesis. Nature 2005;436:725–30.
84. Braig M, Lee S, Loddenkemper C, et al. Oncogene-induced senescence as an initial barrier in lymphoma development. Nature 2005;436:660–5.
85. Bartkova J, Rezaei N, Liontos M, et al. Oncogene-induced senescence is part of the tumorigenesis barrier imposed by DNA damage checkpoints. Nature 2006; 444:633–7.
86. Courtois-Cox S, Genther Williams SM, Reczek EE, et al. A negative feedback signaling network underlies oncogene-induced senescence. Cancer Cell 2006; 10:459–72.
87. Kuilman T, Michaloglou C, Vredeveld LC, et al. Oncogene-induced senescence relayed by an interleukin-dependent inflammatory network. Cell 2008;133: 1019–31.
88. Wajapeyee N, Serra RW, Zhu X, et al. Oncogenic BRAF induces senescence and apoptosis through pathways mediated by the secreted protein IGFBP7. Cell 2008;132:363–74.
89. Wilson EM, Oh Y, Rosenfeld RG. Generation and characterization of an IGFBP-7 antibody: identification of 31kD IGFBP-7 in human biological fluids and Hs578T human breast cancer conditioned media. J Clin Endocrinol Metab 1997;82: 1301–3.
90. Hodi FS, Friedlander P, Corless CL, et al. Major response to imatinib mesylate in KIT-mutated melanoma. J Clin Oncol 2008;26:2046–51.
91. Jiang X, Zhou J, Yuen NK, et al. Imatinib targeting of KIT-mutant oncoprotein in melanoma. Clin Cancer Res 2008;14:7726–32.

Melanoma and Immunotherapy

Alexander M.M. Eggermont, MD, PhD[a],*, Dirk Schadendorf, MD, PhD[b]

KEYWORDS

- Melanoma • Immunotherapy • Cytokines • Antibodies
- Vaccines • Review

About 20% of all primary melanomas will spread. The likelihood of metastatic behavior correlates with prognostic factors such as tumor thickness, mitotic index, presence of ulceration, lymphocyte infiltration, age, gender, and anatomic site.[1] Immunotherapies are developed for melanoma patients in stage IV who have distant metastases and in stage II to III patients in the adjuvant micrometastatic setting, where only a fraction of patients have widespread (microscopic) disease.

IMMUNOTHERAPY DEVELOPMENT IN STAGE IV MELANOMA

Stage IV melanoma with dissemination to distant sites and visceral organs is, with the exception of rare cases of surgery for oligometastatic disease, almost invariably incurable, with a median survival time of only 8 to 9 months and a 3-year survival rate of only 10% to 15%.[1] By and large increased response rates, observed with combinations of chemotherapy and immunotherapy, have not translated into survival benefits. Interestingly, with various immunotherapeutic approaches, long-lasting responses can be observed in a minority of patients (5%–10%), which is too small to affect the survival of the overall population. Unfortunately, it is currently not possible to identify responding patients before treatment decisions.

CYTOKINES
Interferon-α

Interferon-α (IFN-α) is the first recombinant cytokine evaluated for its effects on metastatic melanoma, which showed response rates of 5% to 15% in phase II independent of dose or schedule.[2] In randomized trials, where IFN-α was added to chemotherapeutic regimens, its superiority could not be demonstrated over chemotherapy alone, as is summarized in **Table 1**.[3–10] Thus, IFN-α has not been approved for application in

[a] Department of Surgical Oncology, Erasmus University MC–Daniel den Hoed Cancer Center, 301 Groene Hilledijk, 3075 EA Rotterdam, The Netherlands
[b] Department of Dermatology, University Hospital Essen, Hufelandstr 55, 45122 Essen, Germany
* Corresponding author.
E-mail address: a.eggermont@erasmusmc.nl (A.M.M. Eggermont).

Hematol Oncol Clin N Am 23 (2009) 547–564
doi:10.1016/j.hoc.2009.03.009
0889-8588/09/$ – see front matter © 2009 Elsevier Inc. All rights reserved.

hemonc.theclinics.com

Table 1
Randomized trials with IFN-α–containing regimens

Year (Author)	Regimen	#Pts	Median Survival (Months)	Signif.	Ref.
1991 (Falkson)	D ± IFN	64	9.6 vs 17.6	P<.01	3
1993 (Thomson)	D ± IFN	170	7.6 vs 8.8	NS	4
1994 (Bajetta)	D ± IFN[a]	242	11 vs 11 vs 13	NS	5
1998 (Falkson)	D vs D/IFN vs D/T vs D/IFN/T	258	10 vs 9 vs 8 vs 9.5	NS	6
2000 (Middleton)	D/IFN vs DCBT	105	6.5 vs 6.5	NS	7
2001 (Young)	D ± IFN	61	7.2 vs 4.8	NS	8
2005 (Kaufmann)	TMZ ± IFN	282	8.4 vs 9.7	NS	9
2005 (Vuoristo)	D/nIFN vs DCBT/rIFN vs D/rIFN vs DCBT/rIFN	108	11 vs 10 vs 9 vs 7.5	NS	10

Abbreviations: B, BCNU (carmustine); C, cisplatin; D, dacarbazine; IFN, interferon a; NS, not significant; T, tamoxifen; TMZ, temozolomide; V, vinblastine.
[a] Dose 3 or 9 MIU.

stage IV melanoma. Yet it is frequently used in various schedules for which evidence is lacking. Pegylated IFN-α, an IFN-α formulation with increased bioavailability,[11] showed dose-dependent response rates in the range of 6% to 12% in a recent trial of stage IV melanoma patients.[12]

Interferon-α in the Adjuvant Setting

In contrast, IFN-α has been approved in the adjuvant setting for treatment of high-risk melanoma. Many review articles, systematic reviews, meta-analyses and pooled analyses have been published on the subject.[13–17] Taken together, the data show that, with the exception of ultra–low-dose IFN-α therapy of 1 mU,[18] IFN-α given at 3-5-10 million (flat dose), and when given at high doses (20 mU/m2 induction and 10 mIU/m2 maintenance), has an impact on relapse-free survival (RFS) but not or only a marginal effect on overall survival (OS). High-dose IFN therapy was approved in both United States and Europe for stage IIB to III, but is little used in Europe. Low-dose IFN-α (3 mU, t.i.w., s.c) was approved in Europe and seems more active in stage II melanoma than in advanced stage III. In a meta-analysis, no dose – outcome effect could be established.[15,16] In 2008, long-term adjuvant therapy (5 years) with pegylated-IFNα-2b was reported to have a significant and sustained effect on RFS in stage III melanoma.[19] Interestingly, in this EORTC 18991 trial, the efficacy was evident only in the sentinel node, positive stage III patients compared with macroscopically involved stage III patients. Exactly the same observation was made using regular IFN in the intermediate dose IFN-α trial EORTC 18952 in stage IIB to III.[20] Thus, in the 2 largest adjuvant trials in melanoma, IFN-α was most beneficial in patients with less advanced disease. This is in line with the positive results of the trials with low-dose IFN-α in stage II patients before sentinel node staging was practiced and where results were mainly driven by the supposedly sentinel node-positive patients inside these stage II trials.[21–23]

Identification of patients who are IFN-α sensitive is clearly the priority to achieve more selective use of IFN-α and improve outcome. The presence or emergence of autoimmune antibodies was reported to correlate with improved outcome with high-dose IFN-α treatment.[24] When this was studied in the randomized EORTC 18952 and 18991 trials comparing IFN-α versus observation of the emergence of autoantibodies was not an independent prognostic factor, let alone a predictive factor.[25,26] Thus, unfortunately, in the absence of predictive factors, selective use of IFN-α still needs to be developed. In the EORTC trials 18952 and 18991, it was noted that IFN-α sensitivity was higher in patients with ulcerated primaries. This observation led to the decision to perform the EORTC 18081 trial in patients with ulcerated primaries thicker than 1 mm comparing Pegylated IFN-α-2b to observation, which will be activated in 2009.

Interleukin-2

Interleukin-2 (IL-2) is the only approved cytokine for the treatment of Stage IV melanoma. Analysis of 8 clinical trials of high-dose IL-2 in 270 patients reported a 16% overall response rate.[27] Complete responses occurred in 6% of patients and were long lasting (>5 years) in 4% of patients. IL-2 was approved for stage IV disease, based on a series of phase II studies, by the FDA in 1998 in the United States, but not by the EMEA in Europe because of the absence of phase III trial data. The most effective treatment regimens are the high-dose bolus and high-dose continuous infusion regimens that are associated with serious toxicity, limiting its use to patients in good condition to be treated in specialized centers.[27] Its curative potential makes it an essential component of immunologic strategies in the treatment of metastatic malignant melanoma.[28] Factors of prognostic significance for IL-2–based therapies are development of hypothyroidism, LDH level, ECOG performance status, number and site of metastases, and pretreatment neutrophil count.[29–32] Findeisen and colleagues,[33] recently demonstrated that serum amyloid A and C-reactive Protein are potent independent prognostic factors for poor prognosis. This fits well with the poor prognosis of elevated neutrophil counts in stage IV. Apparently, ongoing inflammatory activity correlates with poor outcome.

Combinations and Biochemotherapy

A long series of randomized trials (**Table 2**) evaluated the efficacy of combining cytokines or combining cytokines with chemotherapy. Combining IFN-α and IL-2 did not improve response rates or survival.[34–46] Biochemotherapy, a combination of IL-2 and/or IFN-α with various chemotherapeutic agents, has also failed to affect survival and has been associated with increased toxicity. Biochemotherapy improves response rates and sometimes progression-free survival rates[36,41,46] but not OS and thus has been largely abandoned.

New Cytokines

IL-15 and IL-21 have a sequence homology with IL-2 and have recently received much attention. IL-15 stimulates proliferation of IL-2–dependent T-cell lines in the presence of neutralizing anti–IL-2 antibodies. It mediates activities similar to IL-2, but differences in alpha subunits lead to differences in in vivo immune functions.[47] IL-21 is produced by activated CD4+ T cells and natural killer cells. Activation of the IL-21 receptor leads to multiple effects on T cells, including proliferation, differentiation, and activation of cytokine and chemokine production. IL-21 has effects on both CD8+ T cells and CD4+ T cells and synergizes with IL-15 in inducing optimal and sustained antigen-specific CD8+ T-cell responses.[48] In contrast to IL-2, IL-21 does not enhance the proliferation of T regulatory cells. IL-21 may therefore promote autoimmunity and anti-tumor immunity in cancer patients. IL-21 is being investigated in clinical phase I to II studies as a single drug in patients with metastatic melanoma.[49,50]

Table 2
Randomized trials of IL-2-containing regimens/biochemotherapy trials

Year (Author)	Regimen	#Pts	Median Survival (Months)	Signif.	Ref.
1993 (Sparano)	IL2 ± IFN	85	10.2 vs 9.7	NS	34
2002 (Agarwala)	IL2 ± Histamine	305	9.1 vs 8.2	NS	35
1997 (Keilholz)	IL2/IFN ± C	133	9 vs 9	NS	36
1998 (Johnston)	CDBT ± IFN/IL2	65	5.5 vs 5.0	NS	37
1999 (Dorval)	C/IL2 ± IFN	117	10.4 vs 10.9	NS	38
1999 (Rosenberg)	CDT ± IFN/IL2	102	15.8 vs 10.7	P<.06	39
2001 (Hauschild)	D/IFN ± IL2	290	11 vs 11	NS	40
2002 (Eton)	CVD ± IFN/IL2	183	9.2 vs 11.9	P<.06	41
2002 (Atzpodien)	D/B/C/T ± IFN/IL2	124	13 vs 12	NS	42
2002 (Ridolfi)	CVD ± IFN/IL2	176	9.5 vs 11.0	NS	43
2005 (Keilholz)	CD/IFN ± IL2	363	9 vs 9	NS	44
2006 (Bajetta)	CVD ± IFN/IL2	139	12 vs 11	NS	45
2008 (Atkins)	CVD ± IFN/IL2	416	8.7 vs 8.4	NS	46

Abbreviations: B, BCNU (carmustine); C, cisplatin; D, dacarbazine; IFN, interferon α; IL2, interleukin-2; NS, not significant; T, tamoxifen; TMZ, temozolomide; V, vinblastine.

ADOPTIVE IMMUNOTHERAPY

Rosenberg and coworkers at the Surgery Branch of the National Cancer Institute (NCI) have developed an evolutionary program in adoptive immunotherapeutic approaches to treat cancer, melanoma in particular, which has demonstrated significant progress in insights and results over the years. Adoptive cell transfer immunotherapy is based on ex vivo activation and expansion of tumor-reactive lymphocytes taken from the tumor-bearing host and their reinfusion back to the patient.[51] The availability of recombinant IL-2 in the 1980s promoted the investigation and use of cell therapy in human cancer with lymphokine activated killer (LAK) cells and IL-2, demonstrating nonspecific antitumor activity.[52] Tumor-infiltrating lymphocytes (TILs) are T cells that can have specific antitumor activity and can be reliably generated from melanoma patients.[53] With such TILs in combination with high-dose IL-2, some 86 patients with metastaatic melanoma were treated in the early 1990s. The overall response rate was 34%, also in patients failing prior high-dose IL-2 therapy.[54]

Conditioning of the Patient by Lymphodepletion

The program went through a major evolution by the introduction of a lymphodepletion conditioning regimen of the host, using fludarabine and cyclophosphamide, before the infusion of T-cells. This allowed for the persistent clonal repopulation of T cells, provided by short-term in vitro selection and expansion procedures, in these cancer patients, 100- to 1000-fold proliferation of transferred cells in vivo, and maintenance of functional activity of T cells and trafficking to tumor sites.[55] Moreover, the preconditioning of the patient eliminates immunosuppressive lymphocyte populations that will compete for IL-2, administered to support the expansion and activation of the transferred T cells. Such competition for IL-2 by competing lymphocyte populations and the abrogative effects on IL-2 + LAK cell therapy had been recognized early on,[56,57] but this "cytokine sink phenomenon" has been clearly demonstrated in various animal models by Gattinoni and colleagues.[58] Dudley and coworkers established also the proof of principle that in this setting the use of T-cell clones against normally expressed "self-antigens" can be effective and that these antigenic targets can be useful for immunotherapy in patients if the autoimmune consequences of such a treatment are not of a major concern.[55] The most recent report by Rosenberg's group shows very impressive response rates varying from 50% to 72% in 93 metastatic melanoma. Complete response rates of 9% to 16%, depending on the combination with which degree of total body irradiation (2 Gy or 12 GY), is of great importance.[59] These treatment regimens, both the clinical as well as the laboratory aspects, are currently still very complex. If simplification by less clonal selection, shorter in vivo expansion of T-cells and lower doses of IL-2 prove to be just as effective as the current protocols, then widespread dissemination of this approach could be achieved.[60] The key role of lymphodepletion does not only demonstrate that immunotherapy has a future but it also demonstrates that concepts such as lymphodepletion may also be quite important for immunotherapeutic strategies in general, including vaccine development strategies.[61]

Other Developments in Adoptive Immunotherapy

Other recent interesting reports on the adoptive transfer of immune cells include a communication by Mackensen and colleagues[62] on Melan-A specific cytolytic T lymphocytes (CTLs) generated by ex vivo stimulation of purified CD8$^+$ peripheral blood lymphocytes (PBLs) with mature Melan-A pulsed Dendritic cells (DCs). They reported responses in 3 of 11 patients after infusion of the T cells with a 6-day course of low-dose IL-2. However, only regression of melanoma lesions was observed in subcutaneous and lymphatic, not in visceral, metastases. Powell and colleagues[63] reported on melanocyte-directed autoimmunity in two out of nine patients with stage IV melanoma who were vaccinated with a GP-100:209-217 peptide stimulated autologous PBMC in combination with high-dose IL-2 after nonmyeloablative chemotherapy. In addition, a report in 2008 demonstrated a durable clinical remission of a patient with refractory metastatic melanoma who was treated with autologous CD4 T-cell clones specific for melanoma-associated antigen NY-ESO-1, isolated and expanded ex vivo; the treatment also led to endogenous responses against melanoma antigens other than NY-ESO-1.[64]

Transduction of T-cell Receptor

Conversion of normal PBLs into antitumor lymphocytes by transduction with genes encoding one of the T-cell receptor (TCR) relevant to tumor cells is yet another experimental development for treating various cancers.[65,66] Rosenbergs' group reported on four tumor responses in 31 patients with metastatic melanoma treated by autologous PBL transduced by MART-1-specific TCR following nonmyeloablative conditioning.

MONOCLONAL ANTIBODIES
Immunoregulatory Antibodies

Anti-CTLA-4
An immune signal will be generated when only an antigen is presented by a major histocompatibility complex (MHC) molecule and a costimulatory molecule; B7.1 or B7.2. binds to CD28 to provide the signal for T-cell activation.[67] After activation, T cells upregulate CTLA4, which competes for binding to B7, resulting in inhibition of TCR signaling, IL-2 gene transcription, and T-cell proliferation. Monoclonal antibodies that bind to CTLA-4 can block the interaction between B7 and CTLA-4. Inhibition of this negative switch may break peripheral tolerance to self-tissues and induce

antitumor responses.[68] Two fully human IgG monoclonal antibodies recognizing CTLA-4, ipilimumab (MDX-010) and tremelimumab (CP-675,206), have been tested, alone or in combination, in phase II/III trials. Comprehensive reviews on clinical development of ipilimumab[69] and tremelimumab[70] were published recently.

Ipilimumab Activity of ipilimumab in patients with metastatic melanoma was examined alone or in combination with chemotherapy or vaccines, and in various dose regimens.

Ipilimumab has been observed to be able to induce long-lasting responses: Seven patients (10%) were still alive 2 to more than 4 years out of 72 chemotherapy-naïve patients, who were treated with ipilimumab (3 mg/kg every 4 weeks for 4 months) alone (median survival, 11.5 months) or in combination with DTIC (median survival 13 months) in a randomized phase II trial.[71] Ipilimumab in combination with a vaccine was assessed in a randomized II study in 56 patients (3 mg/kg every 3 weeks or a 3 mg/kg initial dose of ipilimumab followed by 1 mg/kg every 3 weeks), with both cohorts receiving concomitant vaccination with 2 modified, HLA-A*0201-restricted peptides.[72] The overall response rate was 13%; better clinical responses were observed in patients with grade 3/4 autoimmune toxicity, an observation confirmed in a 139- patient study at the NCI.[73] The most common grade 3/4 immune-related adverse events were colitis/diarrhea and dermatitis that responded to systemic steroids without significantly affecting the efficacy of ipilimumab therapy.[74] These studies suggest that induction of manageable autoimmunity in patients with metastatic melanoma treated with ipilimumab could be a surrogate marker of objective and durable clinical responses.

An induction regimen consisting of 10 mg/kg every 3 weeks for 4 months (Q3Wx4) along with a maintenance treatment of 10 mg/kg ipilimumab every 12 weeks starting at week 24 (Q12W) has emerged as the most effective schedule and been used in most ongoing phase II and phase III clinical trials.[75] This schedule showed clinical activity, in the form of either objective response or stable disease, in 27% of 155 patients with metastatic melanoma who developed progressive disease on a median number of 2 prior therapies.[76] Median OS was 10.2 months and Immune-related grade 3/4 adverse events occurred at 21.9% of patients. Overall positive results of ipilimumab in patients with metastatic melanoma led to the initiation of a pivotal trial in first line comparing dacarbazine ± ipilimumab. Another phase III trial of ipilimumab alone or in combination with a peptide vaccine as a second-line therapy is also ongoing.

Tremelimumab Early phase clinical studies of tremelimumab demonstrated acceptable toxicity (irAEs) and similar efficacy of 10 mg/kg monthly and 15 mg/kg quarterly doses of the antibody with median survival of 10.3 and 11 months, respectively.[77,78] In 246 patients, single-agent tremelimumab (15 mg/kg quarterly, ≥1 dose, 44% of patients ≥2 doses) resulted in a response rate of only 8.3%. However, the duration of the response (183+ to 540+ days) and the median OS of 10.1 months suggested activity.[79] This schedule was evaluated in comparison with standard dacarbazine or temozolomide (TMZ) chemotherapy in previously untreated 324 and 319 patients, respectively. The trial was stopped, based on a second interim analysis, for futility, in March 2008. Median OS by intent to treat was 11.8 months in the tremelimumab arm, and 10.7 months in the chemotherapy arm, with a hazard ratio (chemotherapy over tremelimumab) of 1.04.[80]

Conclusions and the need for new response criteria CTLA-4 monoclonal antibodies constitute a promising direction in the treatment of stage IV melanoma, but the recently reported lack of efficacy of tremelimumab as a single agent in first line suggests that future investigative effort of anti-CTLA-4 agents may focus on combination studies and patients with refractory tumors. Important is the observation that new lesions in patients receiving ipilimumab or tremelimumab may not always indicate progressive disease and treatment failure as defined by modified World Health Organization criteria. Four patterns of response have been observed: (a) response in baseline lesions; (b) stable disease with slow, steady decline in total tumor burden; (c) response after initial increase in total tumor burden; (d) response in index and new lesions after the appearance of new lesions. Importantly in 17 out of 26 patients who developed new lesions after 12 weeks of treatment regression or stabilization of disease was observed.[81] Novel, immune-related response criteria (irRC) that may more accurately describe response to immunotherapy and avoid premature treatment cessation in patients with disease progression before response were presented at American Society of Clinical Oncology 2008. Contrary to mWHO criteria, irRC (a) only consider measurable lesions (>1 cm), (b) define total tumor burden as the sum of index lesions identified at baseline and new lesions detected after baseline, and (c) aim for follow-up after progressive disease to detect late activity.[82]

Anti–PD-1
Another monoclonal antibody that has been developed acts against the programmed death-1 receptor (PD-1R), the ligand of which (PD-1L) can be directly expressed on melanoma cells. PD-1R is a part of the B7:CD28 family of costimulatory molecules that regulate T-cell activation and tolerance, and thus anti–PD-1R can play a role in breaking tolerance.[83,84]

Agonistic antibodies OX44 and anti-CD137 (4-1BB)
The antibodies anti-OX44 and anti-4-1BB have an agonistic action on T-cell activation and the anti-CD25 antibody that targets T-regulatory cells that constitutionally overexpress CD25.[85] It has been demonstrated that combinations of these antibodies can significantly optimize T-cell responses; thus, we are most likely witnessing an emerging field of immunomodulation that holds great promise.[85,86]

   Inducible receptor-like protein 4-1BB is expressed by both $CD4^+$ and $CD8^+$ T cells after activation. Cross-linking of 4-1BB, either by 4-1BB ligand binding or antibody ligation, delivers a costimulatory signal to enhance T-cell activation and proliferation. In a preclinical B-16 mouse melanoma model, a combination of granulocyte monocyte colony-stimulating factor (GM-CSF)-secreting tumor cell immunotherapy and anti-4-1BB monoclonal antibody treatment resulted in rejection of established tumors.[87] In a preclinical B16F10 mouse melanoma model, a combination treatment with anti-$CD4^+$ and anti 4-1BB monoclonal antibodies potentiated the observed anticancer effects.[88] Phase I dose-escalation study of BMS-663,513, an agonist anti-CD137 human monoclonal antibody, in 54 metastatic melanoma patients reported manageable toxicity (up to 15 mg/kg), with fatigue, transaminitis, and neutropenia being the most common adverse events, and clinical activity that justifies its further development both as a single agent and in combination.[89] A large, randomized phase II clinical study with BMS-663,513 in previously treated melanoma patients with stage IV disease has recently finished recruitment.

Anti-integrin monoclonal antibodies
The human monoclonal antibody targeting α_v integrin, CNTO 95,[90] and the chimeric monoclonal antibody Volociximab (M200) recognizing $\alpha5\beta1$ integrin with antiangiogenic properties are currently being evaluated.[91] Results of large phase II trials are awaited to judge whether any of these agents will make it to phase III.

VACCINE DEVELOPMENT IN STAGE IV

The development of an effective therapeutic vaccine for metastatic melanoma continues to be the elusive "holy grail" in a disease where other systemic treatments continue to fail as well, perhaps with the exception of the current adoptive immuno-therapy regiments with lymphodepletion by chemotherapy and total body irradiation at the Surgery Branch of the NCI.[92] Rosenberg and coworkers have pointed out that the optimism about the clinical application of currently available cancer vaccines is based more on surrogate endpoints than on clinical tumor responses. They questioned the validity of this optimism as well as the robustness of the surrogate immuno-monitoring endpoints. In the NCI Surgery Branch experience in 440 patients treated in various vaccine protocols in only 2.6% tumor responses was observed, comparable to the 4.0% response rate reported in 40 studies in 756 patients.[92] It is clear that with these very low response rates, surrogate endpoints for tumor regression are virtu-ally impossible to establish.

Autologous Vaccines

Autologous vaccines are prepared with the patients' own tumor. Vitespen (Onco-phage, formerly HSPPC-96), a tumor-derived, HSP-peptide complex vaccine, was demonstrated to be nontoxic and to induce T-cell activation in a trial with 64 stage IV melanoma patients.[93,94] A phase III trial comparing the vaccine to physician choice therapy in 322 stage IV melanoma patients showed similar OS in both arms.[95] An unscheduled landmark analysis of survival of the selected patients who received more than 10 vaccines showed a benefit in M1a+M1b patients only. Whether these results will be convincing enough for further clinical development is unclear at the moment.

Allogeneic Vaccines

Among a variety of allogeneic cell line-based vaccines that were tested in stage IV disease, Melacine and Canvaxin are the most well known, because they were also evaluated in the adjuvant setting. The key observations and their fate are discussed in the vaccines in the adjuvant setting section.

MAGE-3 Vaccines

A number of clinical trials involving antigens encoded by genes of the MAGE family, particularly MAGE-3, have reported tumor CTL-mediated regressions in melanoma patients.[96] A recombinant MAGE-A3 fusion protein combined with different immuno-logic adjuvants – AS02B or AS15 – has been assessed in the EORTC 16,032 to 18,031 randomized phase II trial as a first-line treatment to 68 patients with unresectable stage III or stage IV M1a melanoma. The combination with AS15 yielded higher anti–MAGE-3 antibody titers, stronger T-cell induction, and some long-lasting clinical responses.[97] A gene signature derived from pretreatment tumor biopsies has been developed and shown to predict clinical benefit.[98] A randomized trial in patients with resected stage IIIB and IIIC melanoma is planned.

Peptide-based Vaccines

Peptide-based vaccines thus far have not lived up to expectations. Initial findings in small studies are often not confirmed by larger studies. Smith and colleagues[99] of the NCI Surgery Branch reported that in 305 patients in whom peptide vaccines were combined with high-dose IL-2, the results were almost identical to those ob-tained in 379 patients treated with IL-2 alone. Only the combination of IL-2 with the immunogenic peptide gp100:209-217(210M) was associated with an increased response rate of 22%. Sosman and colleagues, however, did not observe such an increase for this peptide in 3 phase II trials consisting of 131 patients. They confirmed only the activity of high-dose IL-2.[100] A new interest is stimulated by insights into tissue-specific processing of the immunogenic epitopes of proteins and by the discovery of unusually long cytotoxic T-lymphocyte epitopes that may lead to identification of new targets.[101] Longer peptides harboring particular peptide epitopes allow an adequate epitope processing and consequently a better peptide vaccine efficacy.[102] The first prospective, randomized, clinical trial analyzing peptide vaccination in the adjuvant setting by the ECOG 4697 has recently finished recruitment and will provide a first answer whether peptide vaccination might be effective.

Dendritic Cell-based Vaccines

DCs play a crucial role in the induction of antigen-specific T-cell responses and are considered to be promising adjuvants for vaccine development, and favorable clinical responses have been reported in some patients.[103,104] However, the data on the usefulness of DCs for melanoma immunotherapy remain inconclusive because of a great variety in DC preparation and vaccination protocols, the use of different antigens, and the lack of rigorous criteria for defining clinical responses. In a randomized phase III trial conducted by Schadendorf and colleagues, patients received autologous peptide-loaded DC vaccination or DTIC (850 mg/m^2) at 4-week intervals. Response rates were low (DTIC, 5.5%; DC, 3.8%), and the trial was closed early due to futility.[105]

Vaccination by Intratumoral Gene Transfer

Vaccination by intratumoral gene transfer has been explored for some 15 years, and its efficacy remains to be established. A phase I/II study was recently reported on intratumoral injections of adenovirus-IL-2 (TG1024) in patients with advanced solid tumors including melanoma.[106] When combined with DTIC, responses were reported in 5 of 25 treated melanoma patients.

Some responses have been reported after intratumoral injections of the IL-12 gene in stage IV melanoma patients.[107,108] More interest has been generated by the 28% overall response rate observed in a recent phase II study with intratumoral injections of OncoVEX^{GM-CSF}, an oncolytic herpes simplex virus vector encoding GM-CSF, into 43 stage IIIC and IV patients.[109] Injected tumors routinely responded, often with local complete response, within 2 months of therapy. Importantly, systemic long-term responses were observed independent of the disease stage: 6 CR, 6 PR, and 7 SD of injected tumors. A phase III trial in 360 previously treated, unresectable melanoma patients is planned. Another vaccination trial with intratumoral gene delivery is ongoing in M1a patients with Allovectin-7. This is a plasmid/lipid complex containing the DNA sequences encoding HLA-B7 and β2 microglobulin, which together form an MHC class I. Intratumoral gene therapy may be a promising therapy for patients with metastatic melanoma.

VACCINES IN THE ADJUVANT SETTING

The disappointing results in stage IV melanoma patients are often played down by arguments that the immunosuppressed stage IV patients are unsuitable for vaccine development and that vaccines can only be successfully developed in the adjuvant setting in immunocompetent patients after full resection of their tumor(s). However, it is precisely in this setting that in large adjuvant trials in resected stage II, III, and

IV patients results with adjuvant vaccines have failed, or even worse, have given an indication of being potentially detrimental. There have been at least 25 randomized trials conducted in stage II to III melanoma evaluating chemotherapy, nonspecific immune stimulants such as Bacillus Calmette-Guerin (BCG), Corynebacterium parvum, levamisole, or combinations of these agents with dacarbazine. The trials were almost invariably underpowered and yielded negative results with the exception of the occasional incidental nonrepeatable positive finding in trials involving small numbers of patients.[13] Seven large randomized trials of allogeneic melanoma cell-based vaccines have been conducted, and not one had an impact on survival. Only the Australian trial that investigated an allogeneic tumor cell-based oncolysate showed some impact.[110] In the United States, a trial of the Melacine vaccine in stage II patients showed no benefit for the total study population,[111] but there appeared to be activity in patients with particular HLA types.[112] Unfortunately, a prospective study of the vaccine in patients with the relevant HLA types has never been conducted.

The allogeneic cancer vaccine (Canvaxin) developed from 3 cell lines has been evaluated in large phase III trials because of promising results of a matched pair analysis in the JWCC database.[113] In stage III melanoma 1166 patients and in resected stage IV 496 patients were randomized to Canvaxin plus BCG or placebo plus BCG after surgery. Both trials were closed prematurely by the Independent Data Monitoring Committee (IDMC).[114] There was a survival disadvantage in patients receiving Canvaxin treatment in both studies. The median survival in the stage III study had not been reached, but the 5-year survival was 59% for those receiving the vaccine and 68% for placebo-treated patients. In the stage IV study, the median survival was 32 months for the patients treated with Canvaxin and 39 months for patients receiving placebo, with respective 5-year survival rates of 40% and 45%. Recently, results were reported for the large phase III EORTC 18961 trial in 1314 stage II patients of adjuvant ganglioside vaccine GMK. This vaccine had been reported to be successful in a small randomized trial in the Memorial Sloan Kettering Cancer Center.[115] The EORTC 18961 trial was stopped early by the Independent Data Monitoring Committee because of futility for DFS and for inferior survival in the vaccine arm.[116] This difference in survival at the second interim analysis is quite similar to that observed in the second interim analysis of the ECOG 1694 trial, in which 880 stage IIB to III patients were randomized between high-dose IFN therapy and the GMK vaccine.[117] This trial is now difficult to interpret with respect to the potential detrimental impact observed. It is clear that the results of these large adjuvant trials are a significant setback to the development of a vaccination strategy in melanoma.[61]

SUMMARY

Immunotherapy of melanoma is a very exciting and dynamic field. Yet success is rather elusive because of the tremendous complexity. The advances in basic understanding of the immune system and the host-tumor interactions should ultimately lead to effective treatments.

REFERENCES

1. Balch CM, Buzaid AC, Soong SJ, et al. Final version of the American Joint Committee on Cancer staging system for cutaneous melanoma. J Clin Oncol 2001;19:3635–48.
2. Legha SS. The role of interferon alfa in the treatment of metastatic melanoma. Semin Oncol 1997;24:S24–31.

3. Falkson CI, Falkson G, Falkson HC. Improved results with the addition of interferon alfa- 2b to dacarbazine in the treatment of patients with metastatic malignant melanoma. J Clin Oncol 1991;9:1403–8.
4. Thomson DB, Adena M, McLeod GR, et al. Interferon-alpha 2a does not improve response or survival when combined with dacarbazine in metastatic malignant melanoma: results of a multi-institutional Australian randomized trial. Melanoma Res 1993;3:133–8.
5. Bajetta E, Di Leo A, Zampino MG, et al. Multicenter randomized trial of dacarbazine alone or in combination with two different doses and schedules of interferon alfa-2a in the treatment of advanced melanoma. J Clin Oncol 1994;12:806–11.
6. Falkson CI, Ibrahim J, Kirkwood JM, et al. Phase III trial of dacarbazine versus dacarbazine with interferon alpha-2b versus dacarbazine with tamoxifen versus dacarbazine with interferon alpha-2b and tamoxifen in patients with metastatic malignant melanoma: an Eastern Cooperative Oncology Group Study. J Clin Oncol 1998;16:1743–51.
7. Middleton MR, Lorigan P, Owen J, et al. A randomized phase III study comparing dacarbazine, BCNU, cisplatin and tamoxifen with dacarbazine and interferon in advanced melanoma. Br J Cancer 2000;82:1158–62.
8. Young AM, Marsden J, Goodman A, et al. Prospective randomized comparison of dacarbazine (DTIC) versus DTIC plus interferon-alpha (IFN-alpha) in metastatic melanoma. Clin Oncol (R Coll Radiol) 2001;13:458–65.
9. Kaufmann R, Spieth K, Leiter U, et al. Temozolomide in combination with interferon-alfa versus temozolomide alone in patients with advanced metastatic melanoma: a randomized, phase III, multicenter study from the Dermatologic Cooperative Oncology Group. J Clin Oncol 2005;23:9001–7.
10. Vuoristo MS, Hahka-Kemppinen M, Parvinen LM, et al. Randomized trial of dacarbazine versus bleomycin, vincristine, lomustine and dacarbazine (BOLD) chemotherapy combined with natural or recombinant interferon-alpha in patients with advanced melanoma. Melanoma Res 2005;15:291–6.
11. Bukowski RM, Tendler C, Cutler D, et al. Treating cancer with PEG Intron: pharmacokinetic profile and dosing guidelines for an improved interferon-alpha-2b formulation. Cancer 2002;95:389–96.
12. Dummer R, Garbe C, Thompson JA, et al. Randomized dose-escalation study evaluating peginterferon alfa-2a in patients with metastatic malignant melanoma. J Clin Oncol 2006;24:1188–94.
13. Eggermont AM, Gore M. Randomized adjuvant therapy trials in melanoma: surgical and systemic. Semin Oncol 2007;34:509–15.
14. Lens MB, Dawes M. Interferon alfa therapy for malignant melanoma: a systematic review of randomized controlled trials. J Clin Oncol 2002;20:1818–25.
15. Wheatley K, Ives N, Hancock B, et al. Does adjuvant interferon-alpha for high-risk melanoma provide a worthwhile benefit? A meta-analysis of the randomised trials. Cancer Treat Rev 2003;29:241–52.
16. Wheatley K, Ives N, Eggermont AM, et al. Interferon-α as adjuvant therapy for melanoma: an individual patient data meta-analysis of randomised trials. J Clin Oncol 2007;25 [abstract 8526].
17. Kirkwood JM, Manola J, Ibrahim J, et al. A pooled analysis of eastern cooperative oncology group and intergroup trials of adjuvant high-dose interferon for melanoma. Clin Cancer Res 2004;10:1670–7.
18. Kleeberg UR, Suciu S, Bröcker EB, et al. Final results of the EORTC 18871/ DKG 80-1 randomised phase III trial. rIFN-alpha2b versus rIFN-gamma versus ISCADOR M versus observation after surgery in melanoma patients

with either high-risk primary (thickness >3 mm) or regional lymph node metastasis. Eur J Cancer 2004;40:390–402.

19. Eggermont AM, Suciu S, Santinami M, et al. Adjuvant therapy with pegylated interferon alfa-2b versus observation alone in resected stage III melanoma: final results of EORTC 18991, a randomised phase III trial. Lancet 2008;372:117–26.

20. Eggermont AM, Suciu S, MacKie R, et al. Post-surgery adjuvant therapy with intermediate doses of interferon alfa 2b versus observation in patients with stage IIb/III melanoma (EORTC 18952): randomised controlled trial. Lancet 2005;366: 1189–96.

21. Grob JJ, Dreno B, de la Salmonière P, et al. Randomised trial of interferon alpha-2a as adjuvant therapy in resected primary melanoma thicker than 1.5 mm without clinically detectable node metastases. Lancet 1998;351:1905–10.

22. Pehamberger H, Soyer HP, Steiner A, et al. Adjuvant interferon alfa-2a treatment in resected primary stage II cutaneous melanoma. Austrian Malignant Melanoma Cooperative Group. J Clin Oncol 1998;16:1425–9.

23. Cameron DA, Cornbleet MC, Mackie RM, et al. Adjuvant interferon alpha 2b in high risk melanoma - the Scottish study. Br J Cancer 2001;84:1146–9.

24. Gogas H, Ioannovich J, Dafni U, et al. Prognostic significance of autoimmunity during treatment of melanoma with interferon. N Engl J Med 2006;354:709–18.

25. Bouwhuis M, Suciu S, Kruit W, et al. Prognostic value of autoantibodies (auto-AB) in melanoma patients (pts) in the EORTC 18952 trial of adjuvant interferon (IFN) compared to observation (obs). J Clin Oncol 2007;25 [abstract 8507].

26. Bouwhuis M, Suciu S, Testori A, et al. Prognostic value of autoantibodies (auto-AB) in melanoma stage III patients in the EORTC 18991 phase III randomized trial comparing adjuvant pegylated interferon α2b (PEG-IFN) vs Observation. Eur J Cancer - Supplements 2007;5:11 [abstract 13BA].

27. Atkins MB, Lotze MT, Dutcher JP, et al. High-dose recombinant interleukin 2 therapy for patients with metastatic melanoma: analysis of 270 patients treated between 1985 and 1993. J Clin Oncol 1999;17:2105–16.

28. Petrella T, Quirt I, Verma S, et al. Single-agent interleukin-2 in the treatment of metastatic melanoma: a systematic review. Cancer Treat Rev 2007;33:484–96.

29. Atkins MB, Mier JW, Parkinson DR, et al. Hypothyroidism after treatment with interleukin-2 and lymphokine-activated killer cells. N Engl J Med 1988;318: 1557–63.

30. Keilholz U, Conradt C, Legha SS, et al. Results of interleukin-2-based treatment in advanced melanoma: a case record-based analysis of 631 patients. J Clin Oncol 1998;16:2921–9.

31. Phan GQ, Attia P, Steinberg SM, et al. Factors associated with response to high-dose interleukin-2 in patients with metastatic melanoma. J Clin Oncol 2001;19: 3477–82.

32. Schmidt H, Suciu S, Punt CJ, et al. Pretreatment levels of peripheral neutrophils and leukocytes as independent predictors of overall survival in patients with American Joint Committee on Cancer Stage IV Melanoma: results of the EORTC 18951 Biochemotherapy Trial. J Clin Oncol 2007;25:1562–9.

33. Findeisen P, Zapatka M, Peccerella T, et al. Serum amyloid A as a prognostic marker in melanoma identified by proteomic profiling. J Clin Oncol 2009 [Epub ahead of print].

34. Sparano JA, Fisher RI, Sunderland M, et al. Randomized phase III trial of treatment with high-dose interleukin-2 either alone or in combination with interferon alfa-2a in patients with advanced melanoma. J Clin Oncol 1993;11: 1969–77.

35. Agarwala SS, Glaspy J, O'Day SJ, et al. Results from a randomized phase III study comparing combined treatment with histamine dihydrochloride plus inter-leukin-2 versus interleukin-2 alone in patients with metastatic melanoma. J Clin Oncol 2002;20:125–33.
36. Keilholz U, Goey SH, Punt CJ, et al. Interferon alfa-2a and interleukin-2 with or without cisplatin in metastatic melanoma: a randomized trial of the European Organization for Research and Treatment of Cancer Melanoma Cooperative Group. J Clin Oncol 1997;15:2579–88.
37. Johnston SR, Constenla DO, Moore J, et al. Randomized phase II trial of BCDT [carmustine (BCNU), cisplatin, dacarbazine (DTIC) and tamoxifen] with or without interferon alpha (IFN-alpha) and interleukin (IL-2) in patients with meta-static melanoma. Br J Cancer 1998;77:1280–6.
38. Dorval T, Negrier S, Chevreau C, et al. Randomized trial of treatment with cisplatin and interleukin-2 either alone or in combination with interferon-alpha-2a in patients with metastatic melanoma: a Federation Nationale des Centres de Lutte Contre le Cancer Multicenter, parallel study. Cancer 1999; 85:1060–6.
39. Rosenberg SA, Yang JC, Schwartzentruber DJ, et al. Prospective randomized trial of the treatment of patients with metastatic melanoma using chemotherapy with cisplatin, dacarbazine, and tamoxifen alone or in combination with inter-leukin-2 and interferon alfa-2b. J Clin Oncol 1999;17:968–75.
40. Hauschild A, Garbe C, Stolz W, et al. Dacarbazine and interferon alpha with or without interleukin 2 in metastatic melanoma: a randomized phase III multicentre trial of the Dermatologic Cooperative Oncology Group (DeCOG). Br J Cancer 2001;84:1036–42.
41. Eton O, Legha SS, Bedikian AY, et al. Sequential biochemotherapy versus chemotherapy for metastatic melanoma: results from a phase III randomized trial. J Clin Oncol 2002;20:2045–52.
42. Atzpodien J, Neuber K, Kamanabrou D, et al. Combination chemotherapy with or without s.c. IL-2 and IFN-alpha: results of a prospectively randomized trial of the Cooperative Advanced Malignant Melanoma Chemoimmunotherapy Group (ACIMM). Br J Cancer 2002;86:179–84.
43. Ridolfi R, Chiarion-Sileni V, Guida M, et al. Cisplatin, dacarbazine with or without subcutaneous interleukin-2, and interferon alpha-2b in advanced melanoma outpatients: results from an Italian multicenter phase III randomized clinical trial. J Clin Oncol 2002;20:1600–7.
44. Keilholz U, Punt CJ, Gore M, et al. Dacarbazine, cisplatin, and interferon-alfa-2b with or without interleukin-2 in metastatic melanoma: a randomized phase III trial (18951) of the European Organisation for Research and Treatment of Cancer Melanoma Group. J Clin Oncol 2005;23:6747–55.
45. Bajetta E, Del Vecchio M, Nova P, et al. Multicenter phase III randomized trial of polychemotherapy (CVD regimen) versus the same chemotherapy (CT) plus subcutaneous interleukin-2 and interferon-alpha2b in metastatic melanoma. Ann Oncol 2006;17:571–7.
46. Atkins MB, Hsu J, Lee S, et al. Phase III Trial comparing concurrent biochemo-therapy with cisplatin, vinblastine, dacarbazine, interleukin-2, and interferon alfa-2b with cisplatin, vinblastine, and dacarbazine alone in patients with meta-static malignant melanoma (E3695): a trial coordinated by the Eastern Cooper-ative Oncology Group. J Clin Oncol 2008;26(35):5748–54.
47. Fehniger TA, Cooper MA, Caligiuri MA. Interleukin-2 and interleukin-15: immuno-therapy for cancer. Cytokine Growth Factor Rev 2002;13:169–83.

48. Davis ID, Skak K, Smyth MJ, et al. Interleukin-21 signaling: functions in cancer and autoimmunity. Clin Cancer Res 2007;13:6926–32.

49. Thompson JA, Curti BD, Redman BG, et al. Phase I study of recombinant inter-leukin-21 in patients with metastatic melanoma and renal cell carcinoma. J Clin Oncol 2008;26:2034–9.

50. Frederiksen KS, Lundsgaard D, Freeman JA, et al. IL-21 induces in vivo immune activation of NK cells and CD8(+) T cells in patients with metastatic melanoma and renal cell carcinoma. Cancer Immunol Immunother 2008;57:1439–49.

51. Gattinoni L, Powell DJ Jr, Rosenberg SA, et al. Adoptive immunotherapy for cancer: building on success. Nat Rev Immunol 2006;6:383–93.

52. Mule JJ, Shu S, Schwarz SL, et al. Adoptive immunotherapy of established pulmonary metastases with LAK cells and recombinant interleukin-2. Science 1984;225:1487–9.

53. Rosenberg SA, Spiess P, Lafreniere R. A new approach to the adoptive immu-notherapy of cancer with tumor-infiltrating lymphocytes. Science 1986;233: 1318–21.

54. Rosenberg SA, Yannelli JR, Yang JC, et al. Treatment of patients with metastatic melanoma with autologous tumor-infiltrating lymphocytes and interleukin 2. J Natl Cancer Inst 1994;86:1159–66.

55. Dudley ME, Wunderlich JR, Robbins PF, et al. Cancer regression and autoimmu-nity in patients after clonal repopulation with antitumor lymphocytes. Science 2002;298:850–4.

56. Eggermont AM, Steller EP, Matthews W, et al. Alloimmune cells consume inter-leukin-2 and competitively inhibit the anti-tumour effects of interleukin-2. Br J Cancer 1987;56:97–102.

57. Sugarbaker PH, Matthews W, Steller EP, et al. Inhibitory effects of alloimmune T cells on the generation of cytolytic responses of lymphokine-activated killer cells. J Biol Response Mod 1987;6(4):430–45.

58. Gattinoni L, Finkelstein SE, Klebanoff CA, et al. Removal of homeostatic cytokine sinks by lymphodepletion enhances the efficacy of adoptively transferred tumor-specific CD8+ T cells. J Exp Med 2005;202(7):907–12.

59. Dudley ME, Yang JC, Sherry R, et al. Adoptive cell therapy for patients with metastatic melanoma: evaluation of intensive myeloablative chemoradiation preparative regimens. J Clin Oncol 2008;26(32):5233–9.

60. Tran KQ, Zhou J, Durflinger KH, et al. Minimally cultured tumor-infiltrating lymphocytes display optimal characteristics for adoptive cell therapy. J Immun-other 2008;31(8):742–51.

61. Eggermont AM. Vaccine trials in melanoma—time for reflection. Nat Rev Clin Oncol, in press.

62. Mackensen A, Meidenbauer N, Vogl S, et al. Phase I study of adoptive T-cell therapy using antigen-specific CD8+ T cells for the treatment of patients with metastatic melanoma. J Clin Oncol 2006;24:5060–9.

63. Powell DJ Jr, Dudley ME, Hogan KA, et al. Adoptive transfer of vaccine-induced peripheral blood mononuclear cells to patients with metastatic melanoma following lymphodepletion. J Immunol 2006;177:6527–39.

64. Hunder NN, Wallen H, Cao J, et al. Treatment of metastatic melanoma with autol-ogous CD4+ T cells against NY-ESO-1. N Engl J Med 2008;358:2698–703.

65. Rosenberg SA, Restifo NP, Yang JC, et al. Adoptive cell transfer: a clinical path to effective cancer immunotherapy. Nat Rev Cancer 2008;8:299–308.

66. Morgan RA, Dudley ME, Wunderlich JR, et al. Cancer regression in patients after transfer of genetically engineered lymphocytes. Science 2006;314:126–9.

67. Inman BA, Frigola X, Dong H, et al. Costimulation, coinhibition and cancer. Curr Cancer Drug Targets 2007;7:15–30.
68. Cranmer LD, Hersh E. The role of the CTLA4 blockade in the treatment of malignant melanoma. Cancer Invest 2007;25:613–31.
69. Weber J. Review: anti-CTLA-4 antibody ipilimumab: case studies of clinical response and immune-related adverse events. Oncologist 2007;12: 864–72.
70. Ribas A, Hanson DC, Noe DA, et al. Tremelimumab (CP-675,206), a cytotoxic T lymphocyte associated antigen 4 blocking monoclonal antibody in clinical development for patients with cancer. Oncologist 2007;12:873–83.
71. Hersh EM, Weber JS, Powderly JD, et al. Disease control and long-term survival in chemotherapy-naive patients with advanced melanoma treated with ipilimumab (MDX- 010) with or without dacarbazine. J Clin Oncol 2008;26 [abstract 9022].
72. Attia P, Phan GQ, Maker AV, et al. Autoimmunity correlates with tumor regression in patients with metastatic melanoma treated with anti-cytotoxic T-lymphocyte antigen-4. J Clin Oncol 2005;23:6043–53.
73. Downey SG, Klapper JA, Smith FO, et al. Prognostic factors related to clinical response in patients with metastatic melanoma treated by CTL-associated antigen-4 blockade. Clin Cancer Res 2007;13:6681–8.
74. Beck KE, Blansfield JA, Tran KQ, et al. Enterocolitis in patients with cancer after antibody blockade of cytotoxic T-lymphocyte-associated antigen 4. J Clin Oncol 2006;24:2283–9.
75. Hamid O, Chin K, Li J, et al. Dose effect of ipilimumab in patients with advanced melanoma: results from a phase II, randomized, dose-ranging study. J Clin Oncol 2008;26 [abstract 9025].
76. O'Day SJ, Ibrahim R, DePril V, et al. Efficacy and safety of ipilimumab induction and maintenance dosing in patients with advanced melanoma who progressed on one or more prior therapies. J Clin Oncol 2008;26 [abstract 9021].
77. Ribas A, Antonia S, Sosman J, et al. Results of a phase II clinical trial of 2 doses and schedules of CP-675,206, an anti-CTLA4 monoclonal antibody, in patients (pts) with advanced melanoma. J Clin Oncol 2007;25 [abstract 3000].
78. Gomez-Navarro J, Antonia S, Sosman J, et al. Survival of patients (pts) with metastatic melanoma treated with the anti-CTLA4 monoclonal antibody (mAb) CP-675,206 in a phase I/II study. J Clin Oncol 2007;26 [abstract 8524].
79. Kirkwood JM, Lorigan P, Hersey P, et al. A phase II trial of tremelimumab (CP-675,206) in patients with advanced refractory or relapsed melanoma. J Clin Oncol 2008;26 [abstract 9023].
80. Ribas A, Hauschild A, Kefford R, et al. Phase III, open-label, randomized, comparative study of tremelimumab (CP-675,206) and chemotherapy (temozolomide [TMZ] or dacarbazine [DTIC]) in patients with advanced melanoma. J Clin Oncol 2008;26 [abstract LBA9011].
81. Wolchok JD, Ibrahim R, DePril V, et al. Antitumor response and new lesions in advanced melanoma patients on ipilimumab treatment. J Clin Oncol 2008;26 [abstract 3020].
82. Hodi FS, Hoos A, Ibrahim R, et al. Novel efficacy criteria for antitumor activity to immunotherapy using the example of ipilimumab, an anti-CTLA-4 monoclonal antibody. J Clin Oncol 2008;26 [abstract 3008].
83. Butte M, Keir M, Phamuduy T, et al. Programmed death-1 ligand interacts specifically with the B7-1 costimulatory molecules to inhibit T cell responses. Immunity 2007;27:111–22.

84. Wong RM, Scotland RR, Lau RL, et al. Programmed death-1 blockade enhances expansion and functional capacity of human melanoma antigen-specific CTLs. Int Immunol 2007;19:1223–34.

85. Melero I, Hervas-Stubbs S, Glennie M, et al. Immunostimulatory monoclonal antibodies for cancer therapy. Nat Rev Cancer 2007;7:95–106.

86. Gray JC, French RR, James S, et al. Optimising anti-tumour CD8 T-cell responses using combinations of immunomodulatory antibodies. Eur J Immunol 2008;38:2499–511.

87. Li B, Lin J, Vanroey M, et al. Established B16 tumors are rejected following treatment with GM-CSF-secreting tumor cell immunotherapy in combination with anti-4-1BB mAb. Clin Immunol 2007;125:76–87.

88. Choi BK, Kim YH, Kang WJ, et al. Mechanisms involved in synergistic anticancer immunity of anti-4-1BB and anti-CD4 therapy. Cancer Res 2007;67:8891–9.

89. Sznol M, Hodi FS, Margolin K, et al. Phase I study of BMS-663513, a fully human anti-CD137 agonist monoclonal antibody, in patients (pts) with advanced cancer (CA). J Clin Oncol 2008;26 [abstract 3007].

90. Jayson GC, Mullamitha S, Ton C, et al. Phase I study of CNTO 95, a fully human monoclonal antibody (mAb) to av integrins, in patients with solid tumors. J Clin Oncol 2005;23 [abstract 3113].

91. Linette G, Cranmer L, Hodi S, et al. A multicenter phase II study of volociximab in patients with relapsed metastatic melanoma. J Clin Oncol 2008;26. [abstract 3505].

92. Rosenberg SA, Yang JC, Restifo NP. Cancer immunotherapy: moving beyond current vaccines. Nat Med 2004;10:909–15.

93. Srivastava P. Interaction of heat shock proteins with peptides and antigen presenting cells: chaperoning of the innate and adaptive immune responses. Annu Rev Immunol 2002;20:395–425.

94. Belli F, Testori A, Rivoltini L, et al. Vaccination of metastatic melanoma patients with autologous tumor-derived heat shock protein gp96-peptide complexes: clinical and immunologic findings. J Clin Oncol 2002;20:4169–80.

95. Testori A, Richards J, Whitman E, et al. Phase III comparison of vitespen, an autologous tumor-derived heat shock protein gp96 peptide complex vaccine, with physician's choice of treatment for stage IV melanoma: the C-100-21 Study Group. J Clin Oncol 2008;26:955–62.

96. Coulie PG, Karanikas V, Colau D, et al. A monoclonal cytolytic T-lymphocyte response observed in a melanoma patient vaccinated with a tumor-specific antigenic peptide encoded by gene MAGE-3. Proc Natl Acad Sci U S A 2001;98:10290–5.

97. Kruit WH, Suciu S, Dreno B, et al. Immunization with recombinant MAGE-A3 protein combined with adjuvant systems AS15 or AS02B in patients with unresectable and progressive metastatic cutaneous melanoma: a randomized open-label phase II study of the EORTC Melanoma Group (16032–18031). J Clin Oncol 2008;26 [abstract 9065].

98. Louahed J, Gruselle O, Gaulis S, et al. Expression of defined genes identified by pretreatment tumor profiling: association with clinical responses to the GSK MAGE-A3 immunotherapeutic in metastatic melanoma patients (EORTC 16032–18031). J Clin Oncol 2008;26 [abstract 9045].

99. Smith FO, Downey SG, Klapper JA, et al. Treatment of metastatic melanoma using interleukin-2 alone or in conjunction with vaccines. Clin Cancer Res 2008;14:5610–8.

100. Sosman JA, Carrillo C, Urba WJ, et al. Three phase II cytokine working group trials of gp100 (210M) peptide plus high-dose interleukin-2 in patients with HLA-A2-positive advanced melanoma. J Clin Oncol 2008;26(14):2292–8.

101. Purcell AW, McCluskey J, Rossjohn J. More than one reason to rethink the use of peptides in vaccine design. Nat Rev Drug Discov 2007;6:404–14.

102. Melief CJ, van der Burg SH. Immunotherapy of established (pre)malignant disease by synthetic long peptide vaccines. Nat Rev Cancer 2008;8:351–60.

103. Osada T, Clay TM, Woo CY, et al. Dendritic cell-based immunotherapy. Int Rev Immunol 2006;25:377–413.

104. Thurner B, Haendle I, Roder C, et al. Vaccination with mage-3A1 peptide-pulsed mature, monocyte-derived dendritic cells expands specific cytotoxic T cells and induces regression of some metastases in advanced stage IV melanoma. J Exp Med 1999;190:1669–78.

105. Schadendorf D, Ugurel S, Schuler-Thurner B, et al. Dacarbazine (DTIC) versus vaccination with autologous peptide-pulsed dendritic cells (DC) in first-line treatment of patients with metastatic melanoma: a randomized phase III trial of the DC study group of the DeCOG. Ann Oncol 2006;17:563–70.

106. Dummer R, Rochlitz C, Velu T, et al. Intralesional adenovirus-mediated inter-leukin-2 gene transfer for advanced solid cancers and melanoma. Mol Ther 2008;16:985–94.

107. Heinzerling L, Burg G, Dummer R, et al. Intratumoral injection of DNA encoding human interleukin 12 into patients with metastatic melanoma: clinical efficacy. Hum Gene Ther 2005;16:35–48.

108. Mahvi DM, Henry MB, Albertini MR, et al. Intratumoral injection of IL-12 plasmid DNA–results of a phase I/IB clinical trial. Cancer Gene Ther 2007;14:717–23.

109. Senzer NN, Kaufman HL, Amatruda T, et al. Phase II clinical trial with a second generation, GM-CSF encoding, oncolytic herpesvirus in unresectable meta-static melanoma. J Clin Oncol 2008;26 [abstract 9008].

110. Hersey P, Coates AS, McCarthy WH, et al. Adjuvant immunotherapy of patients with high-risk melanoma using vaccinia viral lysates of melanoma: results of a randomized trial. J Clin Oncol 2002;20:4181–90.

111. Sondak VK, Liu PY, Tuthill RJ, et al. Adjuvant immunotherapy of resected, inter-mediate-thickness, node-negative melanoma with an allogeneic tumor vaccine: overall results of a randomized trial of the Southwest Oncology Group. J Clin Oncol 2002;20:2058–66.

112. Sosman JA, Unger JM, Liu PY, et al. Adjuvant immunotherapy of resected, inter-mediate-thickness, node-negative melanoma with an allogeneic tumor vaccine: impact of HLA class I antigen expression on outcome. J Clin Oncol 2002;20: 2067–75.

113. Hsueh EC, Essner R, Foshag LJ, et al. Prolonged survival after complete resec-tion of disseminated melanoma and active immunotherapy with a therapeutic cancer vaccine. J Clin Oncol 2002;20:4549–54.

114. Morton DL, Mozzillo N, Thompson JF, et al. An international, randomized, phase III trial of Bacillus Calmette-Guerin (BCG) plus allogeneic melanoma vaccine (MCV) or placebo after complete resection of melanoma metastatic to regional or distant sites. J Clin Oncol 2007;25 [abstract 8508].

115. Livingston PO, Wong GY, Adluri S, et al. Improved survival in stage III melanoma patients with GM2 antibodies: a randomized trial of adjuvant vaccination with GM2 ganglioside. J Clin Oncol 1994;12:1036–44.

116. Eggermont AM, Suciu S, Ruka W, et al. EORTC 18961: Post-operative adjuvant ganglioside GM2-KLH21 vaccination treatment vs observation in stage II (T3-T4

N0M0) melanoma: 2nd interim analysis led to an early disclosure of the results. J Clin Oncol 2008;26 [abstract 9004].

117. Kirkwood JM, Ibrahim JG, Sosman JA, et al. High-dose interferon alfa-2b significantly prolongs relapse-free and overall survival compared with the GM2-KLH/QS-21 vaccine in patients with resected stage IIB-III melanoma: results of intergroup trial E1694/S9512/C509801. J Clin Oncol 2001;19:2370–80.

Surgical Management of Melanoma

Jennifer A. Wargo, MD[a,b,*], Kenneth Tanabe, MD[a,b]

KEYWORDS

- Melanoma • Surgery • Margins • Lymphadenectomy
- Sentinel node

Melanoma is an increasing health care problem worldwide. Up to 80,000 cases of melanoma are diagnosed per year[1] and it is the sixth leading cause of cancer death in the United States. The lifetime risk is estimated to be 1 in 75 individuals for the development of melanoma.[1] The incidence of melanoma is increasing significantly at a rate of 4.1% per year, faster than any other malignancy. An average of 18.8 life-years are lost per melanoma death,[2] and it is estimated that 1 American will die from melanoma every hour.[3]

Surgery remains the mainstay of treatment of melanoma, and in most cases it is curative. Several important surgical issues are discussed in this review, including the extent of surgical margins, Mohs micrographic surgery for melanoma in situ, the use of sentinel lymph node biopsy, the usefulness of lymphadenectomy, isolated limb perfusion, and the role of metastasectomy.

SURGICAL TREATMENT OF STAGE I AND II MELANOMA
Prognostic Factors for Stage I and II Melanoma

Most patients present with clinically localized melanoma, and several prognostic factors have been identified for risk stratification in this heterogeneous group. The most important prognostic factors in early stage melanoma are tumor thickness (T1 to T4) and the presence or absence of ulceration. These factors have significant implications on prognosis, as 5-year survival in stage I and II melanomas falls significantly with increasing thickness; 5-year survival dropped from 80% to 55% in the presence of ulceration in a 2006 analysis.[4] Clark level also has prognostic implications in thin melanomas, as tumors extending to Clark level IV are considered T1b regardless of their thickness and are associated with a worse prognosis. However, as additional prognostic factors come to light, Clark level seems less important than many other factors. More recently, the mitotic rate in the primary tumor has been identified as

[a] Department of Surgery, Harvard Medical School, Boston, MA, USA
[b] Division of Surgical Oncology, Department of Surgery, Massachusetts General Hospital, 55 Fruit Street, Boston, MA 02114, USA
* Division of Surgical Oncology, Department of Surgery, Massachusetts General Hospital, 55 Fruit Street, Boston, MA 02114.
E-mail address: ajwargo@partners.org (J.A. Wargo).

Hematol Oncol Clin N Am 23 (2009) 565–581
doi:10.1016/j.hoc.2009.03.002
0889-8588/09/$ – see front matter © 2009 Elsevier Inc. All rights reserved.

an important prognostic factor, possibly even surpassing ulceration in importance in early stage melanoma.[5,6] Mitotic rate will be incorporated in the new version of the American Joint Commission on Cancer (AJCC) staging system, which will be released in 2009.

Margins of Excision for Primary Melanoma

The width of surgical margins depends on the thickness of the lesion and has been defined by a series of prospective randomized clinical trials. Although standard guidelines exist based on these trials, there is still considerable debate about the narrowest efficacious margins for primary melanoma lesions. The earliest recommendations stemmed from studies conducted in the 1950s that demonstrated the presence of atypical melanocytes up to 5 cm from the edge of an excision[7] and provided the basis for "wide local excision." Since this study, there have been numerous studies addressing suitable margins of excision for melanoma. Five of these are prospective, randomized controlled trials (**Table 1**).[8]

A French cooperative group trial was conducted in the 1970s and early 1980s in which patients with primary melanoma tumor thicknesses less than or equal to 2 mm were randomized to one of two treatment arms: patients were treated with either wide excision using 5-cm margins or wide excision using 2-cm margins.[9] No statistically significant differences in local recurrence, distant metastases, or overall survival were observed between the 2 treatment arms. From these data it was concluded that surgical margins could be reduced from 5 cm to 2 cm without any increase in the local recurrence or death rates in patients with melanomas 2 mm or less in thickness. Between 1980 and 1985 the World Health Organization (WHO) Melanoma Program conducted a clinical trial in which patients with melanomas 2 mm or less in thickness were randomized to treatment with wide excision using either a 1-cm surgical margin or a 3-cm surgical margin.[10,11] Six of 612 evaluable patients experienced a local recurrence, and 5 of these 6 patients had been randomized to the narrower margin treatment arm and had primary melanomas measuring between 1.0 and 2.0 mm in thickness (1.0 mm, 1.1 mm, 1.1 mm, 1.9 mm, 1.9 mm). However, no differences in overall survival were observed, leading the investigators to conclude that surgical excision using a 1-cm margin is preferred to that of a 3-cm margin in patients with melanomas 2.0 mm or less in thickness. This conclusion and recommendation has not been universally accepted for patients with melanomas between 1.0 and 2.0 mm in thickness because of the higher incidence of local recurrence in those patients who were treated with a 1-cm margin excision.[9]

Table 1 Prospective randomized trials examining surgical excision margins for primary cutaneous melanoma			
Surgical Trial	Number of Patients	Tumor Thickness (mm)	Surgical Margins (cm)
French Cooperative Study[9]	362	<2	2 vs 5
World Health Organization Melanoma Program[10,11]	612	<2	1 vs 3
Intergoup Melanoma Trial[12,13]	486	1–4	2 vs 4
Swedish Melanoma Study Group[14,15]	989	0.8–2	2 vs 5
United Kingdom Study[16]	774	≥2 mm	1 vs 3

The Intergroup Melanoma Trial was designed to examine the efficacy of 2-cm versus 4-cm surgical margins in patients with "intermediate thickness" melanomas, defined as tumor thickness between 1 mm and 4 mm.[12,13] The 0.4% incidence of local recurrence as a first site of relapse observed in patients treated with 2-cm margins was no different than the 0.9% incidence of local recurrence observed in patients treated with 4-cm margins. Local recurrence at any time was also not different between the 2 groups; 2.1% for patients treated with a 2-cm margin compared with 2.6% for patients treated with a 4-cm margin. No difference in overall survival was observed between the 2 groups. Patients treated with a 4-cm margin required skin grafts more frequently than patients treated with a 2-cm margin (46% vs 11%; $P < .0001$). A multivariate analysis of prognostic factors demonstrated that only the presence of ulceration and location on the head or neck correlated with risk for local recurrence (refer to Table 5 in Balch et al).[13] Based on these results, the investigators concluded that margins of excision can be safely reduced to 2 cm in patients with intermediate thickness melanomas without any adverse impact on local recurrence or overall survival.

The Swedish Melanoma Study Group performed a prospective, randomized multicenter study to evaluate an excision margin of 2 cm versus 5 cm for patients with melanomas measuring between 0.8 and 2.0 mm in thickness.[14,15] Of 989 evaluable patients followed for a median of 11 years, no differences in local recurrence, distant metastases, or overall survival were observed between the 2 groups.

In a prospective study, based in the United Kingdom between 1993 and 2001, patients with melanomas measuring 2 mm or greater in thickness were randomized to undergo wide excision with either 1 cm or 3 cm surgical margins.[16] Lymphatic mapping and sentinel node biopsy were not performed on any of the patients. Time to first local recurrence and in-transit recurrence were originally defined as primary end points; however, because the frequency of these events was lower than expected, at the first interim analysis the investigators increased the total sample size (900 patients) and they chose to combine nodal recurrences with local and in-transit recurrences, thereby creating a new primary endpoint termed "locoregional recurrence." Of the 900 patients enrolled in the study, 774 were eligible and were followed for a median of 5 years, at which time the rate of locoregional recurrences was higher in the patients randomized to 1-cm margins versus 3-cm margins (43% vs 37%, hazard ratio = 1.26; 95% confidence interval, 1.00 to 1.59; $P = .05$). Because patients in this study had not undergone lymphatic mapping and sentinel node biopsy, nodal recurrence was common. The rates of isolated local recurrence (without nodal metastases) were not significantly different between patients with 1-cm and 3-cm surgical margins (3.9% vs 3.4%, respectively). The rate of isolated in-transit metastases (without nodal metastases) was similar (2.6% vs 1.8%). There was no significant difference between the groups in either melanoma-specific or overall survival. The investigators concluded that in patients with melanomas greater than 2 mm in thickness, melanoma cells are left behind in a small number of patients after a 1-cm surgical margin excision, and these cells lead to locoregional recurrences and melanoma-specific death. They make the case that tumor cells in lymphatics may be completely excised using a 3-cm margin but left behind with a 1-cm margin. However, it is clear that "locoregional" recurrences in this trial could have been significantly reduced with implementation of lymphatic mapping and sentinel node biopsy. Moreover, the essentially identical rates of local and in-transit metastases (without nodal metastases) in the 2 groups and the absence of a difference between groups in melanoma-specific or overall survival argue against the investigators' conclusions.

Based on the available data, recommendations suggest that a 0.5-cm margin is adequate for in situ melanoma, whereas margins of 1 cm are suggested for melanomas less than 1.0 mm in thickness. Margins of 1 or 2 cm should be achieved for lesions measuring between 1 and 2 mm in thickness, whereas 2-cm margins should be achieved for melanomas greater than 2 mm in thickness.[17]

Mohs Micrographic Surgery for Melanoma

Mohs micrographic surgery was first described in 1941 in a coordinated effort between a surgeon and pathologist to assess 100% of the surgical margin intraoperatively.[18] It is used most often for other skin cancers such as squamous cell and basal cell carcinomas. Its use in malignant melanoma in situ remains controversial, although some have championed its use in cosmetically sensitive areas such as the head and neck. These lesions often arise in a background of lentigo maligna in chronically sun-damaged skin, and histologic control of surgical margins often requires analysis of paraffin sections. The inability to accurately characterize cells of melanocytic origin on frozen section compromises its accuracy when applied to melanoma. In this technique, margins of 1 to 3 cm are marked around the primary lesion, which is often more accurately defined using a Wood lamp. The clinically visible tumor is first removed in one layer, and a 1-mm section of tissue is taken from this excision to confirm the depth of the lesion by frozen section, with the remainder of the tissue sent for permanent section. The first Mohs layer is then taken using an angled incision so that peripheral and deep margins can be assessed in the same plane during processing, which involves the use of frozen section with hematoxylin and eosin (H&E) and immunostains. This procedure is repeated until the margins are completely cleared. Following this, an additional margin is taken for paraffin-embedded sections and the defect is then repaired. This is a labor-intensive process, although early reports results suggest recurrence rates of less than 1%.[19–22] However, the data are not mature and Mohs remains highly controversial in the treatment of melanoma.

Sentinel Lymph Node Biopsy

Another important issue in the surgical management of melanoma is the use of sentinel lymph node biopsy, which has essentially replaced elective lymph node dissection. Elective lymph node dissection was performed for intermediate thickness melanomas until the 1990s. Several prospective randomized controlled trials comparing elective lymph node dissection with observation of the nodes did not conclusively demonstrate survival benefit in those treated with elective lymph node dissection.[23,24] In addition, more than 80% of patients with clinically negative nodes will not have any histologic evidence of melanoma in the resected nodes,[25] and thus will be subjected to the morbidity of the procedure (paresthesias, wound complications, extremity lymphedema) without any therapeutic benefit.

Sentinel lymph node biopsy for melanoma, introduced by Wong and colleagues in 1990,[26] was first studied in a feline model and has been subsequently developed for clinical use.[27] Primary advantages of this technique are its greater accuracy for detection of micrometastases in regional nodes, and reduced morbidity relative to elective lymph node dissection. Sentinel lymph node biopsy has become a standard approach for intermediate thickness melanomas, and the status of the sentinel node is now considered to be the single most important predictor of survival in these patients.[28]

Sentinel lymph node biopsy is generally performed using preoperative lymphoscintigraphy, in which technetium-99m–labeled sulfur colloid is injected at a dose of up to 0.5 mCi in four quadrants around the primary lesion.[29] Although antimony sulfide is a better compound for mapping because of its superior characteristics for imaging,[30] this agent is not available in the United States. A scintillation camera is then used to document static and dynamic images demonstrating pathways of lymphatic drainage to sentinel nodes, with identifiable lymph nodes apparent within 30 minutes after the injection (**Fig. 1**) and persisting for many hours.[31] This is particularly useful in nonextremity melanomas, as lesions have variable drainage basins that cannot be predicted clinically, and may even drain to contralateral nodes.[32] The greatest accuracy is achieved if radioactive colloid and blue dye are used during sentinel node biopsy.[33] Intraoperative intradermal injection of 1 to 2 mL of isosulfan blue dye in four quadrants around the primary lesion or excision scar facilitates visualization of the sentinel node (**Fig. 2**). A handheld gamma probe is used to identify the area of increased tracer uptake and the sentinel node is identified using the gamma probe and visualization of the blue staining (**Fig. 3**). Each sentinel node identified (typically between one and three) is then excised, embedded in paraffin, and examined histologically. A positive result is defined as the presence of identifiable melanoma cells with either routine H&E stains or by immunohistochemical staining with S100 or HMB-45 (**Fig. 4**). Analysis of sentinel nodes by step sections and immunoperoxidase stains has been demonstrated to be more sensitive than conventional H&E staining of bivalved nodes.[34,35] Frozen section is generally not employed to assess sentinel nodes because of its lack of sensitivity, and the inability to embed previously frozen tissue into paraffin.

The accuracy of sentinel lymph node biopsy has been studied by several groups. Morton and colleagues studied this initially, and reported an 82% identification rate of sentinel nodes using isosulfan blue dye alone, with a false-negative rate of 5% of node-positive basins.[35] This initial assessment of the accuracy of lymphatic mapping involved simultaneous complete lymphadenectomy for comparison of the status of the sentinel node with that of the other lymph nodes. Others have validated these results with long-term clinical follow-up of lymph node basins with negative sentinel nodes, rather than simultaneous complete lymphadenectomy.[28] Many surgeons favor identification of sentinel nodes using isosulfan blue in conjunction with radioactive colloid.[36,37]

Sentinel node biopsy results are important for accurate staging, and for deciding whether to perform completion lymphadenectomy or offer adjuvant therapy. Several studies have demonstrated increased overall survival and disease-free survival interval in sentinel lymph node–negative patients compared with sentinel node–positive patients.[38,39] One of these studies demonstrated a 3-year disease-free survival of 88.5% versus 55.8% in sentinel node–negative versus sentinel node–positive

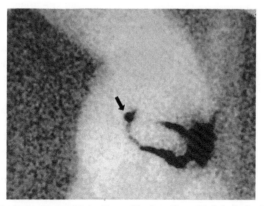

Fig. 1. Lymphoscintigraphy. Dermal injection of technetium-99–labeled sulfur colloid around a melanoma on the back reveals a sentinel node in the axilla.

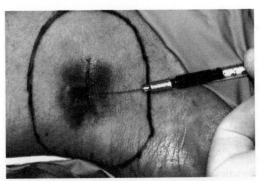

Fig. 2. Injection of isosulfan blue. Intradermal injection of isosulfan blue around a scar from a melanoma biopsy is performed immediately before skin incision in the regional lymph node basin.

patients, with a 58.6% increase in disease-free survival if the sentinel lymph node biopsy was negative.[38]

There is considerable debate regarding the usefulness of sentinel lymph node biopsy for melanoma. More mature data suggest that up to 14% of patients with negative sentinel nodes will develop recurrence of disease within 3 years.[40–42] It has also been suggested that in some patients, microscopic deposits of melanoma identified within sentinel lymph nodes may have remained dormant or been destroyed by the host immune system had the sentinel node not been removed. In the literature regarding micrometastases in sentinel nodes, several groups have demonstrated that small tumor deposits (<0.1 mm) within a sentinel node alter prognosis minimally if at all.[43–47] Others argue that in the absence of a truly effective adjuvant therapy in AJCC stage III patients, sentinel node biopsy should not be performed. Some recommend against sentinel node biopsy, advocating screening of relevant regional lymph node basins by ultrasound with delayed lymphadenectomy performed if clinically occult nodes are identified and verified by cytology.[48] The argument against sentinel node biopsy is further supported by the analysis of the first Multicenter Selective Lymphadenectomy Trial (MSLT-I), which demonstrated no difference in 5-year overall

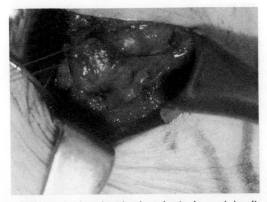

Fig. 3. Identification of the sentinel node. Blue lymphatic channels leading to a blue sentinel node are easily identified in the regional lymph node basin.

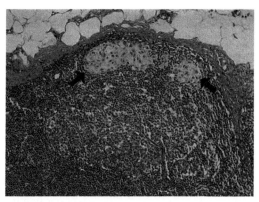

Fig. 4. Histology of the sentinel node. Use of step sections (and immunohistochemical stains that are not shown in this photomicrograph) facilitate detection of small foci of metastatic melanoma.

survival in 1973 stage I melanoma patients randomized to either wide local excision alone or wide local excision with sentinel node biopsy[49] (see later discussion). Additional trials are underway, but until more data are available, sentinel node biopsy remains a standard approach for melanoma patients.

Current indications for sentinel node biopsy include clinically negative nodal basins and primary melanomas greater than 1 mm in thickness. The procedure may also be considered in patients with thin melanomas (0.76–1 mm) in the presence of adverse histologic features, such as ulceration, invasion to Clark level IV, or any mitoses. Sentinel lymph node biopsy should not be performed in the setting of clinically positive nodes, or in patients who would otherwise not be considered for lymphadenectomy.

SURGICAL TREATMENT OF STAGE III MELANOMA
Prognostic Factors for Stage III Melanoma

Stage III melanoma is characterized by the presence of nodal metastases (micro- or macrometastases) with or without in-transit/satellite lesions. The presence of lymph node metastases confers a significantly worse prognosis, with less than half of node-positive patients surviving for 5 years.[42] The number of nodes involved is of prognostic significance, and is reflected in the recent revisions to the AJCC staging system.

In patients with stage III disease, four prognostic factors for survival have been identified: the number of metastatic lymph nodes; microscopic versus macroscopic tumor deposits in lymph nodes; the presence of in-transit or satellite metastases, and the presence of ulceration in the primary lesion.[42] In earlier staging systems, the size of the involved lymph node was believed to be of significance, although this has been disproven.[50] However, macroscopic disease (ie, that which is identified clinically and confirmed histologically) does have a significant impact, with much poorer survival in those with macroscopic as opposed to microscopic disease.[42] In-transit and satellite metastases represent dissemination of tumor by way of the lymphatic channels, and the 5-year survival rate in patients with these findings is similar to that in patients with lymph node metastases. If these findings are present in association with lymph node metastases (N3), the survival rate drops significantly.[42]

Before considering surgical therapy for clinically apparent stage III disease, patients should be evaluated to exclude any evidence of distant disease. Chest radiography, computed tomography (CT) of the chest, abdomen, and pelvis may be performed, especially to follow up on any signs or symptoms of suspected metastases based on history, physical examination, and a detailed review of systems. If inguinal lymphadenopathy is apparent, pelvic CT should be obtained to assess iliac lymph nodes.

Therapeutic and Completion Lymph Node Dissection

Therapeutic lymph node dissection is the term applied to a lymphadenectomy in the setting of clinically palpable nodes. Therapeutic lymphadenectomy is indicated for patients with clinically palpable metastatic melanoma in lymph nodes – even bulky nodal disease – and can be performed with acceptable morbidity and good palliation. Completion lymphadenectomy refers to removing the remaining nodes after sentinel lymph node biopsy, and is recommended for management of the regional lymph node drainage basin in the presence of a positive sentinel node. Some challenge this recommendation, as 4 randomized trials of elective lymph node dissection failed to demonstrate an overall survival benefit (**Table 2**).[51–54] However, most patients in these studies did not have lymph node metastases and thus the trials were not sufficiently powered to detect a small survival benefit.[55] Subgroup analysis of the trials have supported the practice of completion lymph node dissection. For example, in the World Health Organization Trial 14, subgroup analysis demonstrated a significantly improved 5-year survival rate in patients with occult nodal metastases detected by lymph node dissection compared with patients who had delayed lymphadenectomy at the time they developed palpable nodal metastases (48% vs 27%, respectively; $P = .04$).[53]

Nonetheless, the impact of completion lymphadenectomy on overall survival is still a matter of debate. Results from MSLT-I suggest that sentinel node biopsy with immediate completion lymphadenectomy if the sentinel node is positive improves disease-free survival but not overall survival for these patients.[49] In this trial, 1,327 patients with melanomas 1.2 to 3.5 mm in thickness were randomized in a 4:6 ratio to wide excision followed by nodal observation, or to wide excision plus lymphatic mapping and sentinel lymph node biopsy with immediate completion lymphadenectomy if the sentinel node was positive for metastasis (**Fig. 5**). The groups were comparable with regard to distribution of age, gender, anatomic location, thickness, and ulceration. Sentinel nodes were analyzed using H&E stains and immunohistochemistry.

Table 2			
Prospective randomized trials examining elective lymph node dissection for melanoma			
Surgical Trial	Number of Patients	Groups Studied (n)	Tumor Location and Thickness
Mayo Clinic Study[51]	171	No lymphadenectomy (62) Immediate lymphadenectomy (54) Delayed lymphadenectomy (55)	Extremity and trunk Any thickness
WHO Melanoma Group[52]	553	Immediate lymphadenectomy (267) Delayed lymphadenectomy (286)	Extremity only Any thickness
WHO Melanoma Program[53]	240	Immediate lymphadenectomy (122) Delayed lymphadenectomy (118)	Trunk 1.5 mm thickness or greater
Intergroup Melanoma Surgical Trial[54]	740	Immediate lymphadenectomy (379) Delayed lymphadenectomy (361)	Extremity and trunk 1–4 mm thickness

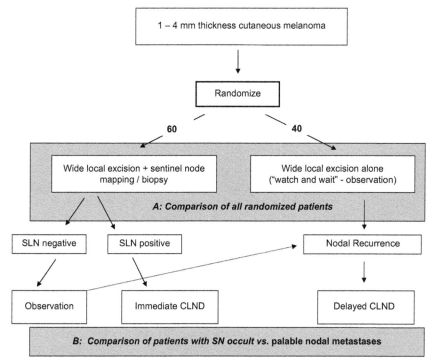

Fig. 5. Multicenter Selective Lymphadenectomy Trial-I (MSLT-I) schema.

Wound complications at the primary site were comparable, although surgical morbidity was significantly greater if the sentinel node biopsy was followed by completion lymphadenectomy.[49] Five-year melanoma-specific survival rates were similar in the two groups (87.1 ± 1.3% and 86.6 ± 1.6%, respectively). The 5-year survival rate of the patients with nodal metastases was higher for those who underwent immediate lymphadenectomy than those in whom lymphadenectomy was delayed (72.3 ± 4.6% vs 52.4 ± 5.9%; hazard ratio for death, 0.51; 95% CI, 0.32 to 0.81; $P = .004$). The strategy of analysis of the subgroup of patients with positive nodes has been criticized.[56]

The value of completion lymphadenectomy for positive sentinel nodes will be addressed in MSLT-II, which will evaluate the therapeutic value of completion lymph node dissection versus sentinel node biopsy alone in patients who have metastasis in the sentinel node. In this trial, patients with positive sentinel nodes are randomized to completion lymphadenectomy versus clinical observation of the nodal basin.

An important factor in assessing the benefit of a completion lymph node dissection following a positive sentinel node biopsy is the likelihood of finding metastases in the remaining nonsentinel nodes. This issue was addressed in a recent series of 658 patients, in which 90 (14%) were found to have a positive sentinel node, with 18 (20%) of that group having evidence of metastases in additional nonsentinel nodes.[57] Although identification of factors predictive for which sentinel node–positive patients will harbor melanoma in remaining regional nodes remains a top priority, it is still not possible to accurately identify which patients comprise the 20% with melanoma in nonsentinel nodes. In addition, it should be recognized that this 20% figure is probably a low estimate; lymph nodes in a completion lymphadenectomy specimen are not generally analyzed with step sections and immunohistochemical staining. They are usually analyzed by H&E staining of sections from a bivalved node.

Completion lymphadenectomy clearly provides prognostic information. The number of positive nodes is associated with survival, is included in AJCC staging,[42] and provides further rationale for completion lymph node dissection for a positive sentinel node.

Another important aspect of surgical management of AJCC stage III melanoma patients is the extent of lymph node dissection required. Investigators at John Wayne Cancer Center recently reviewed their experience with lymph node dissection before the use of sentinel node biopsy, and concluded that the extent of lymph node dissection is more important with higher tumor burden and less important with a lower tumor burden.[58] It is reasonable to recognize that those with micrometastatic disease in a sentinel node and those with bulky nodal disease are different groups of patients. The magnitude of benefit from lymph node dissection may be different in these 2 groups of patients, and the potential benefit must be carefully weighed against the morbidity of the procedure. Several studies are underway that should be able to help address this issue, including MSLT-II.

The Sunbelt Melanoma Trial addressed the role of molecular detection of melanoma-associated gene expression in sentinel nodes. In Protocol B of this study, patients with tumor-negative sentinel lymph node by standard histopathology and immunohistochemistry underwent molecular staging of the sentinel lymph node by reverse transcriptase polymerase chain reaction (RT-PCR) to detect melanoma-specific mRNA (tyrosinase, MART 1, MAGE 3, gp100); patients with positive sentinel lymph node on RT-PCR were randomized to observation versus completion lymphadenectomy versus completion lymphadenectomy plus adjuvant interferon. No differences in disease-free or overall survival were observed in the treatment arms.[59] The value of molecular analysis of sentinel lymph nodes remains to be demonstrated.

Isolated Limb Perfusion

Patients with in-transit metastases have an unfavorable outcome. In-transit metastasis reflects a disseminated stage of disease, with a 5-year survival rate of 25% to 30%. Surgical excision is the mainstay of therapy if the size and number of the lesions permit, although there is no formal recommendation regarding the extent of the surgical margin. Amputation is rarely necessary.

Another therapeutic option for patients with extensive in-transit metastases in an extremity involves the use of isolated limb perfusion (ILP). This technique was introduced in 1958, and has the advantage of achieving high regional concentrations of therapeutic agents and minimizing systemic side effects.[60] The arterial supply and venous drainage are surgically isolated through an open incision, and an oxygenated extracorporeal circuit is used to circulate chemotherapeutic agents for 1 to 1.5 hours (Fig. 6). Melphalan is typically used as a chemotherapeutic agent, and the limb temperature is typically elevated to 39 to 40°C with a tourniquet in place.[61] In patients who have clinically positive nodes, therapeutic lymph node dissection is performed at the same setting just before limb perfusion. Tumor response to isolated limb perfusion can be dramatic. Complete response rate with melphalan alone is 54%,[62] which increases to 91% with the addition of tumor necrosis factor (TNF).[63] These responses are often short-lived, with recurrence rates of 50% within 1 to 1.5 years after limb perfusion,[64] although some patients benefit from a durable remission. Overall 5-year survival after ILP was 32% in a recent series.[64] Recurrences following ILP may be treated with excision, although repeat ILP has also been used with success in patients with extensive disease.[65]

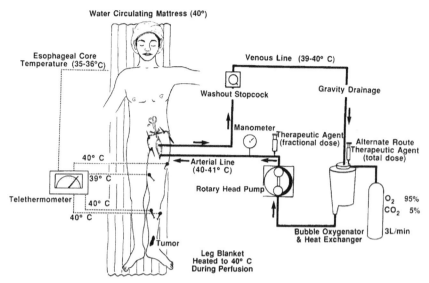

Fig. 6. Isolated limb perfusion. (*From* Klauser JM, Lev-Chelouche D, Meller I, et al. Isolated limb perfusion in the treatment of advanced soft-tissue sarcomas. In: Malawer MM, Sugarbaker PH, editors. Musculoskeletal cancer surgery. Treatment of sarcomas and allied diseases. Kluwer Academic Publishers; 2001. p. 76; with permission.)

Isolated Limb Infusion

Isolated limb perfusion can be effective for in-transit metastases, however it is time- and resource-consuming and can be toxic. One alternative to this approach involves normothermic isolated limb infusion (ILI),[66,67] a technique in which the artery and vein are isolated percutaneously and the limb is isolated using a tourniquet (**Fig. 7**). Melphalan is typically used as a chemotherapeutic agent. One major difference between ILP and ILI is that in ILI blood is circulated at a much lower rate in the isolated extremity and is only circulated for 30 minutes. In addition, a pump oxygenator is not used in ILI and thus the isolated extremity becomes hypoxic, leading to acidosis. In the largest series using ILI, melphalan and dactinomycin chemotherapy was used in 135 patients.[57] In this series there was an overall response rate of 85% with 41% achieving a complete response and 42% achieving a partial response.[66] No randomized controlled trials have compared ILP with ILI, although results from a single institution prospective database were published recently, yielding a higher overall and complete response rate for ILP than ILI (88% vs 44% and 57% vs 30%, respectively).[67]

Although ILI is associated with significantly less morbidity than ILP, the response rates in the United States are lower than those reported from Thompson and colleagues in Australia, and are lower than the response rates observed following isolated limb perfusion.[67,68]

Adjuvant Therapy

Radiotherapy

Adjuvant radiotherapy has been used with some success following therapeutic lymph node dissection in the setting of bulky metastases, multiple positive nodes, or extracapsular spread. Adjuvant radiotherapy has also been used for primary tumors that are difficult to control with surgery alone, including locally recurrent lesions on the head

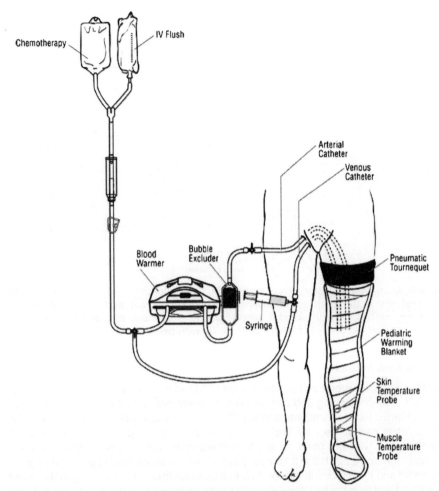

Fig. 7. Isolated limb infusion. (*From* Brady MS, Brown K, Patel A, et al. A phase II trial of isolated limb infusion with melphalan and dactinomycin for regional melanoma and soft tissue sarcoma of the extremity. Ann Surg Oncol 2006;13(8):1126; with permission.)

and neck, extensive perineural invasion, and unresectable, positive deep margins.[69] Published results demonstrate improved locoregional control[70] and a modest survival benefit[71] compared with historical controls.

Other adjuvant therapy
Other forms of adjuvant therapy are in use for patients with resected stage III disease, and include interferon alpha 2b (INFα2b), which currently has FDA approval for adjuvant treatment of stage IIB and stage III melanoma. Although initial studies (Eastern Cooperative Oncology Group [EOCG] trial 1684) demonstrated prolongation of relapse-free interval and overall survival[72] with 1 year of high dose INFα2b, subsequent trials failed to confirm this observation. A metaanalysis of these trials showed no overall survival benefit.[73] Nearly all patients experience adverse effects with interferon therapy including fatigue, neutropenia, headache, fever, and chills.[72] A detailed

description of the use of adjuvant interferon and other experimental adjuvant therapies (including melanoma vaccines) is beyond the scope of this review.

SURGICAL TREATMENT OF STAGE IV MELANOMA
Prognostic Factors for Stage IV Melanoma

For stage IV melanoma, the site of distant metastasis and serum lactate dehydrogenase (LDH) levels seem to have the most value in prognosis, with a far more favorable prognosis in those with cutaneous metastases and a normal serum LDH level. There is a significant difference in 1-year survival rates between those with cutaneous, subcutaneous, or distant nodal metastases (M1) versus those with lung metastases (M2) versus those with any other visceral metastases, or any metastasis with an elevated serum LDH level (M3). Predicted 1-year survival rates for patients in these groups are 59%, 57%, and 41%, respectively.[42]

Metastasectomy

There is a large body of literature supporting resection of metastases from melanoma, with the following factors cited as predictors of better outcome: stage of initial disease, disease-free interval after treatment of the primary melanoma, initial site of metastasis, extent of metastatic disease (single vs multiple sites), and complete resection.[74] This approach can be successful. A recent series reported a 5-year survival rate of 29% following pulmonary metastasectomy and a median survival of 40 months compared with 13 months in those who were not eligible for resection.[75] Similar results have been demonstrated for resection of metastatic lesions in the gastrointestinal tract, with a series reporting a median survival of 47.5 months in patients in whom a complete resection was achieved.[76] This was in sharp contrast to the median survival of 4 weeks in those patients in whom complete resection could not be achieved.[76] The aforementioned factors are of critical importance in deciding whether or not to perform metastasectomy, and patient selection is key. To enhance patient selection for curative procedures, some recommend treating patients with a single-site asymptomatic metastasis with 2 to 3 months of chemotherapy before resection, to assess for disease stabilization or the development of additional metastases.[74] If there is a response to treatment or disease stabilization with no evidence of further metastases, resection is performed.[74]

Preoperative imaging is a critical part of the evaluation of a potential metastasectomy patient, and may include the use of [^{18}F]fluorodeoxyglucose positron emission tomography (FDG-PET) to more accurately detect occult metastatic disease. A recent comparison of FDG-PET with conventional imaging in patients with stage IV melanoma demonstrated a sensitivity of 76% and specificity of 87% for conventional imaging, compared with 79% and 87% for FDG-PET.[77] Sensitivity was 88% and specificity was 91% for combined conventional imaging with FDG-PET.[77] As with any other modality, it is important to understand the limits of the technology to properly apply its use.

Another important indication for metastasectomy is palliation, as most patients with stage IV melanoma will not be candidates for metastasectomy for curative intent. The goal of a palliative procedure is to control identifiable symptoms caused by an advanced malignancy and minimizing morbidity.[74] Classic examples of palliative metastasectomy include resection of bleeding small bowel metastases, resection of ulcerated subcutaneous metastases, and resection of symptomatic brain metastases. A thorough discussion should be held between the surgeon, the patient, and their family to address the goals and expected outcomes as well as potential morbidity of the procedures.

REFERENCES

1. Rigel DS, Friedman RJ, Kopf AW. The incidence of malignant melanoma in the United States: issues as we approach the 21st century. J Am Acad Dermatol 1996;34:839–47.
2. Ries LA, Eisner MP, Kosary CL, editors. SEER cancer statistics review, 1973–1999. Bethesda (MD): National Cancer Institute; 2002. Available at: http://seer.cancer.gov/csr/1973_1999/. Accessed June, 2006.
3. Greenlee RT, Hill-Harmon MB, Murray T, et al. Cancer statistics 2001. CA Cancer J Clin 2001;51:15–36.
4. Crowson AN, Magro CM, Mihm MC Jr. Prognosticators of melanoma, the melanoma report, and the sentinel lymph node. Mod Pathol 2006;19:S71–87.
5. Barnhill RL, Katzen J, Spatz A, et al. The importance of mitotic rate as a prognostic factor for localized cutaneous melanoma. J Cutan Pathol 2005;32:268–73.
6. Francken AB, Shaw HM, Thompson JF, et al. The prognostic importance of tumor mitotic rate confirmed in 1317 patients with primary cutaneous melanoma and long follow-up. Ann Surg Oncol 2004;11:426–33.
7. Wong CK. A study of melanocytes in the normal skin surrounding malignant melanomata. Dermatologica 1970;141:215–25.
8. Lens MB, Nathan P, Bataille V. Excision margins for primary cutaneous melanoma. Updated pool analysis of randomized controlled trials. Arch Surg 2007;142(9):885–91.
9. Ross MI, Balch CM. Surgical treatment of primary melanoma. In: Balch CM, Houghton AN, Sober AJ, et al, editors. Cutaneous melanoma. 3rd edition. St. Louis (MO): Quality Medical Publishing, Inc.; 1998. p. 141–53.
10. Veronesi U, Cascinelli N, Adamus J, et al. Thin stage I primary cutaneous malignant melanoma. Comparison of excision with margins of 1 or 3 cm. N Engl J Med 1988;318(18):1159–62.
11. Veronesi U, Cascinelli N. Narrow excision (1-cm margin). A safe procedure for thin cutaneous melanoma. Arch Surg 1991;126(4):438–41.
12. Balch CM, Urist MM, Karakousis CP, et al. Efficacy of 2-cm surgical margins for intermediate-thickness melanomas (1 to 4 mm). Results of a multi-institutional randomized surgical trial. Ann Surg 1993;218(3):262–7.
13. Balch CM, Soong SJ, Smith T, et al. Long-term results of a prospective surgical trial comparing 2 cm vs. 4 cm excision margins for 740 patients with 1-4 mm melanomas. Ann Surg Oncol 2001;8(2):101–8.
14. Cohn-Cedermark G, Rutqvist LE, Andersson R, et al. Long term results of a randomized study by the Swedish Melanoma Study Group on 2-cm versus 5-cm resection margins for patients with cutaneous melanoma with a tumor thickness of 0.8-2.0 mm. Cancer 2000;89(7):1495–501.
15. Ringborg U, Andersson R, Eldh J, et al. Resection margins of 2 versus 5 cm for cutaneous malignant melanoma with a tumor thickness of 0.8 to 2.0 mm: randomized study by the Swedish Melanoma Study Group. Cancer 1996;77(9):1809–14.
16. Thomas JM, Newton-Bishop J, A'Hern R, et al. Excision margins in high-risk malignant melanoma. [see comment]. N Engl J Med 2004;350(8):757–66.
17. Rigel DS, Carucci JA. Malignant melanoma: prevention, early detection and treatment in the 21st century. CA Cancer J Clin 2000;50:216–36.

18. Mohs FE. Chemosurgery: a microscopically controlled method of cancer excision. Arch Surg 1941;42:279–95.
19. Zitelli JA, Brown C, Hanusa BH. Mohs micrographic surgery for the treatment of primary cutaneous melanoma. J Am Acad Dematol 1997;37:236–45.
20. Bhardwaj SS, Tope WD, Lee PK. Mohs micrographic surgery for lentigo maligna and lentigo maligna melanoma using Mel-5 immunostaining: University of Minnesota experience. Dermatol Surg 2006;32(5):690–6.
21. Bienert TN, Trotter MJ, Arlette JP. Treatment of cutaneous melanoma of the face by Mohs micrographic surgery. J Cutan Med Surg 2003;7(1):25–30.
22. Temple CL, Arlette JP. Mohs micrographic surgery in the treatment of lentigo maligna and melanoma. J Surg Oncol 2006;94(4):287–92.
23. Balch CM. Randomized surgical trials involving elective node dissection for melanoma. Adv Surg 1999;32:64–70.
24. Balch CM, Soong SJ, Bartolucci AA, et al. Efficacy of elective regional node dissection of 1 to 4 mm thick melanomas for patients 60 years of age or older. Ann Surg 1996;224(3):255–63.
25. Beitsch P, Balch C. Operative morbidity and risk factor assessment in melanoma patients undergoing inguinal lymph node dissection. Am J Surg 1992;164:462–5.
26. Wong JH, Cagle LA, Morton DL. Lymphatic drainage of skin to a sentinel lymph node in a feline model. Ann Surg 1991;214(5):637–41.
27. Morton DL, Wen DR, Wong JH, et al. Intraoperative lymphatic mapping and selective lymphadenectomy: technical details of a new procedure for clinical stage I melanoma. Presented at the Annual Meeting of the Society of Surgical Oncology, Washington, DC, March 2000.
28. Gershenwald JE, Colome MI, Lee JE, et al. Patterns of recurrence following a negative sentinel lymph node biopsy in 243 patients with stage I or II melanoma. J Clin Oncol 1998;16:2253–60.
29. Glass EC, Essner R, Morton DL. Kinetics of three lymphoscintigraphic agents in patients with cutaneous melanoma. J Nucl Med 1998;39:1185–90.
30. Thompson JF, Uren RF, Shaw HM, et al. Location of sentinel lymph nodes in patients with cutaneous melanoma: new insights into lymphatic anatomy [see comment]. J Am Coll Surg 1999;189(2):195–204.
31. Essner R, Bostic PJ, Glass EC, et al. Standardized probe-directed sentinel node dissection in melanoma. Surgery 2000;127:26–31.
32. Thompson JF, Uren RF. Lymphatic mapping in management of patients with primary cutaneous melanoma. Lancet Oncol 2005;6:877–85.
33. Morton DL, Thompson JF, Nieweg OE. The sentinel lymph node biopsy procedure: identification with blue dye and a gamma probe. In: Thompson JF, Morton DL, Kroon BB, editors. Textbook of melanoma. London: Martin Dunitz; 2004. p. 323–38.
34. Yu LL, Flotte TJ, Tanabe KK, et al. Detection of microscopic melanoma metastases in sentinel lymph nodes. Cancer 1999;86(4):617–27.
35. Morton DL, Wen DR, Wong JH, et al. Technical details of intraoperative lymphatic mapping for early stage melanoma. Arch Surg 1992;127:392–9.
36. Krag DN, Meijer SJ, Weaver DL, et al. Minimal-access surgery for staging of malignant melanoma. Arch Surg 1995;130:654–8.
37. Leong SP, Steinmetz I, Habib FA, et al. Optimal selective sentinel lymph node dissection in primary malignant melanoma. Arch Surg 1997;132:666–73.
38. Gershenwald JE, Mansfield PF, Lee JE, et al. Role of lymphatic mapping and sentinel lymph node biopsy in patients with thick (>4mm) primary melanoma. Ann Surg Oncol 2000;7:160–5.

39. Gershenwald JE, Thompson W, Mansfield PF, et al. Multi-institutional melanoma lymphatic mapping experience: the prognostic value of sentinel lymph node status in 612 stage I or II melanoma patients. J Clin Oncol 1999;17:976–83.
40. Berk DR. Sentinel lymph node biopsy for cutaneous melanoma: the Stanford experience 1997-2004. Arch Dermatol 2005;141:1016–22.
41. Vuylsteke RJ. Clinical outcome of Stage I/II melanoma patients after selective sentinel lymph node dissection: long-term follow-up results. J Clin Oncol 2003; 21:1057–65.
42. Balch CM, Soong SJ, Gershenwald JE, et al. Prognostic factors analysis of 17,600 melanoma patients: validation of the American Joint Committee on cancer staging system for cutaneous melanoma. J Clin Oncol 2001;19:3622–34.
43. Ranieri JM, Wagner JD, Azuage R, et al. Importance of lymph node tumor burden in melanoma patients staged by sentinel node biopsy. Ann Surg Oncol 2002;9:975–81.
44. Carlson GW, et al. The amount of metastatic melanoma in a sentinel lymph node. Does it have prognostic significance? Ann Surg Oncol 2003;10:575–81.
45. Starz H, et al. Sentinel lymphonodectomy and S-classification: a successful strategy for better prediction and improvement of outcomes in melanoma. Ann Surg Oncol 2005;11(3 Suppl):162S–8S.
46. Spanknebel K, et al. Characterization of micrometastic disease in melanoma sentinel lymph nodes by enhanced pathology: recommendations for standardizing pathological analysis. Am J Surg Pathol 2005;29:412–4.
47. Van Akkooi ACJ, et al. Clinical relevance of melanoma micrometastases (<0.1 mm) in sentinel nodes: are these nodes to be considered negative? Ann Oncol 2006;17:1578–85.
48. Thomas JM. Prognostic false-positivity of the sentinel node in melanoma. Nat Clin Pract Oncol 2008;5(1):18–23.
49. Morton DL, Thompson JF, Cochran AJ, et al. Sentinel-node biopsy or nodal observation in melanoma [see comment] [erratum appears in N Engl J Med. 2006 Nov 2;355(18):1944]. N Engl J Med 2006;355(13):1307–17.
50. Buzaid AC, Tinoco LA, Jendiroba D, et al. Prognostic value of size of lymph node metastases in patients with cutaneous melanoma. J Clin Oncol 1995;13:2361–8.
51. Sim FH, Taylor WF, Pritchard DJ, et al. Lymphadenectomy in the management of stage I malignant melanoma: a prospective randomized study. Mayo Clin Proc 1986;61:697–705.
52. Veronesi U, Adamus J, Bandiera DC, et al. Delayed regional lymph node dissection in stage I melanoma of the skin of the lower extremities. Cancer 1982;49:2420–30.
53. Cascinelli N, Morabito A, Santinami M, et al. Immediate or delayed dissection of regional nodes in patients with melanoma of the trunk: a randomized trial. WHO Melanoma Programme. Lancet 1998;351:793–6.
54. Balch DM, Soong S, Ross MI, et al. Long-term results of a multi-institutional randomized trial comparing prognostic factors and surgical results for intermediate thickness melanomas (1.0 to 4.0 mm). Intergroup Melanoma Surgical Trial. Ann Surg Oncol 2000;7:87–97.
55. McMasters KM, Reintgen DS, Ross MI, et al. Sentinel lymph node biopsy for melanoma: Controversy despite widespread agreement. J Clin Oncol 2001;19:2851–5.
56. Thomas JM. Time for comprehensive reporting of MSLT-1. Lancet Oncol 2006; 7(1):9–11.
57. Cascinelli N, Clemente C, Bifulco C, et al. Do patients with tumor-positive sentinel node constitute a homogenous group? Ann Surg Oncol 2001;8(9 Suppl):35S–7S.
58. Chan AD, Essner R, Wanek LA, et al. Judging the therapeutic value of lymph node dissections for melanoma. J Am Coll Surg 2000;191:16–23.

59. McMasters KM, Ross MI, Reintgen DS, et al. Final results of the sunbelt melanoma trial. J Clin Oncol 2008;26 [May 20 suppl; abstrast 9003].
60. Benckhuijsen C, Kroon BB, van Geel AN, et al. Regional perfusion treatment with melphalan for melanoma in a limb: an evaluation of drug kinetics. Eur J Surg Oncol 1988;14:157–63.
61. Lingam MK, Byrne DS, Aitchison T, et al. A single center's 10-year experience with isolated limb perfusion in the treatment of recurrent malignant melanoma of the limb. Eur J Cancer 1996;32A:1668–73.
62. Vrouenraets BC, Nieweg OE, Kroon BB. Thirty-five years of isolated limb perfusion for melanoma: indications and results. Br J Surg 1996;83:1319–28.
63. Lejeune F, Lienard D, Eggermont A, et al. Rationale for using TNF alpha and chemotherapy in regional therapy of melanoma. J Cell Biochem 1994;56:52–61.
64. Grunhagen DJ, Brunstein F, Graveland WJ, et al. One hundred consecutive isolated limb perfusions with TNF-alpha and Melphalan in melanoma patients with multiple in-transit metastases. Ann Surg 2004;240:939–48.
65. Feldman AL, Alexander HR Jr, Bartlett DL, et al. Management of extremity recurrences after complete responses to isolated limb perfusion in patients with melanoma. Ann Surg Oncol 1999;6:562–7.
66. Lindner P, Doubrovsky A, Kam PC, et al. Prognostic factors after isolated limb infusion with cytotoxic agents for melanoma. Ann Surg Oncol 2002;9:127–36.
67. Beasley GM, Petersen RP, Yoo J, et al. Isolated limb infusion for in-transit malignant melanoma of the extremity: a well-tolerated but less effective alternative to hyperthermic isolated limb perfusion. Ann Surg Oncol 2008;15(8):2195–205.
68. Brady MS, Brown K, Patel A, et al. A phase II trial of isolated limb infusion with melphalan and dactinomycin for regional melanoma and soft tissue sarcoma of the extremity. Ann Surg Oncol 2006;13(8):1123–9.
69. Morris KT, Marquez CM, Holland JM, et al. Prevention of local recurrence after surgical debulking of nodal and subcutaneous melanoma deposits by hypofractionated radiation. Ann Surg Oncol 2000;7(9):680–4.
70. Stevens G, Thompson JF, Firth I, et al. Locally advanced melanoma: results of postoperative hypofractionated radiation therapy. Cancer 2000;88:88–94.
71. Ang KK, Byers RM, Peters LJ, et al. Regional radiotherapy as adjuvant treatment for head and neck malignant melanoma. Arch Otolaryngol Head Neck Surg 1990; 116:169–72.
72. Kirkwood JM, Strawderman MH, Ernstoff MS, et al. Interferon alfa-2b adjuvant therapy of high risk resected cutaneous melanoma: The Eastern Cooperative Oncology Group Trial EST 1684. J Clin Oncol 1996;14:7–17.
73. Wheatley K, Ives N, Hancock B, et al. Does adjuvant interferon-alpha for high-risk melanoma provide a worthwhile benefit? A meta-analysis of the randomised trials. Cancer Treat Rev 2003;29:241–52.
74. Wong SL, Coit DG. Role of surgery in patients with stage IV melanoma. Curr Opin Oncol 2004;16:155–60.
75. Tafra L, Dale PS, Wanek LA, et al. Resection and adjuvant immunotherapy for melanoma metastatic to the lungs and thorax. J Thorac Cardiovasc Surg 1995; 110:119–28.
76. Ollila DW, Essner R, Wanek L, et al. Surgical resection for melanoma metastatic to the gastrointestinal tract. Arch Surg 1996;131:975–9.
77. Finkelstein SE, Carrasquillo JA, Hoffman JM, et al. A prospective analysis of positron emission tomography and conventional imaging for detection of stage IV metastatic melanoma in patients undergoing metastasectomy. Ann Surg Oncol 2004;11(8):731–8.

The History and Future of Chemotherapy for Melanoma

Arvin S. Yang, MD, PhD[a], Paul B. Chapman, MD[a,b], *

KEYWORDS

• Dacarbazine • Temozolomide • Cisplatin • Sorafenib
• Combination chemotherapy

Melanoma is considered a chemotherapy-resistant tumor, but in fact several chemo-therapeutic agents show single-agent activity at the level of 10% to 15%, similar to the efficacy of the chemotherapeutic armamentarium used against other tumor types. Several combination chemotherapy regimens have been tested, but no survival benefit has been demonstrated. Few of these trials have been compared with standard dacarbazine (DTIC) in an adequately powered randomized trial, and even the largest of these trials were only powered to detect unrealistically large improvements in overall survival. In this article, the authors review past chemotherapy trials and the current state of chemotherapy for melanoma. Looking to the future, the authors are encouraged by recent observations that the addition of sorafenib to DTIC (or temozolomide) can increase response rates and survival. The authors suggest that this could form the core on which additional active chemotherapeutic drugs could be added with the hope of developing a regimen that improves overall survival. This paradigm of stepwise addition of active chemotherapeutic drugs has been successful in the development of chemotherapy regimens that improve survival in other solid tumor systems. In colon carcinoma, for example, the current regimens were built on fluorouracil (5FU)/leucovorin, which has similar activity to DTIC in melanoma. This could serve as a model for studies on melanoma.

SINGLE AGENTS AGAINST MELANOMA
Dacarbazine

DTIC has been considered the standard of care for metastatic melanoma since 1972 and can induce objective responses in some patients. It is a pro-drug that requires conversion in the liver to 5-(3-methyl-1-triazeno)imidazole-4-carboxamide (MTIC), the active compound. The typical DTIC dose is 850 to 1,000 mg/m^2 every 3 weeks.

[a] Melanoma/Sarcoma Service, Department of Medicine, Memorial Sloan-Kettering Cancer Center, 1275 York Avenue, New York, NY 10065, USA
[b] Weill Medical College of Cornell University, New York, NY, USA
* Corresponding author. Melanoma/Sarcoma Service, Department of Medicine, Memorial Sloan-Kettering Cancer Center, 1275 York Avenue, New York, NY 10065.
E-mail address: chapmanp@mskcc.org (P.B. Chapman).

Hematol Oncol Clin N Am 23 (2009) 583–597
doi:10.1016/j.hoc.2009.03.006
0889-8588/09/$ – see front matter © 2009 Elsevier Inc. All rights reserved.

hemonc.theclinics.com

Among the 8 randomized trials in which DTIC was used as a comparator arm since 1992, more than 1,000 patients have been treated with DTIC with an overall response rate of 13.4% and median survivals ranging from 5.6 months to 11 months (**Table 1**). Most of the responses were partial although complete responses did occur occasionally. Given the low response rate, it is unrealistic to expect DTIC to have an effect on median survival, but it is likely that there is an effect on survival in the responding patients. In considering the 5 trials in which 1-year survival was reported, the average overall 1-year survival rate was 27% (see **Table 1**). Thus, any new chemotherapy regimen for melanoma should aim for a response rate greater than 13.4%.

Temozolomide

Temozolomide (TMZ) is administered orally and, like DTIC, is a pro-drug that converts to the active compound, MTIC. Unlike DTIC, TMZ does not require the liver for conversion to MTIC. In a randomized trial comparing TMZ given for 5 days every month with DTIC given once every 3 weeks, there was no difference in response rate or survival.[1]

Despite this, TMZ offers 2 potential advantages over DTIC. TMZ readily crosses the intact blood-brain barrier and can then convert to MTIC raising the possibility that TMZ would have enhanced activity against brain metastases. Unfortunately, the objective response rate of melanoma brain metastases to TMZ is low,[2] although there is some indication that treatment with TMZ is associated with a lower incidence of progression of disease in the brain.[3,4]

Another potential advantage of TMZ is that, as an oral agent, continuous dosing is feasible. An extended-dosing schedule of 75 mg/m^2/day for 42 days followed by 14 days off has been used in several clinical trials. This schedule provides 6 weeks of continuous drug exposure and delivers 50% more drug over 2 months compared with the standard schedule of 5 days every month. However, a phase II trial using

Table 1
Efficacy of DTIC in randomized trials since 1992 in which DTIC was the control arm

Trial	Number in DTIC Arm	Number of DTIC Responders	Response Rate to DTIC (%)	Median Overall Survival (mo)	1 y Overall Survival (%)
Cocconi et al[84]	52	12	23	6.7	30
Thomson et al[85]	83	14	17		
Avril et al[27]	117	8	7	5.6	
Chapman et al[56]	116	12	10	6.3	27
Bajetta et al[86]	82	16	20	11	
Falkson et al[87]	69	22	32	10	20
Middleton et al[1]	149	28	19	6.4	22
Bedikian et al[82]	385	29	8	7.8	30
Total	1055	141	13.4[a]		27 (average)

[a] The total DTIC responders/total treated.

extended-dosing TMZ showed only a 12.5% response rate,[5] which is not different from what would be expected with standard-dosing TMZ or with DTIC.

Several investigators have looked into the mechanism of TMZ resistance. One of the methylation targets of TMZ is the O^6 position of guanine, which is repaired by the enzyme methylguanine methyltransferase (MGMT). Loss of MGMT expression, as measured by *MGMT* promoter methylation, has been correlated with an improved response rate to TMZ in glioblastoma[6] and glioma,[7] and with progression-free survival in glioblastoma.[6] However, in melanoma patients, it has not been possible to detect a correlation between response to DTIC or TMZ and loss of MGMT tumor expression.[5,8,9] Efforts to inhibit MGMT have not been successful to date.[10,11] This experience suggests that in melanoma, mechanisms other than MGMT expression are important for TMZ resistance.

Platinum Analogs

Cisplatin

Cisplatin has significant single-agent activity in melanoma ranging from 10% to more than 20%[12-15] with an average of 14.4% (**Table 2**). There is some suggestion that doses of less than 80 mg/m^2 are associated with lower response rates compared with doses of more than 80 mg/m^2, although this has not been tested in a randomized setting. High doses of cisplatin ($\geq$ 150 mg/m^2) have generally not been associated with improved response rates.[16]

Carboplatin

Carboplatin has been tested in 3 phase II clinical trials and found to have a response rate similar to cisplatin in melanoma patients (see **Table 2**). Casper treated 43 patients with 400 mg/m^2 carboplatin every 4 weeks and noted 7 overall responders (16%) with 1 complete response lasting 16 months.[17] Additional phase II testing with the same dosing and schedule demonstrated an 11% overall response rate with 3 out of 27 patients responding with a medium survival of 4.7 months.[18] Similar data were obtained by Evans[19] in a phase II trial, in which 5 out of 26 evaluable (19%) patients responded to 400 mg/m^2 carboplatin every 4 weeks. Currently, carboplatin is administered at a dose calculated to result in an area-under-the-concentration curve (AUC) of 5 or 6 mg min/mL, although there are no single-agent data testing carboplatin using this dosing method for melanoma. Myelosuppression is the main adverse effect; thrombocytopenia is a dose-limiting toxicity.

Nitrosoureas

Carmustine (BCNU), lomustine (CCNU), and fotemustine all have single-agent activity in melanoma (see **Table 2**). BCNU has shown response rates ranging from 10% to 20%.[20-22] Fotemustine, a nitrosourea available in Europe, may be the most active, with response rates over multiple clinical trials averaging 22%.[23-26] In addition, although nitrosoureas are lipid-soluble and cross the blood-brain barrier, only fotemustine was found to have a 25% response rate for cerebral metastasis.[24] In a phase III clinical trial of fotemustine (100 mg/m^2 weekly for 3 weeks) versus DTIC (250 mg/m^2/day for 5 days every 4 weeks), the response rate for fotemustine was 15.2% versus 6.8% for DTIC.[27] The median time to brain metastasis was 22.7 months for fotemustine versus 7.2 months for DTIC. Toxicities associated with nitrosoureas include myelosuppression, which can be prolonged, and gastrointestinal toxicities.

Table 2
Efficacy of other single-agent chemotherapy drugs in melanoma

Agent	No. of Evaluable Melanoma Patients	No. of Responders	Response Rate (%)
Temozolomide	(205)	(27)	(13.2)
Middleton[1]	156	21	13.5
Rietschel[5]	49	6	12.5
Cisplatin	(104)	(15)	(14.4)
Chary[15]	11	3	27
Goodnight[13]	10	1	10
Schilcher[14]	16	4	25
Al-Sarraf[12]	67	7	10
Carboplatin	(96)	(15)	(15.6)
Casper[17]	43	7	16
Chang[18]	27	3	11
Evans[19]	26	5	19
Fotemustine	(314)	(69)	(22)
Calabresi[23]	30	6	20
Jacquillat (brain)[24]	153	37	24.1
Schallreuter[26]	19	9	47.3
Avril[27]	112	17	15.2
BCNU	(119)	(22)	(18.5)
Ramirez[20]	99	19	19
De Vita[21]	20	3	15
Paclitaxel	(122)	(16)	(13.1)
Weirnik[31]	12	4	33
Legha[32]	25	3	12
Einzig[33]	28	4	14
Walker[34]	25	0	0
Bedikian[35]	32	5	15.6
Docetaxel	(105)	(12)	(11.4)
Einzig[28]	35	2	5.7
Bedikian[29]	40	5	12.5
Aamdal[30]	30	5	16.7

Numbers in parentheses are the totals from the trials listed. Response rates in parentheses are the percent total responders among the total number treated.

Taxanes

Docetaxel

Preclinical studies indicate that taxanes disturb the cytoskeleton architecture and stabilize microtubules causing mitotic arrest. Docetaxel showed an average response rate of 11.4% in 3 phase II clinical trials (see **Table 2**). Enzig administered 100 mg/m^2 docetaxel every 3 weeks to chemotherapy naive patients. Two out of 35 (6%) patients responded with 1 complete response. Both these responses lasted longer than 2 years.[28] Using the same dosing and schedule, a second trial was performed at MD Anderson with 5 out of 40 (12.5%) patients responding, with 1 complete response and overall median survival time of 13 months.[29] In a third phase II clinical trial, 38 patients were also treated with 100 mg/m^2 docetaxel every 3 weeks and evaluated after 2 cycles; 5 partial responses were noted in the 30 evaluable patients (17%).[30] In these studies the most common hematological toxicity was neutropenia. Additional toxicities included peripheral neuropathy, fatigue, fluid retention, oral mucositis, and hypersensitivity reactions.

Paclitaxel

Multiple phase I/II trials have been carried out with differing dosing schedules for paclitaxel (see **Table 2**). In a phase I trial with paclitaxel administered at 200 to 275 mg/m^2 over 24 hours every 3 weeks, there were 4 partial responses noted in the 12 patients enrolled.[31] A phase II trial with paclitaxel administered at 250 mg/m^2 over 24 hours every 3 weeks in 25 patients resulted in 3 partial responses (12%); a further 4 patients had durable objective regression although failing to qualify for partial response.[32] An additional 28 evaluable patients were studied in a second phase II study of paclitaxel administered at 250 mg/m^2 over 24 hours. Four patients (14%) had objective responses with 3 complete responses.[33] Weekly paclitaxel has also been tested in phase II clinical trials but with little success. A phase II study with paclitaxel administered at 80 mg/m^2 over 1 hour weekly for 3 weeks every 4-week cycle had no responses in the 25 patients enrolled.[34] However, 8 patients showed stable disease. A phase II trial performed with paclitaxel administered at 90 mg/m^2 on days 1, 5, and 9 every 3 weeks demonstrated a 15.6% response in 5/32 patients.[35] In general, toxicities associated with paclitaxel included neutropenia, peripheral neuropathy, which can be a dose-limiting toxicity, and fatigue.

Chemotherapy Drugs with Little Activity in Melanoma

Some chemotherapy drugs have been tested and found to have little activity against melanoma. In a phase II study, 30 mg/m^2 of melphalan was given to 17 patients with melanoma with a median of 2 cycles administered without any responses.[36] Phase II studies with ifosfamide have also been disappointing. Of 12 metastatic melanoma patients, none responded to 3 g/m^2 ifosfamide administered on days 1 and 2 every 3 weeks.[37] Multiple clinical trials concluded that camptothecans have minimal activity in the treatment of metastatic melanoma. Only 3 patients with metastatic melanoma responded out of 72 (4%) cumulative patients treated in 4 phase I/II clinical trials with irinotectan or topotecan single agent or in combination with docetaxel.[38–41] Combining 4 phase II trials with doxorubicin, only 4 out of 90 (4%) patients with metastatic melanoma responded to liposomal doxorubicin.[42–45]

ADDITION OF ANTIANGIOGENIC DRUGS TO DACARBAZINE OR TEMOZOLOMIDE

Because tumors larger than 1 mm must recruit blood vessels to grow, antiangiogenic drugs were anticipated to have single-agent activity, although in melanoma, these agents have shown fairly limited activity so far. However, one thought was to combine these drugs with active chemotherapy agents. Hwu and colleagues tested whether the activity of extended-dosing TMZ could be enhanced by adding 1 of 2 weak antiangiogenic agents: thalidomide or interferon-α2b. Although these drugs have little activity against melanoma as single agents, phase II trials combining either thalidomide or low-dose interferon-α with extended-dose TMZ demonstrated objective response rates of approximately 30%.[46,47] This result, seen in two trials, was twice the response rate observed with extended-dose TMZ alone (see **Table 2**) and suggested the potential value of the addition of an antiangiogenic drug to TMZ. Subsequent studies with TMZ and thalidomide have reported high rates of thromboembolic events indicating that thalidomide's therapeutic index may be too narrow in melanoma patients.

Sorafenib is a tyrosine kinase inhibitor that has activity against VEGFR and BRAF. Like bevacizumab, thalidomide, and interferon-α, sorafenib has little activity as a single agent in melanoma. However, in a trial of 101 patients with melanoma randomized to DTIC ± sorafenib, the combination of DTIC + sorafenib was associated with a doubling of the response rate, a doubling of the median progression-free survival, and a 50% improvement in progression-free survival at 9 months.[48] With only 101 patients, it is not surprising that this improved response rate and progression-free survival rate were not associated with a detectable improvement in overall survival. Results of trials with TMZ and sorafenib, published only in abstract form to date, show similar results; the addition of sorafenib was associated with a response rate of 26%.[49]

The observations from phase II trials of TMZ combined with thalidomide or interferon-α as well as a randomized trial of DTIC ± sorafenib are consistent with the idea that combining TMZ or DTIC with an antiangiogenic drug can double the objective response rate. With further improvement in the response rate, or with larger trials, an improvement in overall survival should be possible.

COMBINATION CHEMOTHERAPY REGIMENS

Because there are several chemotherapy drugs that have single-agent activity in melanoma (discussed earlier), there is rationale for combining drugs into combination regimens. Many of the combination regimens tested in melanoma have combined DTIC with immunologic agents (eg, interferon, interleukin-2), hormones (eg, tamoxifen), or novel biologic agents such as bcl-2 antisense each of which individually have shown little single-agent activity. In this section, some of the common combinations of cytotoxic chemotherapeutic regimens used in melanoma are discussed and the few phase III randomized trials that have been published are highlighted.

Dacarbazine/Carmustine/Cisplatin/Tamoxifen (Dartmouth Regimen)

This regimen was first described in 1984 and a 55% response rate was observed in 20 melanoma patients.[50] A subsequent series of single institution studies confirmed high response rates of 40% to 50%.[51-54] Some reports suggested that the addition of tamoxifen was important for the high response rate even though tamoxifen has no single-agent activity in melanoma; other reports did not agree.[55] A multi-institutional, phase III randomized trial compared the Dartmouth regimen directly to single-agent DTIC in 240 patients with metastatic melanoma.[56] The response rate was 18.5% in the combination chemotherapy cohort compared with 10.2% in the DTIC cohort. Although this difference was not statistically significant ($P = .09$), there was a statistically significant increase in response rate associated with the combination regimen among the cohort of patients with M1a or M1b disease. There was no significant difference in survival in this trial powered to detect a 50% improvement in median overall survival.

Subsequently, a smaller randomized trial was reported that compared this combination to DTIC/interferon-α.[57] This trial showed a higher response rate in the experimental and control arms (26.4% versus 17.3%) but the difference was not statistically significant. The trial also failed to show a statistically significant improvement in overall or 1-year survival.

Cisplatin/Vinblastine/Dacarbazine

Cisplatin/vinblastine/dacarbazine (CVD), a combination chemotherapy regimen developed at the MD Anderson Cancer Center, consists of 3-week cycles of cisplatin

20 mg/m^2/day × 4; vinblastine 2 mg/m^2/day × 4, and DTIC 800 mg/m^2 on day 1. In a single institution phase II trial with 50 evaluable patients, a response rate of 40% was achieved with an estimated 1-year survival of 50%.[58] In a randomized trial against biochemotherapy in which CVD was the control arm, the same investigators reported that CVD showed an objective response rate of 27% and an estimated 1-year survival of approximately 40%.[59] This single institution experience shows that the regimen is associated with a response rate 2 to 3 times higher than with DTIC and a 1-year survival rate twice as high as DTIC. Of course, it is difficult to control for patient selection bias and there has been no peer-reviewed published study comparing the CVD regimen to DTIC.

Carboplatin/Paclitaxel

Preclinical studies support synergistic actions between cisplatin and paclitaxel,[60] and this combination has shown some clinical activity in melanoma in chemotherapy-naive patients. A combination of carboplatin at an AUC of 7.5 and paclitaxel at 175 mg/m^2 over 3 hours was administered to 17 patients in a phase II trial.[61] There was a 20% response rate with 3 partial responders in the 15 evaluable patients, with a median survival of 9 months. Grade III or IV hematological toxicities occurred in 11/15 (73%) of those treated during the clinical study. A larger phase II study for second line therapy revealed few responses.[62] In this randomized trial, paclitaxel monotherapy was administered at 100 mg/m^2 weekly for 6 weeks then 2 weeks off, versus paclitaxel 80 mg/m^2 and carboplatin 200 mg/m^2 weekly for 6 weeks and 2 weeks off. Forty patients were enrolled and overall response rates were less than 10% for both arms. More recently, albumin-bound paclitaxel has also been tested with carboplatin in a phase I trial with 3 out of 10 treated patients obtaining a partial response.[63]

Recently, sorafenib has been tested in combination with carboplatin and paclitaxel. A phase I trial with 38 patients (24 with melanoma, most having progressed after prior therapy) received sorafenib either 100, 200, or 400 mg twice daily on days 2 to 19 of a 21-day cycle with carboplatin at AUC 6 and paclitaxel at 225 mg/m^2 administered on day 1.[64] The overall response was 10 out of 24 treated patients with 1 complete response. These encouraging response rates prompted 2 phase III trials of carboplatin and paclitaxel with or without sorafenib. The first trial treated 270 patients who had previously progressed on systemic chemotherapy with paclitaxel at 225 mg/m^2 and carboplatin at AUC 6 once every 3 weeks with or without sorafenib at 400 mg twice daily on days 2 to 19. There was no difference in progression-free survival, which was the primary endpoint, or in response rate.[65] The control group (no sorafenib) showed a response rate of 11% with a median progression-free survival of 17.4 weeks; the median overall survival was 42 weeks. The cohort receiving sorafenib had essentially identical outcomes. That the addition of sorafenib to carboplatin/paclitaxel did not improve response rate contrasts with the original observations in the phase I trial[64] and with the observations of McDermott who showed that sorafenib doubled the response rate to DTIC.[48] This difference may be explained by the different chemotherapy regimens or by the fact that the DTIC/sorafenib patients were chemotherapy-naive. A second, larger phase III cooperative group trial randomizing previously untreated melanoma patients to carboplatin and paclitaxel with or without sorafenib has finished accrual and is awaiting the results of overall survival as the primary endpoint.

Myeloablative Chemotherapy Regimens with Autologous Bone Marrow Rescue

The concept of combination chemotherapy has been pushed to the extreme by several investigators who explored the use of myeloablative chemotherapy using alkylating agents at potentially lethal doses followed by autologous bone marrow rescue.[66–77] Among 263 evaluable patients with metastatic melanoma in 12 studies, there was an overall response rate of 52% with individual trials showing response rates ranging from 22% to 61% (**Fig. 1**). There were 33 reported complete responders (12.5% complete response rate) but the duration of the complete response was generally short. Few complete responders maintained a complete response longer 12 months.[67,69] This experience confirms that alkylating agents can induce responses in up to half of melanoma patients if the doses are sufficiently high. However, complete responses remain infrequent and are generally short-lived.

Phase III Trials of Combination Chemotherapy in Melanoma

Although many phase III trials have been published comparing combination therapy with DTIC, this article focuses only on the trials comparing combination chemotherapy with DTIC. Of the combination chemotherapy regimens tested in melanoma over the past 30 years, there are only three published randomized trials comparing with DTIC that have accrued at least 50 patients in each cohort. As noted earlier, the Dartmouth regimen was compared with DTIC and showed an increased objective response rate but no overall survival benefit.[56] The trial was sufficiently powered to detect a 50% improvement in survival.

A second randomized trial was a 3-armed trial in which patients were treated with either DTIC/Bacillus Calmette-Guerin (BCG) (N = 130), or DTIC/bleomycin/hydroxy-urea/BCG (N = 161), or the combination without BCG (N = 95).[78] Patients receiving combination chemotherapy had a 29% response rate compared with an 18% response rate in the DTIC cohort, which was a statistically significant difference; BCG had no detectable effects on response. With this number of patients, the trial was sufficiently powered to detect a median survival difference of approximately 50%. Perhaps not surprisingly, there was no overall survival difference observed although responders showed significantly improved survival over nonresponders.

A third trial compared DTIC with DTIC + vindesine.[79] In that trial, 9/51 (18%) patients treated with DTIC responded compared with 15/59 (25%) of patients treated with the combination. The difference was not statistically significant nor was the

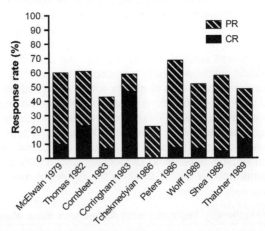

Fig. 1. Response rates of trials using myeloablative chemotherapy followed by autologous bone marrow rescue.

difference in median survival, although again, responders showed significantly improved median survival over nonresponders (11.7 versus. 3.4 months; $P < .0001$).

These 3 randomized trials showed that combination chemotherapy induced objective responses more frequently than DTIC although the response rates were still less than 30%. Neither of the 2 trials that looked at overall survival was able to detect a benefit in median overall survival, but neither was powered to detect a difference of less than 50%. It seems unlikely that chemotherapy regimens with objective response rates this low would be associated with a 50% improvement in median overall survival. It is possible that these regimens can improve median overall survival by a smaller margin, but much larger studies would have been needed to detect this.

ADJUVANT CHEMOTHERAPY FOR MELANOMA

The role of adjuvant chemotherapy in melanoma has been recently reviewed.[80] In other tumor types in which adjuvant chemotherapy has been shown to improve median overall survival, the magnitude of improvement ranged from 4% to 35%. Thus, adjuvant trials in melanoma should be powered to detect small improvements in overall survival. To detect even a 30% improvement in survival with 80% power, a 2-arm adjuvant trial would need more than 500 patients. In addition, active adjuvant chemotherapy regimens generally have activity in the metastatic setting of at least 20%. Thus, the guiding principles for developing adjuvant chemotherapy in melanoma should be a regimen associated with at least a 20% response rate.

Given the requirements of a treatment regimen with at least a 20% response rate and a clinical trial design with at least 500 patients, there has not yet been a realistic test of adjuvant chemotherapy in melanoma patients. The trial that comes closest to an adequate test was reported by Veronesi and colleagues[81] published 25 years ago. In this 4-arm study, 761 patients were randomized to DTIC, BCG, DTIC + BCG, or observation after complete surgical resection. There was no survival difference at 3 years. Even this trial does not meet the requirements of adequate statistical power or of an adequately active treatment regimen. Although this is the largest adjuvant chemotherapy trial on melanoma, it only had the power to detect a benefit of at least 50% improvement in survival – clearly outside what has ever been seen in other tumor types. As noted earlier, the response rate of DTIC in the metastatic setting is less than 20%.

Other adjuvant chemotherapy trials have been reported but these were so underpowered as to be uninformative. Adjuvant chemotherapy trials in melanoma should not be carried out unless they use a regimen with at least a 20% response rate in the metastatic setting and are adequately powered to be able to detect improvements in overall survival as small as 30%.

THE FUTURE

DTIC (or TMZ) remains the standard chemotherapy treatment of metastatic melanoma although it is not known if there is a small overall survival benefit associated with treatment. Combination chemotherapy regimens can induce objective responses in a higher proportion of patients than DTIC alone although the 2 largest randomized trials did not detect an overall survival benefit compared with DTIC. Because these trials were powered only to detect a large difference in survival (>50%), it remains possible that combination chemotherapy can improve survival by a smaller margin. However, larger studies with at least 400 patients per cohort would be needed to detect these small benefits. One option to develop combination chemotherapy regimens that improve overall survival would be to conduct randomized trials using active combinations with a sufficient number of patients to detect a realistic improvement in survival. Studies of this size have been difficult to conduct on melanoma. Indeed, the largest randomized trial ever conducted on melanoma had a total of 771 patients.[82] Therefore, although current combination chemotherapy regimens might be associated with a small improvement in overall survival, it seems unlikely that the melanoma community will be able to conduct a trial large enough to test this hypothesis.

Another option would be to develop a combination treatment with a higher response rate that would be expected to improve overall survival to a level more easily detected. The experience with metastatic colon cancer may be useful. Since the 1960s, 5FU had been the standard therapy, which, like DTIC, induced responses in less than 15% of patients but was not believed to improve overall survival. The addition of leucovorin, a drug with no single-agent activity itself, almost doubled the objective response rate but it still was not clear if this improved overall survival. This may be analogous to the recent observations that addition of sorafenib to DTIC or to TMZ can double the response rate in metastatic melanoma but may not affect overall survival. Building on 5FU/leucovorin, the colon cancer community added chemotherapy drugs that had 10% single-agent activity: oxaliplatin or irinotecan. This further increased the response rate to the point that a benefit in overall survival could be demonstrated. However, to detect these improvements, the randomized trials had 695 and 795 patients, respectively. In the melanoma field, we might build on the results with DTIC/sorafenib by adding either cisplatin or carboplatin. This stepwise approach could lead us to a combination chemotherapy regimen that improves overall survival but larger randomized trials than in the past must be run to detect important improvements in overall survival.

A third option is to focus on responders. Most investigators have observed that patients who respond to therapy live longer. Many have rejected these observations arguing that this observation could be explained by selection bias and that patients who tolerate and respond to therapy are more likely to live longer anyway. However, survival improvement among responders has been reported in several randomized chemotherapy trials[78,79,83] in which this bias would not exist. There are long-term survivors among responders, which is not seen in untreated patients.

This cohort of responding patients should be studied to understand why they respond to treatment. There are currently many genetic tools that allow us to genotype tumors (or patients) before therapy and then see which genetic changes correlate with response to treatment. This approach is being used with so-called "targeted therapy" agents and is beginning to be used for chemotherapy in other tumor types. Instead of considering the small proportion of melanoma patients who respond to treatment as statistical aberrations, they should be viewed as consistent but low frequency events worthy of study that could give us clues leading to improved therapy.

REFERENCES

1. Middleton MR, Grob JJ, Aaronson N, et al. Randomized phase III study of temozolomide versus dacarbazine in the treatment of patients with advanced metastatic malignant melanoma. J Clin Oncol 2000;18:158–66.
2. Margolin K, Atkins B, Thompson A, et al. Temozolomide and whole brain irradiation in melanoma metastatic to the brain: a phase II trial of the Cytokine Working Group. J Cancer Res Clin Oncol 2002;128:214–8.
3. Atkins MB, Gollob JA, Sosman JA, et al. A phase II pilot trial of concurrent biochemotherapy with cisplatin, vinblastine, temozolomide, interleukin 2, and IFN-alpha 2B in patients with metastatic melanoma. Clin Cancer Res 2002;8:3075–81.

4. Paul MJ, Summers Y, Calvert AH, et al. Effect of temozolomide on central nervous system relapse in patients with advanced melanoma. Melanoma Res 2002;12: 175–8.

5. Rietschel P, Wolchok JD, Krown S, et al. Phase II study of extended-dose temozolomide in patients with melanoma. J Clin Oncol 2008;26:2299–304.

6. Hegi ME, Diserens A-C, Gorlia T, et al. MGMT gene silencing and benefit from temozolomide in glioblastoma. N Engl J Med 2005;352:997–1003. 10.1056/NEJMoa043331.

7. Paz MF, Yaya-Tur R, Rojas-Marcos I, et al. CpG island hypermethylation of the DNA repair enzyme methyltransferase predicts response to temozolomide in primary gliomas. Clin Cancer Res 2004;10:4933–8.

8. Ma S, Egyhazi S, Ueno T, et al. O6-methylguanine-DNA-methyltransferase expression and gene polymorphisms in relation to chemotherapeutic response in metastatic melanoma. Br J Cancer 2003;89:1517–23.

9. Middleton MR, Lunn JM, Morris C, et al. O6-methylguanine-DNA methyltransferase in pretreatment tumour biopsies as a predictor of response to temozolomide in melanoma. Br J Cancer 1998;78:1199–202.

10. Ranson M, Hersey P, Thompson D, et al. Randomized trial of the combination of lomeguatrib and temozolomide compared with temozolomide alone in chemotherapy naive patients with metastatic cutaneous melanoma. J Clin Oncol 2007;25:2540–5.10.1200/JCO.2007.10.8217.

11. Gajewski TF, Sosman J, Gerson SL, et al. Phase II trial of the O6-alkylguanine DNA alkyltransferase inhibitor O6-benzylguanine and 1,3-bis(2-chloroethyl)-1-_nitrosourea in advanced melanoma. Clin Cancer Res 2005;11:7861–5.

12. Al-Sarraf M, Fletcher W, Oishi N, et al. Cisplatin hydration with and without mannitol diuresis in refractory disseminated malignant melanoma: a Southwest Oncology Group study. Cancer Treat Rep 1982;66:31–5.

13. Goodnight JE Jr, Moseley HS, Eilber FR, et al. cis-Dichlorodiammineplatinum(II) alone and combined with DTIC for treatment of disseminated malignant melanoma. Cancer Treat Rep 1979;63:2005–7.

14. Schilcher RB, Wessels M, Niederle N, et al. Phase II evaluation of fractionated low and single high dose cisplatin in various tumors. J Cancer Res Clin Oncol 1984; 107:57–60.

15. Chary KK, Higby DJ, Henderson ES, et al. Phase I study of high-dose cis-dichlorodiammineplatinum(II) with forced diuresis. Cancer Treat Rep 1977;61: 367–70.

16. Steffens T, Bajorin D, Chapman P, et al. A phase II trial of high dose cisplatin and dacarbazine. Cancer 1991;68:1230–7.

17. Casper ES, Bajorin D. Phase II trial of carboplatin in patients with advanced melanoma. Invest New Drugs 1990;8:187–90.

18. Chang A, Hunt M, Parkinson DR, et al. Phase II trial of carboplatin in patients with metastatic malignant melanoma. A report from the Eastern Cooperative Oncology Group. Am J Clin Oncol 1993;16:152–5.

19. Evans LM, Casper ES, Rosenbluth R. Phase II trial of carboplatin in advanced malignant melanoma. Cancer Treat Rep 1987;71:171–2.

20. Ramirez G, Wilson W, Grage T, et al. Phase II evaluation of 1,3-bis(2-chloroethyl)-1-nitrosourea (BCNU; NSC-409962) in patients with solid tumors. Cancer Chemother Rep 1972;56:787–90.

21. De Vita VT, Carbone PP, Owens AH Jr, et al. Clinical trials with 1,3-bis(2-chloroethyl)-1-nitrosourea, NSC-409962. Cancer Res 1965;25:1876–81.

22. Luce JK. Chemotherapy of malignant melanoma. Cancer 1972;30:1604–15.

23. Calabresi F, Aapro M, Becquart D, et al. Short report: multicenter phase II trial of the single agent fotemustine in patients with advanced malignant melanoma. Ann Oncol 1991;2:377–8.
24. Jacquillat C, Khayat D, Banzet P, et al. Final report of the French multicenter phase II study of the nitrosourea fotemustine in 153 evaluable patients with disseminated malignant melanoma including patients with cerebral metastases. Cancer 1990;66:1873–8.
25. Kleeberg UR, Engel E, Israels P, et al. Palliative therapy of melanoma patients with fotemustine. Inverse relationship between tumour load and treatment effectiveness. A multicentre phase II trial of the EORTC-Melanoma Cooperative Group (MCG). Melanoma Res 1995;5:195–200.
26. Schallreuter KU, Wenzel E, Brassow FW, et al. Positive phase II study in the treatment of advanced malignant melanoma with fotemustine. Cancer Chemother Pharmacol 1991;29:85–7.
27. Avril MF, Aamdal S, Grob JJ, et al. Fotemustine compared with dacarbazine in patients with disseminated malignant melanoma: a phase III study. J Clin Oncol 2004;22:1118–25.
28. Einzig AI, Schuchter LM, Recio A, et al. Phase II trial of docetaxel (Taxotere) in patients with metastatic melanoma previously untreated with cytotoxic chemotherapy. Med Oncol 1996;13:111–7.
29. Bedikian AY, Weiss GR, Legha SS, et al. Phase II trial of docetaxel in patients with advanced cutaneous malignant melanoma previously untreated with chemotherapy. J Clin Oncol 1995;13:2895–9.
30. Aamdal S, Wolff I, Kaplan S, et al. Docetaxel (Taxotere) in advanced malignant melanoma: a phase II study of the EORTC Early Clinical Trials Group. Eur J Cancer 1994;30A:1061–4.
31. Wiernik PH, Schwartz EL, Einzig A, et al. Phase I trial of taxol given as a 24-hour infusion every 21 days: responses observed in metastatic melanoma. J Clin Oncol 1987;5:1232–9.
32. Legha SS, Ring S, Papadopoulos N, et al. A phase II trial of taxol in metastatic melanoma. Cancer 1990;65:2478–81.
33. Einzig AI, Hochster H, Wiernik PH, et al. A phase II study of taxol in patients with malignant melanoma. Invest New Drugs 1991;9:59–64.
34. Walker L, Schalch H, King DM, et al. Phase II trial of weekly paclitaxel in patients with advanced melanoma. Melanoma Res 2005;15:453–9.
35. Bedikian AY, Plager C, Papadopoulos N, et al. Phase II evaluation of paclitaxel by short intravenous infusion in metastatic melanoma. Melanoma Res 2004;14:63–6.
36. Hochster H, Strawderman MH, Harris JE, et al. Conventional dose melphalan is inactive in metastatic melanoma: results of an Eastern Cooperative Oncology Group Study (E1687). Anticancer Drugs 1999;10:245–8.
37. Negretti E, Ferrari L, Bonfante V, et al. Phase II study with ifosfamide in advanced malignant melanoma. Tumori 1988;74:163–5.
38. Dumez H, Awada A, Piccart M, et al. A phase I dose-finding clinical pharmacokinetic study of an oral formulation of irinotecan (CPT-11) administered for 5 days every 3 weeks in patients with advanced solid tumours. Ann Oncol 2006;17:1158–65.
39. Tas F, Camlica H, Kurul S, et al. Combination chemotherapy with docetaxel and irinotecan in metastatic malignant melanoma. Clin Oncol (R Coll Radiol) 2003;15:132–5.
40. Janik JE, Miller LL, Korn EL, et al. A prospective randomized phase II trial of GM-CSF priming to prevent topotecan-induced neutropenia in chemotherapy-naive

patients with malignant melanoma or renal cell carcinoma. Blood 2001;97: 1942–6.

41. Kraut EH, Walker MJ, Staubus A, et al. Phase II trial of topotecan in malignant melanoma. Cancer Invest 1997;15:318–20.

42. Vorobiof DA, Rapoport BL, Mahomed R, et al. Phase II study of pegylated liposomal doxorubicin in patients with metastatic malignant melanoma failing standard chemotherapy treatment. Melanoma Res 2003;13:201–3.

43. Smylie MG, Wong R, Mihalcioiu C, et al. A phase II, open label, monotherapy study of liposomal doxorubicin in patients with metastatic malignant melanoma. Invest New Drugs 2007;25:155–9.

44. Fink W, Zimpfer-Rechner C, Thoelke A, et al. Clinical phase II study of pegylated liposomal doxorubicin as second-line treatment in disseminated melanoma. Onkologie 2004;27:540–4.

45. Ellerhorst JA, Bedikian A, Ring S, et al. Phase II trial of doxil for patients with metastatic melanoma refractory to frontline therapy. Oncol Rep 1999;6: 1097–9.

46. Hwu WJ, Krown SE, Menell JH, et al. Phase II study of temozolomide plus thalidomide for the treatment of metastatic melanoma. J Clin Oncol 2003;21:3351–6.

47. Hwu WJ, Panageas KS, Menell JH, et al. Phase II study of temozolomide plus pegylated interferon-alpha-2b for metastatic melanoma. Cancer 2006;106:2445–51.

48. McDermott DF, Sosman JA, Gonzalez R, et al. Double-blind randomized phase II study of the combination of sorafenib and dacarbazine in patients with advanced melanoma: a report from the 11715 Study Group. J Clin Oncol 2008;26:2178–85.

49. Amaravadi R, Schuchter LM, McDermott DF, et al. Updated results of a randomized phase II study comparing two schedules of temozolomide in combination with sorafenib in patients with advanced melanoma. Proc Am Soc Clin Oncol 2007;25:8527.

50. Del Prete SA, Maurer LH, O'Donnell J, et al. Combination chemotherapy with cisplatin, carmustine, dacarbazine, and tamoxifen in metastatic melanoma. Cancer Treat Rep 1984;68:1403–5.

51. McClay EF, Mastrangelo MJ, Berd D, et al. Effective combination chemo/ hormonal therapy for malignant melanoma: experience with three consecutive trials. Int J Cancer 1992;50:553–6.

52. Saba HI, Cruse CW, Wells KE, et al. Treatment of stage IV malignant melanoma with dacarbazine, carmustine, cisplatin, and tamoxifen regimens: a University of South Florida and H. Lee Moffitt Melanoma Center Study. Ann Plast Surg 1992;28:65–9.

53. Richards JM, Gilewski TA, Ramming K, et al. Effective chemotherapy for melanoma after treatment with interleukin-2. Cancer 1992;69:427–9.

54. Lattanzi SC, Tosteson T, Chertoff J, et al. Dacarbazine, cisplatin and carmustine, with or without tamoxifen, for metastatic melanoma: 5-year follow-up. Melanoma Res 1995;5:365–9.

55. Rusthoven JJ, Quirt IC, Iscoe NA, et al. Randomized, double-blind, placebo-controlled trial comparing the response rates of carmustine, dacarbazine, and cisplatin with and without tamoxifen in patients with metastatic melanoma. National Cancer Institute of Canada Clinical Trials Group. J Clin Oncol 1996;14: 2083–90.

56. Chapman PB, Einhorn LH, Meyers ML, et al. Phase III multicenter randomized trial of the Dartmouth regimen versus dacarbazine in patients with metastatic melanoma. J Clin Oncol 1999;17:2745–51.

57. Middleton MR, Lorigan P, Owen J, et al. A randomized phase III study comparing dacarbazine, BCNU, cisplatin and tamoxifen with dacarbazine and interferon in advanced melanoma. Br J Cancer 2000;82:1158–62.
58. Legha SS, Ring S, Papadopoulos N, et al. A prospective evaluation of a triple-drug regimen containing cisplatin, vinblastine, and dacarbazine (CVD) for metastatic melanoma. Cancer 1989;64:2024–9.
59. Eton O, Legha SS, Bedikian AY, et al. Sequential biochemotherapy versus chemotherapy for metastatic melanoma: results from a phase III randomized trial. J Clin Oncol 2002;20:2045–52.
60. Jekunen AP, Christen RD, Shalinsky DR, et al. Synergistic interaction between cisplatin and taxol in human ovarian carcinoma cells in vitro. Br J Cancer 1994; 69:299–306.
61. Hodi FS, Soiffer RJ, Clark J, et al. Phase II study of paclitaxel and carboplatin for malignant melanoma. Am J Clin Oncol 2002;25:283–6.
62. Zimpfer-Rechner C, Hofmann U, Figl R, et al. Randomized phase II study of weekly paclitaxel versus paclitaxel and carboplatin as second-line therapy in disseminated melanoma: a multicentre trial of the Dermatologic Co-operative Oncology Group (DeCOG). Melanoma Res 2003;13:531–6.
63. Stinchcombe TE, Socinski MA, Walko CM, et al. Phase I and pharmacokinetic trial of carboplatin and albumin-bound paclitaxel, ABI-007 (Abraxane) on three treatment schedules in patients with solid tumors. Cancer Chemother Pharmacol 2007;60:759–66.
64. Flaherty KT, Schiller J, Schuchter LM, et al. A phase I trial of the oral, multikinase inhibitor sorafenib in combination with carboplatin and paclitaxel. Clin Cancer Res 2008;14:4836–42.
65. Hauschild A, Agarwala SS, Trefzer U, et al. Results of a phase III, randomized, placebo-controlled study of sorafenib in combination with carboplatin and paclitaxel as second-line treatment in patients with unresectable stage III or stage IV melanoma. J Clin Oncol, in press.
66. McElwain TJ, Hedley DW, Gordon MY, et al. High dose melphalan and non-cryopreserved autologous bone marrow treatment of malignant melanoma and neuroblastoma. Exp Hematol 1979;7(Suppl 5):360–71.
67. Thomas MR, Robinson WA, Glode LM, et al. Treatment of advanced malignant melanoma with high-dose chemotherapy and autologous bone marrow transplantation. Preliminary results–Phase I study. Am J Clin Oncol 1982;5:611–22.
68. Cornbleet MA, McElwain TJ, Kumar PJ, et al. Treatment of advanced malignant melanoma with high-dose melphalan and autologous bone marrow transplantation. Br J Cancer 1983;48:329–34.
69. Lazarus HM, Herzig RH, Wolff SN, et al. Treatment of metastatic malignant melanoma with intensive melphalan and autologous bone marrow transplantation. Cancer Treat Rep 1985;69:473–7.
70. Wolff SN, Herzig RH, Fay JW, et al. High-dose thiotepa with autologous bone marrow transplantation for metastatic malignant melanoma: results of phase I and II studies of the North American Bone Marrow Transplantation Group. J Clin Oncol 1989;7:245–9.
71. Shea TC, Antman KH, Eder JP, et al. Malignant melanoma. Treatment with high-dose combination alkylating agent chemotherapy and autologous bone marrow support. Arch Dermatol 1988;124:878–84.
72. Peters WP, Eder JP, Henner WD, et al. High-dose combination alkylating agents with autologous bone marrow support: a Phase 1 trial. J Clin Oncol 1986;4: 646–54.

73. Tchekmedyian NS, Tait N, Van Echo D, et al. High-dose chemotherapy without autologous bone marrow transplantation in melanoma. J Clin Oncol 1986;4: 1811–8.
74. Slease RB, Benear JB, Selby GB, et al. High-dose combination alkylating agent therapy with autologous bone marrow rescue for refractory solid tumors. J Clin Oncol 1988;6:1314–20.
75. Antman K, Eder JP, Elias A, et al. High-dose combination alkylating agent preparative regimen with autologous bone marrow support: the Dana-Farber Cancer Institute/Beth Israel Hospital experience. Cancer Treat Rep 1987;71:119–25.
76. Thatcher D, Lind M, Morgenstern G, et al. High-dose, double alkylating agent chemotherapy with DTIC, melphalan, or ifosfamide and marrow rescue for metastatic malignant melanoma. Cancer 1989;63:1296–302.
77. Corringham R, Gilmore M, Prentice H, et al. High-dose melphalan with autologous bone marrow transplant treatment of poor prognosis tumors. Cancer 1983;52:1783–7.
78. Costanzi JJ, Al-Sarraf M, Groope C, et al. Combination chemotherapy plus BCG in the treatment of disseminated malignant melanoma: A Southwest Oncology Group study. Med Pediatr Oncol 1982;10:251–8.
79. Ringborg U, Rudenstam CM, Hansson J, et al. Dacarbazine versus dacarbazine-vindesine in disseminated malignant melanoma: a randomized phase II study. Med Oncol Tumor Pharmacother 1989;6:285–9.
80. Shah GD, Chapman PB. Adjuvant therapy of melanoma. Cancer J 2007;13: 217–22.
81. Veronesi U, Adamus J, Aubert C, et al. A randomized trial of adjuvant chemotherapy and immunotherapy in cutaneous melanoma. N Engl J Med 1982;307: 913–6.
82. Bedikian AY, Millward M, Pehamberger H, et al. Bcl-2 antisense (oblimersen sodium) plus dacarbazine in patients with advanced melanoma: the Oblimersen Melanoma Study Group. J Clin Oncol 2006;24:4738–45.
83. Costanza ME, Nathanson L, Schoenfeld D, et al. Results with methyl-CCNU and DTIC in metastatic melanoma. Cancer 1977;40:1010–5.
84. Cocconi G, Bella M, Calabresi F, et al. Treatment of metastatic malignant melanoma with dacarbazine plus tamoxifen. N Engl J Med 1992;327:516–23.
85. Thomson DB, Adena M, McLeod GR, et al. Interferon-alpha 2a does not improve response or survival when combined with dacarbazine in metastatic malignant melanoma: results of a multi-institutional Australian randomized trial. Melanoma Res 1993;3:133–8.
86. Bajetta E, Di Leo A, Zampino MG, et al. Multicenter randomized trial of dacarbazine alone or in combination with two different doses and schedules of interferon alfa-2a in the treatment of advanced melanoma. J Clin Oncol 1994;12:806–11.
87. Falkson CI, Ibrahim J, Kirkwood JM, et al. Phase III trial of dacarbazine versus dacarbazine with interferon alpha-2b versus dacarbazine with tamoxifen versus dacarbazine with interferon alpha-2b and tamoxifen in patients with metastatic malignant melanoma: an Eastern Cooperative Oncology Group study. J Clin Oncol 1998;16:1743–51.

Drug Targeting of Oncogenic Pathways in Melanoma

Leslie A. Fecher, MD[a],*, Ravi K. Amaravadi, MD[b],
Lynn M. Schuchter, MD[a], Keith T. Flaherty, MD[b]

KEYWORDS

- Melanoma • Drug • Molecular • MAPK
- Microphthalmia-associated transcription factor • Cell cycle
- Apoptosis • Angiogenesis • BRAF • KIT • PI3K

TARGETED THERAPY IN MELANOMA

Melanoma continues to be one of the most aggressive and morbid malignancies once metastatic. Overall survival for advanced unresectable melanoma has not changed over the past several decades. However, the presence of some long-term survivors of metastatic melanoma highlights the heterogeneity of this disease and the potential for improved outcomes. Current research is uncovering the molecular and genetic scaffolding of normal and aberrant cell function. Many of the essential mechanisms that permit proliferation, migration, resistance to apoptosis, and escape from immune surveillance are coopted by cancer through somatic genetic changes. The specific alterations that give rise to aberrant signal transduction are often shared by diverse cancer histologies; however, there are some genetic events that cluster in a subset of cancer. Melanoma is a prime model for therapeutic investigation based on molecular and genetic changes. With the discovery of activating BRAF mutations and aberrant MAPK pathway function, a new era in melanoma oncology began. However, the critical role that other pathways play and how they interact with the mitogen-activated protein (MAP) kinase pathway is becoming evident. These pathways include

Conflicts of interest: Ongoing trials sponsored by Novartis, Schering Plough, Plexxicon, Glaxo-Smith-Kline, Geminex, Ardea Biosciences, Exelexis, Tigris, Pfizer, Bayer, Onyx, and AVAX technologies. Dr. Flaherty has served as consultant to Novartis, Schering Plough, Bayer, and Onyx Pharmaceuticals.
Funding Support: P50-CA093372-08 (Fecher, Amaravadi, Flaherty, and Schuchter), K23-CA104884-02 (Flaherty), K23-CA120862-01 (Amaravadi).
[a] Department of Medicine, Division of Hematology and Oncology, Abramson Cancer Center, University of Pennsylvania, 3400 Spruce Street, 16 Penn Tower, Philadelphia, PA 19104, USA
[b] Department of Medicine, Division of Hematology and Oncology, Abramson Cancer Center, University of Pennsylvania, 3400 Spruce Street, 12 Penn Tower, Philadelphia, PA 19104, USA
* Corresponding author.
E-mail address: leslie.fecher@uphs.upenn.edu (L. A. Fecher).

Hematol Oncol Clin N Am 23 (2009) 599–618
doi:10.1016/j.hoc.2009.03.004
0889-8588/09/$ – see front matter © 2009 Elsevier Inc. All rights reserved.

phosphatidylinositol- 3-kinase (PI3K), c-KIT, microphthalmia-associated transcription factor (MITF), and cyclin-dependent kinases (CDKs) **(Fig. 1)**. Of equal interest in therapeutics are the processes that are driven by these oncogenes: cell cycle, angiogenesis, and apoptosis. With the dismal prognosis of advanced disease, systemic therapies with limited impact, and often accessible metastases for correlative studies, exploration of relevant pathways and molecules and their therapeutic targeting is feasible and imperative.

A small subset of patients experience dramatic clinical benefit from available therapies. It is imperative to understand what factors identify these patients. Prospectively, new therapies must be developed in a fashion that matches patients' underlying tumor biology with therapy. Only in this way will advances be made for the entire melanoma patient population. Although successes have been seen with single agents, given the genetic complexity of melanoma, combinatorial therapy (within and across therapeutic categories) will likely prove most successful. Combinatorial therapy will permit simultaneous targeting of multiple oncogenic paths with additive or synergistic impact. Similarly, this approach offers the hope of overcoming potential compensatory mechanisms that would otherwise mediate resistance to therapy.

Improved molecular and genetic profiling within melanoma, similar to that being realized for other cancers, will soon allow individualization of therapy based on tumor and host profiling. With the evolution in molecular therapeutics, the definitions of response that evolved in the era of cytotoxic chemotherapy are being challenged. Measures of disease control such as metabolic response and progression-free

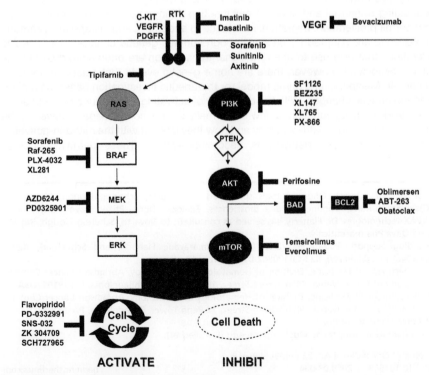

Fig. 1. Signaling pathways and current agents.

survival (PFS) are increasingly seen as more meaningful surrogates for overall survival (OS) than tumor regression early in the course of therapy. Seemingly simple mechanisms of action for selective targeted therapy may not be so straightforward to analyze in humans, requiring the development of correlative studies to assess on-target and off-target effects in tumor cells, the tumor microenvironment, and the host. The known oncogenic pathways in melanoma and the attempts to develop therapy for them are discussed in this review. The targeting of certain cellular processes, downstream of the common genetic alterations, for which the issues of target and drug validation are somewhat distinct, are also highlighted.

TARGETING THE MAPK PATHWAY

The MAP kinase pathway has been the focus of targeted therapy development in melanoma for two reasons: the central role that this pathway seems to play in the pathophysiology of numerous cancers and the identification of activating mutations in this pathway in most melanomas.

NRAS was identified as an oncogene in melanoma more than 15 years ago.[1] In the largest cohorts studied to date, the prevalence of NRAS mutation is at least 15% to 20%.[2] It is NRAS that harbors mutations in melanoma, never KRAS or HRAS, whereas these isoforms are commonly mutated in other cancers. Roughly 20% of all cancers harbor RAS mutations, and the development of effective agents that target RAS is highly desirable and elusive. RAS is a GTPase, as opposed to an ATPase, which distinguishes it from the family of kinases for which targeted therapies have been successfully developed for cancers other than melanoma. Furthermore, the GTPase activity of mutated RAS is actually less than the wild-type forms, making inhibitors of the GTPase activity unappealing.[3,4] After it was discovered that the RAS proteins require prenylation for membrane localization and activation, attention was turned to developing drugs to block this post-translational modification.[5,6] However, a key limitation of this approach is that numerous proteins are isoprenylated, raising concerns that the off-target effects of such drugs would constrain their therapeutic index. RAS proteins are farnesylated and geronylated, and inhibitors of farnesyltransferases and geronyltransferases have been developed. Farnesyltranserase inhibitors (FTIs) are the first to have entered clinical testing. In preclinical models, FTIs can prevent RAS membrane localization and activation, and are associated with cytotoxicity in RAS mutant tumors.[7,8] In clinical trials, single-agent activity has not been observed in cancers that are known to harbor RAS mutations.[9] Only one phase II trial has been undertaken with a single-agent FTI in metastatic melanoma.[10] Fourteen patients were treated with R115777 as the first stage of a Simon two-stage phase II design. The absence of responses in those patients led to termination of the trial. Of note, the patients' tumors were not analyzed for NRAS mutation status. Given the prevalence of these mutations in melanoma, it is possible that none of these patients harbored NRAS mutation, by chance alone. It has yet to be demonstrated that tolerable drug exposure with an FTI significantly inhibits RAS. Whereas the possibility exists that more potent FTIs could prove effective, the concerns of dose-limiting off-target effects remain. Geronyltransferase inhibitors are in early clinical trials.

Targeting BRAF and MEK have been the focus of targeted therapy in melanoma. Because NRAS inhibition remains a challenge, there is evidence that blocking downstream effector pathways may be beneficial. The MAP kinase pathway has clearly been implicated in cancer pathophysiology in the setting of RAS mutations.[11] However, the PI3 kinase pathway, RAL-GDS signaling, and other RAS effector pathways may be also critical. Downstream of RAS lies BRAF, which harbors mutations in most melanomas.[12] The presence of BRAF mutations in melanoma supports the hypothesis that the MAP kinase pathway activity may be the key consequence of NRAS mutations. Notably, NRAS and BRAF mutations are mutually exclusive in melanoma.[13] BRAF is a serine-threonine kinase that phosphorylates MEK and, thereby, activates the MAP kinase pathway. Being hyperactivated in the setting of mutations in the kinase domain (particularly the most common V600E mutation), BRAF is a clear target for kinase inhibitors.[14] Although BRAF-selective kinase inhibitors were lacking, MEK inhibition has been considered a strategy for blocking pathway activation downstream of BRAF.

Each of the MEK inhibitors that have entered clinical trials are fairly selective, allosteric inhibitors of MEK 1 and MEK 2.[15] The first MEK inhibitor to enter phase II testing, CI-1040, was never evaluated in metastatic melanoma, as it was developed in the years before the discovery of BRAF mutations. In fact, 4 tumor histologies were included in the phase II evaluation of this agent, with colon cancer being the only in which BRAF mutations occur (15% of all cases).[16] Notably, a cohort of pancreatic cancer patients was enrolled and KRAS mutations are nearly ubiquitous in that tumor type. The lack of single-agent activity terminated the development of that agent. Some effort was made to perform serial tumor biopsies in patients enrolled on the phase I trial of CI-1040 and greater than 90% inhibition of the MAP kinase pathway was demonstrated for most patients, although their RAS and BRAF mutation status was unknown.[17] Two MEK inhibitors with improved pharmacokinetic properties have entered clinical development: AZD6244 and PD0325901. PD0325901 has only completed phase I testing, whereas AZD6244 was evaluated in a large phase II trial in melanoma.[18,19] In the PD0325901 trial, most patients enrolled had metastatic melanoma. Serial tumor biopsies were performed before and after 2 weeks of treatment to investigate inhibition of ERK phosphorylation, downstream of BRAF and MEK. At the higher doses administered, in most patients the tumors showed >90% inhibition of MEK phosphorylation. In this setting, two melanoma patients experienced objective responses, one with a BRAF mutation and the other with an NRAS mutation. It should be emphasized that there is no experimental evidence to support a threshold level of phosphor-ERK activity, below which one can reliably observe antitumor activity in BRAF or NRAS mutant melanoma. In the phase II trial of AZD6244, 100 patients with melanoma were treated, of whom 45 were found, in retrospect, to harbor BRAF mutation and 18 had an NRAS mutation. Five of the BRAF mutant patients (12%) and none of the NRAS mutant patients had objective responses. This trial established the proof-of-concept that a selective inhibition of MAP kinase pathway signaling can have activity in BRAF mutant melanoma, although the efficacy was limited to a small subset of BRAF mutant patients.

The development of selective BRAF inhibitors was a more protracted process in that the first truly selective BRAF inhibitor did not enter phase I testing until 2006, 4 years after the discovery of BRAF mutation. Sorafenib was the first BRAF inhibitor to be clinically available, but has greater potency for c-Raf and VEGF receptor 2.[20] Our group and others conducted clinical trials with single-agent sorafenib in melanoma and in combination with cytotoxic chemotherapies. Clinical efficacy with single-agent therapy appeared to be even less than with the MEK-selective agent, AZD6244.[21,22] In addition, the dose-limiting toxicities appeared related to VEGF receptor inhibition, as hand-foot syndrome was a limiting effect and that is a side effect of several other VEGF receptor inhibitors that lack RAF inhibitor activity.[23] Our group performed serial tumor biopsies in patients with metastatic melanoma receiving single-agent sorafenib and found less than 90% inhibition of ERK phosphorylation in all cases.[22] This left open the possibility that more potent and selective BRAF inhibitors might be efficacious. RAF-265, XL281, and PLX4032 were each developed to be more selective inhibitors of BRAF than sorafenib, and are in the advanced stages of phase I clinical trials.

TARGETING THE PI3K PATHWAY

Activated by RTKs or G-protein coupled receptors, including RAS, the phosphatidylinositol-3-kinase (PI3K) signaling pathway has been implicated in cancer pathophysiology due to its role in cell growth, proliferation, motility, and survival.[24] More recently, a role in chemoresistance also has come to light.[25,26] PI3K phosphorylates phosphatidylinositol-4,5-biphosphate (PIP2) to phosphatidylinositol-3,4,5-triphosphate (PIP3), which in turn leads to phosphorylation and activation of Akt (protein kinase B) by way of PDK-1. The substrates for Akt phosphorylation are numerous. Akt supports cell growth and proliferation by way of activation of the mammalian target of rapamycin (mTOR), a serine/threonine kinase that promotes transcription and translation.[27] Akt inhibition of GSK-3β, forkhead transcription factors, and the cyclin-dependent kinase (CDK) inhibitor, p27, promotes cell cycle progression and cell survival.[28–30] Whereas the antiapoptotic influences of Akt are exerted by way of phosphorylation of MDM2, bcl-associated death promoter (BAD), and caspase-9.[31–33] PTEN (phosphatase and tensin homolog deleted on chromosome 10), a tumor suppressor, negatively regulates Akt and the PI3K pathway, promoting cell cycle arrest and apoptosis and inhibiting MAPK signaling and migration.[34]

In melanoma, PI3K pathway activation is manifest by functional loss of PTEN or Akt overexpression.[34,35] Mutations of PI3K are rare in primary melanomas or melanoma metastases.[36,37] Akt3 overexpression has been documented in primary and metastatic melanomas and may correlate with tumor progression.[35,38] In vitro, siRNA knockdown of Akt3 led to apoptosis in melanoma cell lines. In vivo, tumor growth attributed to increased angiogenesis and generation of superoxide was seen after Akt overexpression was induced in melanoma xenografts.[39] Recently, mTOR activation, measured by phosphorylated ribosomal protein S6 expression, was noted to be greater in melanomas compared with benign melanocytic lesions.[40] Treatment of melanoma cell lines showing mTOR activation with rapamycin inhibted growth. Loss of functional PTEN in melanoma can be accomplished in a variety of ways including mutation, allelic loss/deletion, and silencing.[34,41,42] In vitro and in vivo, replacement of functional PTEN in PTEN-deficient melanoma cells suppresses growth.[34] Activating mutations in BRAF are often accompanied by PTEN loss, whereby activation of the two pathways seems to act in concert in melanoma progression and possibly in melanoma initiation.[13,43–45]

In vitro and in animal models, various PI3K pathway inhibitors have demonstrated antitumor activity and synergy with chemotherapy.[46] Specific PI3K or Akt inhibitors have been lacking for clinical development until recently. Due to prohibitive toxicities from nonselective PI3K inhibitors, research has focused on mTOR inhibitors. The recent influx of small-molecule PI3K and dual PI3K/mTOR inhibitors, such as SF1126, BGT226, BEZ235, XL147, and XL765, has resulted in several single-agent phase I and I/II studies in advanced solid tumors. PX-866, a derivative of wortmannin, showed promise in preclinical studies and a phase I trial of this oral agent also recently opened to accrual.[47] As PI3K inhibitors are developed in melanoma, it is worth noting that RAS mutations seem to predict resistance to PX-866 in human tumor xenografts, regardless of PI3K pathway aberrations.[48]

Temsirolimus (CCI-779) and everolimus (RAD-001), mTOR inhibitors, have shown minimal activity as single agents in melanoma.[49,50] However, given the potential cooperation between the MAPK and PI3K pathways in melanoma biology, there is particular interest in combining mTOR inhibitors with other targeted agents. Combination MAPK and PI3K inhibition with various drugs suppressed growth and invasion in melanoma cells in vitro.[43,51] Rapamycin in combination with sorafenib decreased melanoma cell growth and induced cell death in monolayer cultures, and suppressed invasive growth in organotypic cultures and completely down-regulated bcl-2 and mcl-1 protein levels.[52] The ongoing Southwest Oncology Group (SWOG) randomized phase II study, S0438, is assessing sorafenib in combination with either temsirolimus or R115777, an FTI, in treatment-naive stage IV melanoma. Additional studies combining temsirolimus with sorafenib alone or with bevacizumab in unresectable advanced melanoma are ongoing. Future studies combining PI3K pathway inhibitors with specific MAPK inhibitors, such as PLX4032 or MEK inhibitors, will be better suited to evaluate the activity of this strategy in melanoma given the nonselective nature of sorafenib as a Raf inhibitor. Combining agents to attack multiple molecular targets, either in the same pathway (vertical) or parallel pathways (horizontal) may produce sustained responses and prevent emergence of resistance. Several studies are being undertaken with perifosine, the inhibitor of Akt activation, alone and in combination with other molecular and cytotoxic agents in melanoma. Although no objective responses have been observed with single-agent perifosine in patients with metastatic melanoma unselected for PI3K pathway activity,[53] selecting patients and combining with other agents may improve outcomes.

The PI3K pathway also seems to mediate resistance to chemotherapy in melanoma, in particular to cisplatin.[25,26] Significantly enhanced growth inhibition of melanoma cells in monolayer cultures was seen when a PI3K inhibitor, wortmannin, LY294002, or rapamycin, was administered in combination with cisplatin or temozolomide, compared with either agent alone.[54] In addition, increased apoptosis, associated with significant decreases in mcl-1 and bcl-2 protein levels and suppression of invasive growth, was noted for these combinations in three-dimensional cultures. Interestingly, the combination of various MAPK inhibitors with chemotherapy did not augment growth inhibition. Finally, antitumor activity was increased in a human melanoma mouse xenograft treated with temsirolimus in combination with cisplatin or dacarbazine (DTIC).[55,56] However, the addition of DTIC to rapamycin in the same xenograft model did not increase antitumor activity.[57] A recently opened phase II study of everolimus in combination with temozolomide in unresectable stage IV melanoma will provide insight into this potential chemosensitization strategy.

TARGETING C-KIT

Following the identification of *V600E BRAF*, the finding of c-KIT (CD117) aberrations in melanoma[58] caused another stir in the melanoma community given the possible application of an effective, readily available, and well-tolerated therapeutic agent. Whether c-KIT plays a part in melanoma initiation or progression has been unclear despite its well-established role in normal melanocyte development.[59] c-KIT, a receptor tyrosine kinase, influences multiple signal transduction pathways including, but not limited to, the MAPK and PI3K pathways and MITF following activation by stem cell factor ligand.[59,60] Variable c-KIT protein expression has been demonstrated in melanoma; and mutations had been found infrequently when melanoma was analyzed as a single entity.[61–63] However, c-KIT mutation or amplification seems to be present in a subset of the less prevalent histologic subtypes of melanoma.[58,64–67] Array comparative genomic hybridization (CGH) showed c-KIT aberrations in 28% of chronic sun-damaged (CSD) melanomas, 36% of acral melanomas, and 39% of mucosal melanomas.[58] If limited to mutations only, the incidence ranges decrease to 2% to 17% of cutaneous (not selected for CSD), 11% to 23% of acral, and 15% to 22% of mucosal melanomas.

Mutation and allelic amplification of c-KIT have been demonstrated in other tumors, including gastrointestinal stromal tumors (GIST).[68,69] Overwhelming therapeutic success with imatinib, a tyrosine kinase inhibitor of c-KIT, and PDGFR, has been seen in most GIST patients, even those without mutations in either c-KIT or PDGFR.[70] Imatinib does not show clinical benefit in melanoma patients unselected for c-KIT mutation or amplification.[71–73] Currently, there are several ongoing studies seeking to determine if imatinib does provide clinical benefit in select subsets of melanoma patients, and if c-KIT mutation or amplification or protein expression predicts clinical benefit. These trials are exploring imatinib alone and in combination with a cytotoxic agent.[74,75] Some studies require prospective genotyping and protein expression, whereas others are performing this retrospectively. Melanomas with increased copy number or mutation have shown increased c-KIT protein expression.[58,63,64] However, the evidence is not consistent that elevated protein expression correlates with aberrant KIT genotype or with clinical response to imatinib in melanoma.[65,71,74] Inconsistent correlation of c-KIT protein expression with the presence of c-KIT mutations, and poor correlation of protein expression with imatinib responsiveness has already been demonstrated in GIST.[76,77]

There are now a few case reports of dramatic responses in melanoma patients treated with imatinib.[71,74,75,78] As the relationship between individual c-KIT mutations or amplification and responsiveness to imatinib has not been established in melanoma, data are being extrapolated from GIST studies. In GIST, exon 11 mutations, localized to the juxtamembrane region of the receptor, are the most common and demonstrate imatinib responsiveness in vitro and in vivo.[68] Other aberrations documented in GIST include deletions, substitutions/point mutations, duplications, insertions, and complex mutations that typically involve the regulatory or kinase domains. The first reported response in melanoma was from a phase II study of imatinib in unselected melanoma patients. A patient with metastatic acral melanoma experienced a near complete response (CR).[71] Retrospective analysis revealed high protein staining and alternative splicing in exon 15, which resulted in deletion of serine codon 715. As this same alternative splicing was seen in 4 other nonresponding patients, this is not predicative of imatinib sensitivity. Another case report describes a dramatic partial response (PR) in a patient with metastatic anorectal mucosal melanoma treated with imatinib 400 mg daily.[75] Genotyping revealed a 7-codon duplication in exon 11 and strong uniform staining on immunohistochemistry. During treatment, the tumor deceased in size and in fluorodeoxyglucose (FDG) avidity. Most recently, a CR was reported in a patient with metastatic anorectal mucosal melanoma treated with imatinib.[78] This patient was found to have a K642E mutation, present on exon 13 and well known in GIST, and amplification of the mutated allele. Of great interest is that after the patient developed recurrent disease following a dose reduction in imatinib secondary to hematologic toxicity, a second CR was achieved with an increased dose of imatinib. Finally, a sustained CR was seen in a patient with metastatic cutaneous melanoma treated with imatinib in combination with temozolomide.[74] On retrospective analysis, no mutation was detected in exons 9, 11, 13, or 17. This response may be explained by a c-KIT mutation outside of the exons examined or a c-KIT aberration other than a mutation, or that the CR was attributable to treatment with temozolomide. In this same ongoing study, another patient with two c-KIT mutations demonstrated significant regression of liver metastases. Soon after, the patient developed metastases of the central nervous system on treatment.

Another possible explanation for a lack of response to imatinib in melanoma may be because imatinib binds the ATP binding site of inactive conformation of c-KIT.[70] Therefore, mutations that stabilize the active formation of c-KIT will be resistant to imatinib therapy. Dasatinib (Sprycel), a second generation c-KIT inhibitor, may be more relevant as it binds the active and inactive formations of c-KIT.[79] There are three ongoing studies on dasatinib in melanoma: a phase II Eastern Collaborative Oncology Group (ECOG) protocol of the single agent in CSD, mucosal, or acral lentiginous melanoma with retrospective analysis of c-KIT amplifications or mutations; a single-agent phase II trial in unselected melanoma patients; and a phase I/II study of dasatinib in combination with DTIC in unselected melanoma patients.

TARGETING THE CELL CYCLE AND CYCLIN-DEPENDENT KINASES

Cell cycle control is often dysregulated in cancer. Cyclin-dependent kinases are the positive regulators of the cell cycle, whereby interaction of these serine/threonine kinases with their respective cyclins permits cell cycle progression. CDK4/6 followed by CDK2 facilitate cell cycle progression from G1 to S phase by way of their interactions with cyclin D and cyclin E, respectively.[80] CDK2 interacts with cyclin A to facilitate S phase progression and impacts the timing of S phase entry.[81] Finally, CDK1 interacts with cyclin A and cyclin B to mediate the G2 to M transition. The role of the cell cycle in melanoma is well known because of the variably penetrant p16INK4a (CDKN2A) germline mutation described in familial melanoma.[82] p16INK4a, an intrinsic cyclin-dependent kinase inhibitor, acts as a tumor suppressor and prevents cycle progression from G1 to S phase by blocking cyclin D/CDK4 phosphorylation and inactivation of retinoblastoma (Rb). The Rb pathway is frequently disrupted in sporadic and familial melanomas, be it through mutation, deletion, or hypermethylation of p16INK4a, cyclin D1 overexpression or amplification, or CDK4 overexpression, amplification or rarely mutation.[83–85] In additional, increasing CDK2 and cyclin E expression has been documented with melanoma progression[86] and treatment of melanoma cell lines with various CDK2 inhibitors decreased growth and/or caused G1 arrest.[87] Dysregulation of the cell cycle in conjunction with other signaling pathway aberrations seems to play a role in therapeutic resistance.[88–90]

Several novel, selective small-molecule CDK inhibitors are under investigation and are potentially of great relevance in melanoma. PD-0332991, an orally bioavailable, highly selective and potent CDK4/6 inhibitor, demonstrated G1 arrest in Rb+ tumor cells and significant tumor regression or growth delay in murine xenografts.[91,92] The first-in human phase I dose escalation trial of PD-0332991 in Rb+ tumors, including melanoma, demonstrated good tolerability at 2 dosing schedules.[93] With myelosuppression as a dose-limiting toxicity (DLT) for one schedule and no maximum tolerated dose (MTD) identified for the other schedule, other reported adverse events included anemia, nausea, vomiting, diarrhea, constipation, and fatigue. Prolonged stable disease (greater than 10–20 cycles) was seen with both dosing schedules and included three patients with melanoma. Another novel small-molecule inhibitor, SCH 727965, potently inhibits CDK2 in addition to CDK1, -5, -7, and -9.[94,95] In vitro, treatment with SCH 727965 inhibited DNA synthesis and caused cell cycle arrest and apoptosis. In tumor xenograft models, treatment produced tumor growth inhibition and regression that was enhanced by combination with cytotoxics. Two phase I studies of SCH 727965 in advanced malignancies have been conducted with differing schedules. The results of one of these studies has been presented and neutropenic infection was identified as the DLT with other reported adverse events including nausea/vomiting and transient elevation of liver function tests, with stable disease

(SD) as the best response.[96] Other promising agents that target multiple CDKs under early clinical investigation include SNS-032 (BMS- 387032), which inhibits CDK2, -7, and -9,[97] AG-024322, which targets CDK1, -2, and -4,[98] and ZK 304709, a multitargeted inhibitor of CDK1, -2, -4, -7, and -9, VEGFR 1, 2, and 3, and PDGFR-b.[99,100] The pan-CDK inhibitor, flavopiridol, demonstrated SD in 7 of 16 (duration 1.8–9.2 months) patients in a phase II study on metastatic melanoma.[101] The demonstration of prolonged SD is similar to that being seen with the newer selective agents. Restoring cell cycle control with these emerging agents will likely have a role in melanoma, most likely as an adjunct to other agents.

TARGETING MICROPHTHALMIA-ASSOCIATED TRANSCRIPTION FACTOR/EPIGENETICS

MITF is one of the latest molecules proposed as a melanoma oncogene.[102] MITF expression is influenced by multiple pathways including a-melanocyte stimulating hormone (MSH), c-KIT/MAPK, and Wnt/b-catenin.[103] Required for melanocyte development, MITF regulates the transcription of a variety of genes impacting essential functions including, but not limited to, differentiation by way of pigment production,[104] cell fate and survival by way of regulation of bcl-2 and p21,[105,106] and cell cycle progression by way of regulation of CDK2 and p16INK4a.[87,107] In melanoma cell lines, significant MITF copy gains were documented and accompanied by V600E BRAF and p16 pathway inactivation.[102] In human cutaneous primary melanomas and melanoma metastases, MITF amplification was seen in 10% to 20%, was absent in nevi, and correlated with decreased survival. In vitro studies demonstrated cooperation between MITF overexpression and mutant V600E BRAF in transforming melanocytes. These findings highlight the heterogeneity of aberrations seen across melanoma and cooperativity amongst pathway aberrations in melanoma initiation and progression.

While the exact role of MITF in melanoma initiation and progression continues to be unraveled, its potential as a therapeutic target cannot be overlooked. Direct inhibition of transcription factors is difficult. However, suppressed MITF expression and cell growth were produced in melanoma cell lines and in mouse xenografts in response to treatment with a variety of histone deacetylase inhibitors (HDACi).[108] HDACi prevent the removal of acetyl groups from histones, thus impacting chromatin conformation and gene transcription.[109] However, there are also multiple nonhistone proteins targeted by HDACi that play a role in their antitumor activity. SAHA and MS-275 are two of the best studied HDACi to date. SAHA was recently approved for the treatment of progressive, persistent, or refractory cutaneous T cell lymphoma.[110] Common side effects included diarrhea, fatigue, nausea, and anorexia, and anemia and thrombocytopenia. A phase II study of SAHA in advanced unresectable melanoma incorporated posttreatment gene expression profiles as potential predictive markers of response in addition to standard response criteria. Prolonged stable disease was seen with either of two dosages and schedules of MS-275 in a small-randomized phase II study for efficacy and safety in pretreated metastatic melanoma.[111] Although no objective responses were seen, the duration of stable disease ranged from 8 to 48 weeks and the treatment was well tolerated with only mild to moderate nausea and hypophosphatemia most commonly reported. Further investigation of HDACi in combination with other agents, particularly cytotoxic chemotherapy, in melanoma may be warranted as HDACi have shown additive or synergistic antitumor activity with a variety of agents, and increased MITF copy number in melanoma cell lines demonstrated correlation with chemoresistance.[102,109]

TARGETING APOPTOSIS SIGNALING

Apoptosis is defined as irreversible cell death associated with loss of mitochondrial membrane potential, release of cytochrome *c*, and activation of caspases (**Fig. 2**). Caspases along with downstream activated nucleases and lipases are the executors of cell suicide. The gatekeepers of the decision to undergo apoptosis are B cell lymphoma/leukemia 2 (Bcl2) and the Bcl-2–related family of pro- and antiapoptotic proteins. These proteins all contain multiple hydrophobic protein domains called Bcl-2 homology (BH) domains. This protein family can be subdivided into three groups: (1) the prosurvival Bcl-2 subfamily including Bcl-2, Bcl-xL, Bcl-w, Mcl-1, and A1; (2) the proapoptotic effector Bax subfamily, which includes Bax, Bak, and Bok; (3) the proapoptotic facilitators, the BH3-only subfamily: Bad, Bid, Bik, Blk, Hrk, BNIP3, and BimL.

Bcl-2

The structure of Bcl-2 consists of four BH domains and a transmembrane domain localizing the protein to the mitochondria and endoplasmic reticulum. Overexpression of Bcl-2 in melanoma cells potentiates chemotherapy resistance.[112,113] Recent evidence suggests that mutant BRAF and CRAF signaling may lead to ERK-dependent[114] and ERK-independent prosurvival signals by directly engaging Bcl-2 family members.[115] Because the function of Bcl-2 depends on physical interactions rather than kinase activity, drug development of Bcl-2 inhibitors has lagged behind the drug development of kinase inhibitors. Natural compounds such as tea polyphenols and gossypol have been explored as potential Bcl-2 inhibitors,[116] but were found to have many other mechanisms of anticancer activity. The first targeted therapy against Bcl-2 was the antisense molecule oblimersen (Genasence). Oblimersen consists of antisense DNA that binds to native Bcl-2 mRNA leading to its degradation. Oblimersen was developed and tested in a wide variety of malignancies.[117] A large randomized phase III trial of oblimersen with dacarbazine versus dacarbazine alone failed to identify an overall survival benefit for oblimersen with chemotherapy.[118] A subset analysis revealed a survival difference in patients without an elevated lactate dehydrogenase level. Some of the reasons postulated for why such a promising drug failed to deliver

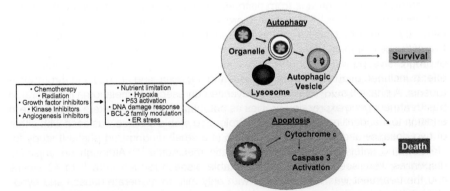

Fig. 2. Numerous reports have recently identified autophagy in cells exposed to stresses that were traditionally thought to induce apoptosis. Stresses such as chemotherapy, radiation, kinase inhibitors, or growth factor withdrawal affect critical regulators such as p53 or Akt that in turn regulate apoptosis. Increasing evidence suggests that these same regulators are also important regulators of autophagy.

as profound an effect as expected from the results of preclinical studies are: (1) drug instability; (2) inadequate target inhibition; (3) the presence of intrinsic resistance mechanisms; (4) the target is not as critical to melanoma biology as previously believed. Human pathology evidence indicates that expression levels of Bcl-2 may not correlate with disease severity. In one study, increased levels of Bcl-2 conferred a favorable prognosis in uveal melanomas.[119] In another study, high levels of Bcl-2 expression were observed in nevi, but low levels of Bcl-2 expression were observed in metastatic melanoma lesions.[120]

Given the central role of Bcl-2 in preventing cell death, new drugs have been developed that target Bcl-2. Small-molecule inhibitors of Bcl-2 have been developed and are currently entering clinical trials. ABT-737, and the orally available analog ABT-263, mimic the BH domain and tightly bind to Bcl-2, Bcl-xL, and Bcl-w. Preclinical evidence demonstrated tumor regression across a variety of malignancies. In preclinical studies on melanoma, single-agent ABT-737 treatment did not result in significant tumor cell death, but if combined with either a proteasome inhibitor[121] or an MEK inhibitor,[122] synergistic cell death was seen. These studies suggest that the role of Bcl-2 inhibitors in the treatment of melanoma may be in combination with other targeted therapies.

Bcl-2-Related Family Members

One of the concerns with targeting Bcl-2 is that other prosurvival Bcl-2 family members may compensate for drug-induced Bcl-2 loss of function. Studies on chronic lymphocytic leukemia, another disease in which Bcl-2 has been identified as an important therapeutic target, have determined that overexpression of Bcl-xL and BCL2A1 contributes to resistance to ABT-737.[123] The antiapoptotic factor, Mcl-1, is overexpressed in dysplastic nevi, and in primary and metastatic melanomas, compared with normal nevi.[124,125] Overexpression of Mcl-1 has also been identified as a mechanism of resistance to ABT-737.[126] In contrast to ABT-737, the small-molecule inhibitor, obatoclax mesylate, is a pan-Bcl-2-family inhibitor. This drug has potent activity against Mcl-1. In certain melanoma cell lines, Mcl-1 was found to be a more important contributor to drug resistance than Bcl-2 or Bcl-xL.[127] The next generation of clinical trials in melanoma will hopefully include combination regimens of novel Bcl-2 inhibitors and other targeted therapies.

Beyond Apoptosis: Targeting Autophagy in Melanoma

Besides changes in Bcl-2 and Mcl-1, there are a host of additional signaling defects that can contribute to defective apoptosis in melanoma. While investigating the general stress responses available to cancer cells defective in apoptosis, Thompson and others have uncovered a new resistance mechanism to cancer therapies: autophagy (see **Fig. 2**). The execution of apoptosis begins with Bax and Bak, which form oligomeric pores in the mitochondria on activation. When cells genetically deficient in Bax and Bak were deprived of an essential growth factor, they were able to survive this stress by undergoing autophagy,[128] the process of intracellular self-eating characterized by the sequestration of mitochondria and long-lived proteins in autophagic vesicles followed by the destruction of vesicle contents through fusion with the lysosome.

Autophagic vesicles are closely related to melanosomes, and preliminary evidence indicates melanoma cells are especially reliant on this process to survive the metabolic and therapeutic stresses they encounter (R. Amaravadi, unpublished data, 2008). Autophagy is often activated in parallel with apoptosis, but unlike apoptosis it is a reversible process that cells can rely on to clear drug-induced intracellular damage. Most cancer therapies have been found to activate autophagy in cell culture and mouse models of cancer.[129] Although there is still a great deal to be learned about the role of autophagy in cancer biology, efforts at therapeutically inhibiting drug-induced autophagy in the hope of augmenting the efficacy of existing therapies are underway. The decades-old drug, chloroquine, and its more modern derivative, hydroxychloroquine, can inhibit autophagy by deacidifying the lysosome. Based on preclinical evidence that hydroxychloroquine can augment the efficacy of chemotherapy and targeted therapies in a wide variety of cancer models,[129,130] clinical trials combining hydroxychloroquine with chemotherapy or targeted therapies have been launched. As the molecular biology of autophagy becomes better understood, more specific autophagy inhibitors will likely be developed.

TARGETING ANGIOGENESIS

The successful development of VEGF signaling inhibitors in other cancers raises the possibility that this approach might be efficacious in melanoma. However, only renal cell carcinoma seems susceptible to single-agent therapy with a monoclonal antibody against VEGF (bevacizumab) or a VEGF receptor tyrosine kinase inhibitor (sorafenib or sunitinib).[131–133] The addition of bevacizumab to cytotoxic chemotherapy has improved outcomes in colon, non–small cell lung, and breast cancer, but not in pancreatic cancer.[134–137] It is clear that melanoma is not akin to renal cell carcinoma, as neither bevacizumab or sorafenib have significant single-agent activity in phase II trials.[21,22,138] There are data to support the possibility that the addition of either of these agents to chemotherapy may prolong progression-free survival compared with chemotherapy alone, but this has not yet been established with certainty.[139–140] The results of 2 ongoing clinical trials will give much greater insight into this question (http://nci.nih.gov/search/ResultsClinicalTrials). A randomized phase II trial has been completed comparing carboplatin, paclitaxel, and bevacizumab to carboplatin and paclitaxel alone in 200 patients with metastatic melanoma. A much larger, phase III trial is fully accrued and compares carboplatin, paclitaxel, and sorafenib to carboplatin and paclitaxel alone in 824 patients, with overall survival as the primary endpoint. Both trials are expected to report results in 2009.

PROSPECTS FOR IMPROVED OUTCOMES

Progress in unraveling the nuances of melanoma initiation and progression continues at a rapid pace. Our understanding of melanoma biology has evolved significantly in the last decade with a greater understanding of the influences on the cell cycle, the finding of activating BRAF mutations, the potential role of c-KIT, and glimpses into other relevant molecules and pathways and their interplay. To understand the contribution of each individual class of agents, novel response criteria are being explored. With the advent of molecular agents, cytostatic effects and prolonged disease stabilization are being recognized as true manifestations of clinical benefit in addition to traditional tumor response criteria. In the future, molecular parameters, in tissue or imaging, will likely be incorporated into standard response criteria. Only in this way will the building blocks be established for multidrug targeted therapy regimens.

The lack of improvement of survival with systemic therapies to date is well known in the melanoma community. The metaanalysis by Korn and colleagues proposed a reevaluation of phase II trial design and endpoints in an effort to facilitate the movement of promising novel therapies or regimens into phase III trials.[141] There are a host of promising targeted therapies in various stages of clinical development. Single agent evaluation must precede combinatorial strategies. For each agent, it is essential to establish that the intended molecular effect is being achieved, even in the absence of clinical efficacy. This will permit an armamentarium of validated targeted drugs to enter the arena of combination testing. In melanoma, multiple pathways and cellular processes combine to create a tumor with remarkable resistance to conventional cytotoxic agents. The hope is that combinations of targeted agents that counter the key oncogenic events in an individual patient's melanoma will circumvent this tumor's formidable defenses.

REFERENCES

1. van 't Veer LJ, Burgering BM, Versteeg R, et al. N-ras mutations in human cutaneous melanoma from sun-exposed body sites. Mol Cell Biol 1989;9(7):3114–6.
2. Edlundh-Rose E, Egyházi S, Omholt K, et al. NRAS and BRAF mutations in melanoma tumours in relation to clinical characteristics: a study based on mutation screening by pyrosequencing. Melanoma Res 2006;16(6):471–8.
3. McGrath JP, Capon DJ, Goeddel DV, et al. Comparative biochemical properties of normal and activated human ras p21 protein. Nature 1984;310:644–9.
4. Sweet RW, Yokoyama S, Kamata T, et al. The product of ras is a GTPase and the T24 oncogenic mutant is deficient in this activity. Nature 1984;311:273–5.
5. Schafer WR, Kim R, Sterne R, et al. Genetic and pharmacological suppression of oncogenic mutations in ras genes of yeast and humans. Science 1989;245:379–85.
6. Schafer WR, Trueblood CE, Yang CC, et al. Enzymatic coupling of cholesterol intermediates to a mating pheromone precursor and to the ras protein. Science 1990;249:1133–9.
7. Kohl NE, Omer CA, Conner MW, et al. Inhibition of farnesyltransferase induces regression of mammary and salivary carcinomas in ras transgenic mice. Nat Med 1995;1:792–7.
8. Nagasu T, Yoshimatsu K, Rowell C, et al. Inhibition of human tumor xenograft growth by treatment with the farnesyl transferase inhibitor B956. Cancer Res 1995;55:5310–4.
9. Downward J. Targeting RAS signalling pathways in cancer therapy. Nat Rev Cancer 2003;3:11–22.
10. Gajewski TF, Niedzwiecki D, Johnson J, et al. Phase II study of the farnesyltransferase inhibitor R115777 in advanced melanoma: CALGB 500104. J Clin Oncol 2006 ASCO Annual Meeting Proceedings Part I. vol. 24, No. 18S (June 20 Supplement), 2006:8014.
11. Dent P, Reardon DB, Morrison DK, et al. Regulation of Raf-1 and Raf-1 mutants by Ras-dependent and Ras-independent mechanisms in vitro. Mol Cell Biol 1995;15(8):4125–35.
12. Davies H, Bignell GR, Cox C, et al. Mutations of the BRAF gene in human cancer. Nature 2002;417(6892):949–54.
13. Tsao H, Goel V, Wu H, et al. Genetic interaction between NRAS and BRAF mutations and PTEN/MMAC1 inactivation in melanoma. J Invest Dermatol 2004;122(2):337–41.
14. Wan PT, Garnett MJ, Roe SM, et al. Mechanism of activation of the RAF-ERK signaling pathway by oncogenic mutations of B-RAF. Cell 2004;116(6):855–67.
15. Sebolt-Leopold JS, Herrera R. Targeting the mitogen-activated protein kinase cascade to treat cancer. Nat Rev Cancer 2004;4(12):937–47.
16. Rinehart J, Adjei AA, Lorusso PM, et al. Multicenter phase II study of the oral MEK inhibitor, CI-1040, in patients with advanced non-small-cell lung, breast, colon, and pancreatic cancer. J Clin Oncol 2004;22(22):4456–62.

17. Lorusso PM, Adjei AA, Varterasian M, et al. Phase I and pharmacodynamic study of the oral MEK inhibitor CI-1040 in patients with advanced malignancies. J Clin Oncol 2005;23(23):5281–93.
18. Dummer R, Robert C, Chapman PB, et al. AZD6244 (ARRY-142886) vs temozolomide (TMZ) in patients (pts) with advanced melanoma: An open-label, randomized, multicenter, phase II study. J Clin Oncol 2008;26(20 suppl):9033 [abstract].
19. Lorusso P, Krishnamurthi S, Rinehart JR, et al. A phase 1-2 clinical study of a second generation oral MEK inhibitor, PD 0325901 in patients with advanced cancer. (June 1 Supplement), 2005. ASCO Annual Meeting Proceedings Part I. J Clin Oncol 2005;vol. 23(No. 16S):3011.
20. Wilhelm SM, Carter C, Tang L, et al. BAY 43-9006 exhibits broad spectrum oral antitumor activity and targets the RAF/MEK/ERK pathway and receptor tyrosine kinases involved in tumor progression and angiogenesis. Cancer Res 2004; 64(19):7099–109.
21. Eisen T, Ahmad T, Flaherty KT, et al. Sorafenib in advanced melanoma: a Phase II randomised discontinuation trial analysis. Br J Cancer 2006;95(5):581–6.
22. Flaherty KT, Redlinger M, Schuchter LM, et al. Phase I/II, pharmacokinetic and pharmacodynamic trial of BAY 43-9006 alone in patients with metastatic melanoma. (June 1 Supplement), 2005. ASCO Annual Meeting Proceedings Part I. J Clin Oncol 2005;vol. 23(No. 16S):3037.
23. Faivre S, Delbaldo C, Vera K, et al. Safety, pharmacokinetic, and antitumor activity of SU11248, a novel oral multitarget tyrosine kinase inhibitor, in patients with cancer. J Clin Oncol 2006;24(1):25–35.
24. Vivanco I, Sawyers CL. The phosphatidylinositol 3-kinase AKT pathway in human cancer. Nat Rev Cancer 2002;2:489–501.
25. Belyanskaya LL, Hopkins-Donaldson S, Kurtz S, et al. Cisplatin activates Akt in small cell lung cancer cells and attenuates apoptosis by survivin upregulation. Int J Cancer 2005;117:755–63.
26. Ohta T, Ohmichi M, Hayasaka T, et al. Inhibition of phosphatidylinositol 3-kinase increases efficacy of cisplatin in in vivo ovarian cancer models. Endocrinology 2006;147:1761–9.
27. Hay N, Sonenberg N. Upstream and downstream of mTOR. Genes Dev 2004;18: 1926–45.
28. Burgering BM, Kops GJ. Cell cycle and death control: long live forkheads. Trends Biochem Sci 2002;27:352–60.
29. Diehl JA, Cheng M, Roussel MF, et al. Glycogen synthase kinase-3beta regulates cyclin D1 proteolysis and subcellular localization. Genes Dev 1998;12: 3499–511.
30. Viglietto G, Motti ML, Bruni P, et al. Cytoplasmic relocalization and inhibition of the cyclin-dependent kinase inhibitor p27(Kip1) by PKB/Akt-mediated phosphorylation in breast cancer. Nat Med 2002;8:1136–44.
31. Cardone MH, Roy N, Stennicke HR, et al. Regulation of cell death protease caspase-9 by phosphorylation. Science 1998;282:1318–21.
32. Datta SR, Dudek H, Tao X, et al. Akt phosphorylation of BAD couples survival signals to the cell-intrinsic death machinery. Cell 1997;91:231–41.
33. Mayo LD, Donner DB. A phosphatidylinositol 3-kinase/Akt pathway promotes translocation of Mdm2 from the cytoplasm to the nucleus. Proc Natl Acad Sci USA 2001;98:11598–603.
34. Wu H, Goel V, Haluska FG. PTEN signaling pathways in melanoma. Oncogene 2003;22:3113–22.

35. Stahl JM, Sharma A, Cheung M, et al. Deregulated Akt3 activity promotes development of malignant melanoma. Cancer Res 2004;64:7002–10.
36. Curtin JA, Stark MS, Pinkel D, et al. PI3-kinase subunits are infrequent somatic targets in melanoma. J Invest Dermatol 2006;126:1660–3.
37. Omholt K, Krockel D, Ringborg U, et al. Mutations of PIK3CA are rare in cutaneous melanoma. Melanoma Res 2006;16:197–200.
38. Dhawan P, Singh AB, Ellis DL, et al. Constitutive activation of Akt/protein kinase B in melanoma leads to up-regulation of nuclear factor-kappaB and tumor progression. Cancer Res 2002;62:7335–42.
39. Govindarajan B, Sligh JE, Vincent BJ, et al. Overexpression of Akt converts radial growth melanoma to vertical growth melanoma. J Clin Invest 2007;117:719–29.
40. Karbowniczek M, Spittle CS, Morrison T, et al. mTOR is activated in the majority of malignant melanomas. J Invest Dermatol 2008;128:980–7.
41. Mirmohammadsadegh A, Marini A, Nambiar S, et al. Epigenetic silencing of the PTEN gene in melanoma. Cancer Res 2006;66:6546–52.
42. Zhou XP, Gimm O, Hampel H, et al. Epigenetic PTEN silencing in malignant melanomas without PTEN mutation. Am J Pathol 2000;157:1123–8.
43. Smalley KS, Haass NK, Brafford PA, et al. Multiple signaling pathways must be targeted to overcome drug resistance in cell lines derived from melanoma metastases. Mol Cancer Ther 2006;5:1136–44.
44. Curtin J, Fridlyand J, Kageshita T, et al. Distinct sets of genetic alterations in melanoma. N Engl J Med 2005;353:2135–47.
45. Dankort D, et al. Braf(V600E) cooperates with Pten loss to induce metastatic melanoma. Nat Genet 2009 [Epub ahead of print].
46. Yap TA, Garrett MD, Walton MI, et al. Targeting the PI3K-AKT-mTOR pathway: progress, pitfalls, and promises. Curr Opin Pharmacol 2008;8:393–412.
47. Ihle NT, Williams R, Chow S, et al. Molecular pharmacology and antitumor activity of PX-866, a novel inhibitor of phosphoinositide-3-kinase signaling. Mol Cancer Ther 2004;3:763–72.
48. Ihle NT, Lemos R Jr, Wipf P, et al. Mutations in the phosphatidylinositol-3-kinase pathway predict for antitumor activity of the inhibitor PX-866 whereas oncogenic Ras is a dominant predictor for resistance. Cancer Res 2009;69:143–50.
49. Margolin K, Longmate J, Baratta T, et al. CCI-779 in metastatic melanoma: a phase II trial of the California Cancer Consortium. Cancer 2005;104:1045–8.
50. Rao RD, Allred JB, Windschitl HE, et al. N0377: results of NCCTG phase II trial of the mTOR inhibitor RAD-001 in metastatic melanoma. J Clin Oncol 2007;25:8530 [abstract].
51. Meier F, Busch S, Lasithiotakis K, et al. Combined targeting of MAPK and AKT signalling pathways is a promising strategy for melanoma treatment. Br J Dermatol 2007;156:1204–13.
52. Lasithiotakis KG, Sinnberg TW, Schittek B, et al. Combined inhibition of MAPK and mTOR signaling inhibits growth, induces cell death, and abrogates invasive growth of melanoma cells. J Invest Dermatol 2008;128:2013–23.
53. Ernst DS, Eisenhauer E, Wainman N, et al. Phase II study of perifosine in previously untreated patients with metastatic melanoma. Invest New Drugs 2005;23:569–75.
54. Sinnberg T, Lasithiotakis K, Niessner H, et al. Inhibition of PI3K-AKT-mTOR signaling sensitizes melanoma cells to cisplatin and temozolomide. J Invest Dermatol 2008 [Epub ahead of print].
55. Thallinger C, Poeppl W, Pratscher B, et al. CCI-779 plus cisplatin is highly effective against human melanoma in a SCID mouse xenotransplantation model. Pharmacology 2007;79:207–13.

56. Thallinger C, Werzowa J, Poeppl W, et al. Comparison of a treatment strategy combining CCI-779 plus DTIC versus DTIC monotreatment in human melanoma in SCID mice. J Invest Dermatol 2007;127:2411–7.
57. Thallinger C, Skorjanec S, Soleiman A, et al. Orally administered rapamycin, dacarbazine or both for treatment of human melanoma evaluated in severe combined immunodeficiency mice. Pharmacology 2008;82:233–8.
58. Curtin JA, Busam K, Pinkel D, et al. Somatic activation of KIT in distinct subtypes of melanoma. J Clin Oncol 2006;24:4340–6.
59. Grichnik JM. Kit and melanocyte migration. J Invest Dermatol 2006;126:945–7.
60. Hemesath TJ, Price ER, Takemoto C, et al. MAP kinase links the transcription factor Microphthalmia to c-Kit signalling in melanocytes. Nature 1998;391:298–301.
61. Janku F, Novotny J, Julis I, et al. KIT receptor is expressed in more than 50% of early-stage malignant melanoma: a retrospective study of 261 patients. Melanoma Res 2005;15:251–6.
62. Willmore-Payne C, Holden JA, Hirschowitz S, et al. BRAF and c-kit gene copy number in mutation-positive malignant melanoma. Hum Pathol 2006;37:520–7.
63. Willmore-Payne C, Holden JA, Tripp S, et al. Human malignant melanoma: detection of BRAF- and c-kit-activating mutations by high-resolution amplicon melting analysis. Hum Pathol 2005;36:486–93.
64. Antonescu CR, Busam KJ, Francone TD, et al. L576P kit mutation in anal melanomas correlates with kit protein expression and is sensitive to specific kinase inhibition. Int J Cancer 2007;121(2):257–64.
65. Beadling C, Jacobson-Dunlop E, Hodi FS, et al. KIT gene mutations and copy number in melanoma subtypes. Clin Cancer Res 2008;14:6821–8.
66. Rivera RS, Nagatsuka H, Gunduz M, et al. C-kit protein expression correlated with activating mutations in KIT gene in oral mucosal melanoma. Virchows Arch 2008;452:27–32.
67. Satzger I, Schaefer T, Kuettler U, et al. Analysis of c-KIT expression and KIT gene mutation in human mucosal melanomas. Br J Cancer 2008;99:2065–9.
68. Lasota J, Miettinen M. Clinical significance of oncogenic KIT and PDGFRA mutations in gastrointestinal stromal tumours. Histopathology 2008;53:245–66.
69. Sleijfer S, Wiemer E, Seynaeve C, et al. Improved insight into resistance mechanisms to imatinib in gastrointestinal stromal tumors: a basis for novel approaches and individualization of treatment. Oncologist 2007;12:719–26.
70. Buchdunger E, Cioffi CL, Law N, et al. Abl protein-tyrosine kinase inhibitor STI571 inhibits in vitro signal transduction mediated by c-kit and platelet-derived growth factor receptors. J Pharmacol Exp Ther 2000;295:139–45.
71. Kim KB, Eton O, Davis DW, et al. Phase II trial of imatinib mesylate in patients with metastatic melanoma. Br J Cancer 2008;99:734–40.
72. Ugurel S, Hildenbrand R, Zimpfer A, et al. Lack of clinical efficacy of imatinib in metastatic melanoma. Br J Cancer 2005;92:1398–405.
73. Wyman K, Atkins MB, Prieto V, et al. Multicenter Phase II trial of high-dose imatinib mesylate in metastatic melanoma: significant toxicity with no clinical efficacy. Cancer 2006;106:2005–11.
74. Fecher LA, Nathanson K, Flaherty KT, et al. Phase I/II of imatinib and temozolomide in advanced unresectable melanoma. J Clin Oncol 2008;26:9059 [abstract].
75. Hodi FS, Friedlander P, Corless CL, et al. Major response to imatinib mesylate in KIT-mutated melanoma. J Clin Oncol 2008;26:2046–51.
76. Chirieac LR, Trent JC, Steinert DM, et al. Correlation of immunophenotype with progression-free survival in patients with gastrointestinal stromal tumors treated with imatinib mesylate. Cancer 2006;107:2237–44.

77. Medeiros F, Corless CL, Duensing A, et al. KIT-negative gastrointestinal stromal tumors: proof of concept and therapeutic implications. Am J Surg Pathol 2004; 28:889–94.

78. Lutzky J, Bauer J, Bastian BC. Dose-dependent, complete response to imatinib of a metastatic mucosal melanoma with a K642E KIT mutation. Pigment Cell Melanoma Res 2008;21:492–3.

79. Schittenhelm MM, Shiraga S, Schroeder A, et al. Dasatinib (BMS-354825), a dual SRC/ABL kinase inhibitor, inhibits the kinase activity of wild-type, juxtamembrane, and activation loop mutant KIT isoforms associated with human malignancies. Cancer Res 2006;66:473–81.

80. Schwartz GK, Shah MA. Targeting the cell cycle: a new approach to cancer therapy. J Clin Oncol 2005;23:9408–21.

81. Berthet C, Aleem E, Coppola V, et al. Cdk2 knockout mice are viable. Curr Biol 2003;13:1775–85.

82. Hussussian CJ, Struewing JP, Goldstein AM, et al. Germline p16 mutations in familial melanoma. Nat Genet 1994;8(1):15–21.

83. Sauter ER, Yeo UC, von Stemm A, et al. Cyclin D1 is a candidate oncogene in cutaneous melanoma. Cancer Res 2002;62:3200–6.

84. Li W, Sanki A, Karim RZ, et al. The role of cell cycle regulatory proteins in the pathogenesis of melanoma. Pathology 2006 Aug;38(4):287–301.

85. Zuo L, Weger J, Yang Q, et al. Germline mutations in the p16INK4a binding domain of CDK4 in familial melanoma. Nat Genet 1996;12(1):97–9.

86. Georgieva J, Sinha P, Schadendorf D. Expression of cyclins and cyclin dependent kinases in human benign and malignant melanocytic lesions. J Clin Pathol 2001;54:229–35.

87. Du J, Widlund HR, Horstmann MA, et al. Critical role of CDK2 for melanoma growth linked to its melanocyte-specific transcriptional regulation by MITF. Cancer Cell 2004;6:565–76.

88. Bhatt KV, Hu R, Spofford LS, et al. Mutant B-RAF signaling and cyclin D1 regulate Cks1/S-phase kinase-associated protein 2-mediated degradation of p27Kip1 in human melanoma cells. Oncogene 2007;26:1056–66.

89. Smalley KS, Lioni M, Dalla Palma M, et al. Increased cyclin D1 expression can mediate BRAF inhibitor resistance in BRAF V600E-mutated melanomas. Mol Cancer Ther 2008;7:2876–83.

90. Smalley KS, Contractor R, Nguyen TK, et al. Identification of a novel subgroup of melanomas with KIT/cyclin-dependent kinase-4 overexpression. Cancer Res 2008;68:5743–52.

91. Fry DW, Harvey PJ, Keller PR, et al. Specific inhibition of cyclin-dependent kinase 4/6 by PD 0332991 and associated antitumor activity in human tumor xenografts. Mol Cancer Ther 2004;3:1427–38.

92. Toogood PL, Harvey PJ, Repine JT, et al. Discovery of a potent and selective inhibitor of cyclin-dependent kinase 4/6. J Med Chem 2005;48:2388–406.

93. O'Dwyer PJ, LoRusso P, DeMichele A, et al. A phase I dose escalation trial of daily oral CDK 4/6 inhibitor PD-0332991. J Clin Oncol 2007;25:3550 [abstract].

94. Wang Y, et al. SCH 727965, a novel small cyclin-dependent kinase inhibitor, has potent anti-tumor activity in a wide-spectrum of human tumor xenograft models. AACR 2008 [abstract 1594].

95. Parry D, et al. In vitro and in vivo characterization of SCH727965 a novel potent cyclin dependent kinase inhibitor. AACR 2007 [abstract 4371].

96. Shapiro GI, et al. A phase I dose escalation study of the safety, pharmacokinetics and pharmacodynamics of the novel cyclin-dependent kinase inhibitor

SCH 727965 administered every 32 weeks in subjects with advanced malignancies. ASCO 2008 [abstract 3532].

97. Heath EI, Bible K, Martell RE, et al. A phase 1 study of SNS-032 (formerly BMS-387032), a potent inhibitor of cyclin-dependent kinases 2, 7 and 9 administered as a single oral dose and weekly infusion in patients with metastatic refractory solid tumors. Invest New Drugs 2008;26:59–65.

98. Brown AP, Courtney CL, Criswell KA, et al. Toxicity and toxicokinetics of the cyclin-dependent kinase inhibitor AG-024322 in cynomolgus monkeys following intravenous infusion. Cancer Chemother Pharmacol 2008;62:1091–101.

99. Ahmed S, Molife R, Shaw H, et al. Phase I dose-escalation study of ZK 304709, an oral multitarget tumor growth inhibitor (MTGI), administered for 14 days of a 28-day cycle. J Clin Oncol 2006;24:2076 [abstract].

100. Graham J, Wagner K, Plummer R, et al. Phase I dose-escalation study of novel oral multitarget tumor growth inhibitor (MTGI) ZK 304709 administered daily for 7 days of a 21-day cycle to patients with advanced solid tumors. J Clin Oncol 2006;24:2073 [abstract].

101. Burdette-Radoux S, Tozer RG, Lohmann RC, et al. Phase II trial of flavopiridol, a cyclin dependent kinase inhibitor, in untreated metastatic malignant melanoma. Invest New Drugs 2004;22:315–22.

102. Garraway LA, Widlund HR, Rubin MA, et al. Integrative genomic analyses identify MITF as a lineage survival oncogene amplified in malignant melanoma. Nature 2005;436:117–22.

103. Levy C, Khaled M, Fisher DE. MITF: master regulator of melanocyte development and melanoma oncogene. Trends Mol Med 2006;12:406–14.

104. Hemesath TJ, Steingrimsson E, McGill G, et al. Microphthalmia, a critical factor in melanocyte development, defines a discrete transcription factor family. Genes Dev 1994;8:2770–80.

105. Carreira S, Goodall J, Aksan I, et al. Mitf cooperates with Rb1 and activates p21Cip1 expression to regulate cell cycle progression. Nature 2005;433:764–9.

106. McGill GG, Horstmann M, Widlund HR, et al. Bcl2 regulation by the melanocyte master regulator Mitf modulates lineage survival and melanoma cell viability. Cell 2002;109:707–18.

107. Loercher AE, Tank EM, Delston RB, et al. MITF links differentiation with cell cycle arrest in melanocytes by transcriptional activation of INK4A. J Cell Biol 2005;168:35–40.

108. Yokoyama S, Feige E, Poling LL, et al. Pharmacologic suppression of MITF expression via HDAC inhibitors in the melanocyte lineage. Pigment Cell Melanoma Res 2008;21:457–63.

109. Xu WS, Parmigiani RB, Marks PA. Histone deacetylase inhibitors: molecular mechanisms of action. Oncogene 2007;26:5541–52.

110. Olsen EA, Kim YH, Kuzel TM, et al. Phase IIb multicenter trial of vorinostat in patients with persistent, progressive, or treatment refractory cutaneous T-cell lymphoma. J Clin Oncol 2007;25:3109–15.

111. Hauschild A, Trefzer U, Garbe C, et al. Multicenter phase II trial of the histone deacetylase inhibitor pyridylmethyl-N-{4-[(2-aminophenyl)-carbamoyl]-benzyl}-carbamate in pretreated metastatic melanoma. Melanoma Res 2008;18:274–8.

112. Iervolino A, Trisciuoglio D, Ribatti D, et al. Bcl-2 overexpression in human melanoma cells increases angiogenesis through VEGF mRNA stabilization and HIF-1-mediated transcriptional activity. FASEB J 2002;16:1453–5.

113. Trisciuoglio D, Desideri M, Ciuffreda L, et al. Bcl-2 overexpression in melanoma cells increases tumor progression-associated properties and in vivo tumor growth. J Cell Physiol 2005;205:414–21.

114. Sheridan C, Brumatti G, Martin SJ. Oncogenic B-RafV600E inhibits apoptosis and promotes ERK-dependent inactivation of Bad and Bim. J Biol Chem 2008;283:22128–35.
115. Smalley KS, Xiao M, Villanueva J, et al. CRAF inhibition induces apoptosis in melanoma cells with non-V600E BRAF mutations. Oncogene 2009;28:85–94.
116. Zeitlin BD, Zeitlin IJ, Nor JE. Expanding circle of inhibition: small-molecule inhibitors of Bcl-2 as anticancer cell and antiangiogenic agents. J Clin Oncol 2008; 26:4180–8.
117. Oblimersen: augmerosen, BCL-2 antisense oligonucleotide—Genta, G 3139, GC 3139, oblimersen sodium. Drugs R D 2007;8:321–34.
118. Bedikian AY, Millward M, Pehamberger H, et al. Bcl-2 antisense (oblimersen sodium) plus dacarbazine in patients with advanced melanoma: the Oblimersen Melanoma Study Group. J Clin Oncol 2006;24:4738–45.
119. Chana JS, Wilson GD, Cree IA, et al. c-myc, p53, and Bcl-2 expression and clinical outcome in uveal melanoma. Br J Ophthalmol 1999;83:110–4.
120. Saenz-Santamaria MC, Reed JA, McNutt NS, et al. Immunohistochemical expression of BCL-2 in melanomas and intradermal nevi. J Cutan Pathol 1994;21:393–7.
121. Miller LA, Goldstein NB, Johannes WU, et al. BH3 mimetic ABT-737 and a proteasome inhibitor synergistically kill melanomas through Noxa-dependent apoptosis. J Invest Dermatol 2009 Apr;129(4):964–71.
122. Cragg MS, Jansen ES, Cook M, et al. Treatment of B-RAF mutant human tumor cells with a MEK inhibitor requires Bim and is enhanced by a BH3 mimetic. J Clin Invest 2008;118:3651–9.
123. Vogler M, Butterworth M, Majid A, et al. Concurrent upregulation of BCL-XL and BCL2A1 induces ~1000-fold resistance to ABT-737 in chronic lymphocytic leukemia. Blood 2008;doi:10.1182/blood-2008-08-173310.
124. Wong RP, Khosravi S, Martinka M, et al. Myeloid leukemia-1 expression in benign and malignant melanocytic lesions. Oncol Rep 2008;19:933–7.
125. Zhuang L, Lee CS, Scolyer RA, et al. Mcl-1, Bcl-XL and Stat3 expression are associated with progression of melanoma whereas Bcl-2, AP-2 and MITF levels decrease during progression of melanoma. Mod Pathol 2007;20:416–26.
126. Konopleva M, Contractor R, Tsao T, et al. Mechanisms of apoptosis sensitivity and resistance to the BH3 mimetic ABT-737 in acute myeloid leukemia. Cancer Cell 2006;10:375–88.
127. Wolter KG, Verhaegen M, Fernandez Y, et al. Therapeutic window for melanoma treatment provided by selective effects of the proteasome on Bcl-2 proteins. Cell Death Differ 2007;14:1605–16.
128. Lum JJ, Bauer DE, Kong M, et al. Growth factor regulation of autophagy and cell survival in the absence of apoptosis. Cell 2005;120:237–48.
129. Amaravadi RK, Thompson CB. The roles of therapy-induced autophagy and necrosis in cancer treatment. Clin Cancer Res 2007;13:7271–9.
130. Amaravadi RK, Yu D, Lum JJ, et al. Autophagy inhibition enhances therapy-induced apoptosis in a Myc-induced model of lymphoma. J Clin Invest 2007; 117:326–36.
131. Escudier B, Eisen T, Stadler WM, et al. Sorafenib in advanced clear-cell renal-cell carcinoma. N Engl J Med 2007;356(2):125–34.
132. Motzer RJ, Michaelson MD, Redman BG, et al. Activity of SU11248, a multitargeted inhibitor of vascular endothelial growth factor receptor and platelet-derived growth factor receptor, in patients with metastatic renal cell carcinoma. J Clin Oncol 2006;24(1):16–24.

133. Yang JC, Haworth L, Sherry RM, et al. A randomized trial of bevacizumab, an anti-vascular endothelial growth factor antibody, for metastatic renal cancer. N Engl J Med 2003;349(5):427–34.
134. Hurwitz H, Fehrenbacher L, Novotny W, et al. Bevacizumab plus irinotecan, fluorouracil, and leucovorin for metastatic colorectal cancer. N Engl J Med 2004; 350(23):2335–42.
135. Kindler HL, Niedzwiecki D, Hollis D, et al. A double-blind, placebo-controlled, randomized phase III trial of gemcitabine (G) plus bevacizumab (B) versus gemcitabine plus placebo (P) in patients (pts) with advanced pancreatic cancer (PC): a preliminary analysis of Cancer and Leukemia Group B (CALGB). J Clin Oncol 2007;25(1):4508.
136. Miller K, Wang M, Gralow J, et al. Paclitaxel plus bevacizumab versus paclitaxel alone for metastatic breast cancer. N Engl J Med 2007;357(26):2666–76.
137. Sandler A, Gray R, Perry MC, et al. Paclitaxel-carboplatin alone or with bevacizumab for non-small-cell lung cancer. N Engl J Med 2006;355(24):2542–50.
138. Varker KA, Biber JE, Kefauver C, et al. A randomized phase 2 trial of bevacizumab with or without daily low-dose interferon alfa-2b in metastatic malignant melanoma. Ann Surg Oncol 2007;14(8):2367–76.
139. McDermott DF, Sosman JA, Hodi FS, et al. Randomized phase II study of dacarbazine with or without sorafenib in patients with advanced melanoma. J Clin Oncol 2007;34:275.
140. Perez DG, Suman VJ, Fitch TR, et al. Phase 2 trial of carboplatin, weekly paclitaxel, and biweekly bevacizumab in patients with unresectable stage IV melanoma: a North Central Cancer Treatment Group study, N047A. Cancer 2009; 115(1):119–27.
141. Korn EL, Liu PY, Lee SJ, et al. Meta-analysis of phase II cooperative group trials in metastatic stage IV melanoma to determine progression-free and overall survival benchmarks for future phase II trials. J Clin Oncol 2008;26(4):527–34.

Index

Note: Page numbers of article titles are in **boldface** type.

A

ABCD criteria, in early detection of melanoma, 487

Access, to dermatologic care, improving access to skilled examinations, 520–521
  sociologic and structural barriers to, 519–520

Adjuvant therapy, for stage III melanoma, 575–577
    other, 577
    radiotherapy, 575–577
    vaccines in, for stage IV melanoma patients, 555–556

Adoptive immunotherapy, for melanoma, 550–551
    conditioning by lymphodepletion, 550–551
    other developments in, 551
    transduction of T-cell receptor, 551

Age, risk of melanoma mortality according to, 517

Angiogenesis inhibitors, endogenous, in melanoma, 431–432

Angiogenesis, tumor, in melanoma, **431–416**
  antiangiogenesis treatments in patients with, 439–441
  principles of, 431–439
      angiogenic factors and endogenesis inhibitors, 431–432
      bone marrow-derived cells and premetastatic niche, 437–438
      cancer-associated fibroblasts, 438–439
      endothelial progenitor cells, 435
      hematopoietic progenitor cells, 434
      pericytes and mesenchymal stem cells, 436–437
      role of myeloid cells, 432–433
  targeting of, in melanoma therapy, 610

Anti-CD137 agonistic antibody, in melanoma immunotherapy, 553

Anti-CTLA-4 monoclonal antibodies, in melanoma immunotherapy, 551–553

Anti-integrin monoclonal antibodies, in melanoma immunotherapy, 553

Anti-OX44 agonistic antibody, in melanoma immunotherapy, 553

Anti-PD-1 monoclonal antibodies, in melanoma immunotherapy, 553

Antiangiogenesis treatments, in patients with melanoma, 439–441

Antiangiogenic drugs, with dacarbazine or temozolomide in melanoma chemotherapy, 587–588

Apoptosis signaling, targeting of, in melanoma therapy, 608–610

Atypical melanocytic tumors, severely, histopathology and diagnosis of, 470–471

Autologous bone marrow rescue, myeloablative chemotherapy regimens with, for melanoma, 589–590

Autologous vaccines, for melanoma, 554

Autophagy, targeting of, in melanoma therapy, 609–610

Hematol Oncol Clin N Am 23 (2009) 619–631
doi:10.1016/S0889-8588(09)00098-7
0889-8588/09/$ – see front matter